Questions and answers in orthopaedics

MOSBY'S REVIEW SERIES

Questions and answers in orthopaedics

For students, interns, residents, and board aspirants

Edited by

FLOYD G. GOODMAN, B.S., M.D.

Chief, Section of Orthopaedic Surgery, Ingham Medical Center;
Assistant Clinical Professor, Department of Surgery,
Michigan State University College of Human Medicine;
Attending Staff, E. W. Sparrow Hospital,
Lansing, Michigan

GEORGE R. SCHOEDINGER, III, B.S., M.D.

Assistant in Clinical Orthopaedic Surgery,
Washington University School of Medicine,
St. Louis, Missouri

THIRD EDITION

with 1688 review questions
(multiple choice, single answer; multiple choice, multiple answers;
situation and progressive thought; true or false; list)
with answers and references

THE C. V. MOSBY COMPANY

Saint Louis   1977

THIRD EDITION

Copyright © 1977 by The C. V. Mosby Company

All rights reserved. No part of this book may be reproduced in any manner without written permission of the publisher.

Previous editions copyrighted 1966, 1971

Printed in the United States of America

Distributed in Great Britain by Henry Kimpton, London

The C. V. Mosby Company
11830 Westline Industrial Drive, St. Louis, Missouri 63141

Library of Congress Cataloging in Publication Data

Goodman, Floyd G
  Questions and answers in orthopaedics.

  (Mosby's review series)
  Bibliography: p.
  1. Orthopedia—Examinations, questions, etc.
I. Schoedinger, George R., joint author. II. Title.
[DNLM: 1. Orthopedics—Examination questions. WE17
G653q]
RD732.5.G66 1977   617'.3'0076   77-8188
ISBN 0-8016-1900-9

CB/CB/CB 9 8 7 6 5 4 3 2 1

Contributors

WILLIAM H. ANDERSON, Jr., M.D.

Medical Director, E. W. Sparrow Hospital Rehabilitation Services, Lansing, Michigan; Diplomate of the American Board of Physical Medicine and Rehabilitation

VIRGINIA M. BADGER, M.D.

Assistant Professor of Orthopaedic Surgery, Washington University School of Medicine, St. Louis, Missouri

JAMES M. BULLOCK, B.S., M.D.

Assistant Clinical Professor, Department of Surgery, Michigan State University College of Human Medicine; Attending Staff, Michigan State University Health Center, E. W. Sparrow Hospital, Ingham Medical Center, Lansing, Michigan

JOHN GLANCY, C.O.

Assistant Professor of Orthotics and Director, Division of Orthotics, Department of Orthopaedic Surgery, Indiana Medical College, School of Medicine of Purdue University, Indianapolis, Indiana

FLOYD G. GOODMAN, B.S., M.D.

Chief, Section of Orthopaedic Surgery, Ingham Medical Center; Assistant Clinical Professor, Department of Surgery, Michigan State University College of Human Medicine; Attending Staff, E. W. Sparrow Hospital, Lansing, Michigan

JOHN D. KENNEY, M.D.

Clinical Instructor in Orthopaedic Surgery, St. Louis University, St. Louis, Missouri

GEORGE R. SCHOEDINGER, III, B.S., M.D.

Assistant in Clinical Orthopaedic Surgery, Washington University School of Medicine, St. Louis, Missouri

GEORGE O. SERTL, M.D.

Missouri Baptist and St. Luke's Hospitals, St. Louis, Missouri

NEWTON B. WHITE, M.D.

Instructor in Orthopaedic Surgery, St. Louis University, St. Louis, Missouri

Preface TO THIRD EDITION

Our present technologic age, with computer systems, supersonic air travel, and nearly instantaneous space communication, provides new primary knowledge and spin-off that influences medical diagnosis and treatment almost daily. Orthopaedic horizons have likewise broadened; the age of the "general orthopaedist" who tackles all musculoskeletal problems from the occiput to the toenails is fading rapidly. New subspecialties are established almost yearly, witnessed by satellite associations and societies dealing with arthroscopy, biomechanics, implants, the hand, the hip, the foot, spinal cord injury, and pain, to name a few. In contrast, however, the basic metabolic pathways at the cellular level of the osteoblast and fibroblast are oblivious to this "outside" technology and remain unchanged over thousands of years.

The challenge to orthopaedic education then becomes one of gaining insight and understanding down to the cellular level of the neuromusculoskeletal system and, with present-day technology, influencing that behavior to our advantage in disease and repair processes. This edition, with the aid of contributors from many aspects of orthopaedic care, comes close to total review and should therefore be of greater value than ever before to the student, resident, and practicing orthopaedist in meeting that challenge.

Special thanks and appreciation are extended to Cheryl Klebba, a University of Michigan student, and Dr. Rod Justin, who, as a medical student, aided in the manuscript preparation of this edition.

F. G. G.
G. R. S., III

Preface TO FIRST EDITION

The purpose of this publication is to breed unrest and discontent within the mind of its reader; to point out the areas of his ignorance; and to give him discomfort until he has exhausted the available literature to understand, not just the answers, but the problems of orthopaedics.

It came to our attention early in training that even in the best of educational programs some segments of orthopaedics are covered more thoroughly than others. The American Academy of Orthopaedic Surgeons Intraining Examinations have been of value in pointing out those areas in which the training programs and the individual residents need reinforcements. The American Board of Orthopaedic Surgery Examinations point out these discrepancies also, but this is a woeful and disappointing time to learn that one's preparation has been inadequate and that one's standards of personal excellence have been set too low.

Thus the major responsibility continues to fall on the shoulders of the student, intern, or resident to evaluate repeatedly his learning experience and to drive continually to broaden his knowledge and understanding of the whole field.

The sections of subject material covered in this book are meant to be identical to the sections outlined in the Intraining Examination. The questions have been designed, not specifically as testing questions, but as learning questions. Thus, where permissible, many are asked in the "negative" for the value of placing several correct answers at the disposal of the reader instead of several wrong ones. Care has been taken to avoid the time-consuming "key answer" type question in which A is marked if answers 2 and 4 are correct, B is marked if only answers 3 and 4 are correct, etc. The five question types utilized give sufficient variation so that the question will fit the material asked. The list and the situation or progressive thought types of questions are of special significance as they are now finding a place on the Orthopaedic Board Examinations.

An attempt is made to substantiate the subject material of each question from the literature. When conflicting views exist, we have attempted to key the references so that an overall insight might be gained.

We wish to liken the subject of orthopaedics to a well-bred, corn-fed Angus steer and this publication to an integral part, his tail. He who in the pursuit of the animal settles only for the tail indeed will have but a meager portion. He who grasps the tail, worries with it persistently and exhausts the references will likewise exhaust the animal and ultimately capture and devour the tasty beast bit by bit, at his leisure.

We wish to express our appreciation to those people who have taken time from already busy schedules to assist in the preparation of this manuscript: Carol Fellhauer, Ruth Mueller, Joan Raftery, Anita Rodriquez, and Carol Simmons; to the Orthopaedic Teaching Staff at Barnes Hospital, and especially to Nancy Ann Goodman for her help and encouragement.

F. G. G.

G. R. S., III

Contents

SECTION 1

Adult orthopaedics

GEORGE O. SERTL, M.D.

MULTIPLE CHOICE, SINGLE ANSWER (answers on pp. 272-273)

Select the *one* answer that will best complete or answer each of the following statements or questions.

1. Which of the following is the most frequent site of pseudarthrosis in a triple arthrodesis?
   a. Calcaneal cuboid
   b. Talo navicular   Ref. 43, p. 1525
   c. Talocalcaneal
   d. All approximately equal

2. Which of the following is a cause of peroneal spastic flatfoot?
   a. Rheumatoid arthritis
   b. Tuberculosis of tarsal joints   Ref. 43, p. 1804
   c. Tarsal coalition
   d. All of the above

3. Which of the following is correct with regard to treatment of acute hematogenous osteomyelitis from *Staphylococcus aureus?*
   a. 50% of strains will be resistant to penicillin G
      in the primary episode.
   b. 60% of strains will be resistant in recurrent   Ref. 8, 21:2, 1972
      attack.
   c. Methicillin is the most effective penicillinase-
      resistant penicillin against staphylococci.
   d. Methicillin is strongly bound to plasma proteins
      and therefore has a long in vivo half-life.

4. Which of the following surgical procedures is the treatment of choice for hallux rigidus in a young active adult?
   a. Mitchell
   b. Keller   Ref. 43, p. 1823
   c. McBride
   d. McKeever

1

5. The Kidner procedure is indicated in which of the following circumstances?
   a. Never in a child under 10 years of age
   b. Painful peroneal spastic flatfoot   **Ref. 43, p. 1797**
   c. Prehallux syndrome
   d. Painful rigid pes planus with normal peroneals
6. Preiser's disease is associated with which one of the following?
   a. Lunate
   b. Second metatarsal   **Ref. 43, p. 956**
   c. Tarsal navicular
   d. Carpal navicular
7. With regard to the cephalosporins, which of the following is correct?
   a. The patient with a penicillin hypersensitivity
      should not be treated with a cephalosporin.
   b. Cephaloridine should not be used in patients   **Ref. 8, 21:4, 1972**
      with renal dysfunction.
   c. There is no cross-allergenicity of penicillin and
      cephalosporins.
   d. Cephalexin does not give an adequate
      minimal inhibitory concentration
      against resistant staphylococci when
      given every 6 hours
8. Which of the following is *not* a cause of a cavus foot?
   a. Poliomyelitis
   b. Charcot-Marie-Tooth disease   **Ref. 43, p. 1535**
   c. Spina bifida
   d. All of the above are causes of cavus feet
9. Aseptic necrosis of the talus following a fracture through the neck together with subtalar subluxation or dislocation occurs in approximately what percent?
   a. 20%
   b. 40%   **Ref. 127, 52-A:991, 1970**
   c. 60%
   d. 80%
10. A dorsal bunion:
    a. Is usually caused by trauma
    b. Is caused by imbalance between the tibialis   **Ref. 43, p. 1544**
       posterior and the peroneus longus
    c. Is present only in weight bearing in the early
       stages.
    d. None of the above.
11. With regard to the tarsal tunnel syndrome:
    a. Symptoms are not related to activity.
    b. The diagnosis can be confirmed by EMG.   **Ref. 43, p. 1733**
    c. The onset of the syndrome is usually acute.   **Ref. 132, 5-1:109, 1974**
    d. Pain is usually burning and localized to the
       dorsum of the foot.
    e. Tinel's sign is rarely helpful.

12. Which of the following is a characteristic of a psychosocial or psycho-physiologic diagnosis?
    a. Patient frequently awakens
    b. Complaints usually centered on one body system   Ref. 8, 21:14, 1972
    c. Symptoms usually present for over 2 years despite adequate medical treatment
    d. Patient usually from family with few medical problems
13. Which one of the following is *not* considered a reflex sympathetic dystrophy?
    a. Posttraumatic painful osteoporosis
    b. Sudeck's atrophy   Ref. 8, 21:21, 1972
    c. Chronic traumatic edema
    d. Spreading neuralgia
    e. All are considered under this term
14. Which of the following is *not* found in the tibial collateral syndrome?
    a. History of injury, swelling, or locking is absent.
    b. Pain is increased by weight bearing.   Ref. 43, p. 920
    c. Pain is aggravated by forced valgus.
    d. Pain is aggravated by forced internal rotation of the tibia on the femur.
15. Incision and drainage should be considered earlier in which joint for septic arthritis?
    a. Hip
    b. Shoulder   Ref. 43, p. 964
    c. Ankle
    d. Knee
    e. Wrist
16. The pain similar to that of a ruptured disc can be produced by pressure on the:
    a. Posterior longitudinal ligament
    b. Annulus fibrosis   Ref. 43, p. 1036
    c. Nerve root
    d. All of the above
    e. None of the above
17. Which of the following is correct in regard to treatment of chronic tendinitis of the shoulder?
    a. Spontaneous recovery is rather unusual.
    b. Pendulum exercises help to prevent adhesive capsulitis.   Ref. 8, 20:86, 1971
    c. ASA and heat are of no help in relieving pain.
    d. Acromionectomy is not beneficial in those not responding to conservative measures.
18. With regard to cervical discs, which is *not* true regarding rupture?
    a. Lumbar disc surgery is twenty-five times more common than is cervical disc surgery.

b. It occurs more frequently in younger people   **Ref. 43, pp. 1045, 1051**
   (second or third decade).
c. Lesions of the sixth disc space are three times
   more frequent than in the fifth disc space.
d. It is more frequent in men.
e. Results of surgical procedure are better than
   in lumbar disc surgery.

19. In a patient with a midline herniated cervical disc, which of the follow-
    ing is *not* true?
    a. Patient rarely complains of pain or stiffness of
       the neck.
    b. The first symptom is often similar to Lher-   **Ref. 43, p. 1051**
       mitte's sign of multiple sclerosis.
    c. Equilibrium may be grossly disturbed.
    d. Sense of pain and temperature are frequently
       lost and help localize the level of the lesion.
    e. All are true.

20. Which of the following is *not* found in diagnosing adhesive capsulitis
    of the shoulder?
    a. Inactivity a causative factor in 50% of cases
    b. Pain located at the deltoid area with referral   **Ref. 8, 20:88, 1971**
       down the arm
    c. Limitation of passive range of motion
    d. Tenderness of the rotator cuff

21. With regard to tuberculosis of the foot, which of the following is true?
    a. It may occur at any age.
    b. It may present as isolated foci in the os calcis   **Ref. 43, p. 1089**
       or talus.
    c. In multiple infections the most important
       weight-bearing joints are most commonly
       affected.
    d. Lesions of the subtalar joint are treated by
       triple arthrodesis.
    e. All of the above.

22. Paraplegia is most often associated with tuberculosis of the dorsal spine
    because:
    a. Tuberculosis is more common in the dorsal spine
    b. The spinal canal is smallest in the dorsal area   **Ref. 43, p. 1114**
    c. There is a natural tendency to kyphosis in this area
    d. The spinal cord terminates below the level of
       the first lumbar vertebra
    e. All of the above

23. In a Charnley compression arthrodesis of the ankle, the talar pin should
    be in what position with respect to the tibial pin?
    a. Anterior
    b. Posterior   **Ref. 43, p. 1128**
    c. In the same line
    d. Does not make any difference

24. Which of the following is *not* a contraindication to an intertrochanteric osteotomy of the hip?
    a. Advanced osteoarthritis with less than 50° of flexion
    b. Rheumatoid hip joint   **Ref. 8, 20:195, 1971**
    c. Fixed adduction deformity in varus osteotomy
    d. Fixed abduction deformity in valgus osteotomy
    e. All contraindications

25. In fusions of the spine, which of the following is *not* correct?
    a. In the Albee method the spinous processes are fused into one continuous bony ridge.
    b. In the Hibbs method the neural arches are   **Ref. 43, p. 1163** fused by overlapping numerous bony flaps from adjacent bone.
    c. Cancellous bone incorporates more rapidly than does cortical bone into a solid fusion.
    d. Pseudarthrosis is two to three times more common in bone bank than in autogenous bone.
    e. All are correct.

26. The most serviceable position for shoulder fusion is:
    a. Abduction 50°, internal rotation 25°, flexion 25°
    b. Abduction 25°, internal rotation 25°, flexion 25°   **Ref. 43, p. 1186**
    c. Abduction 50°, internal rotation 10°, flexion 25°
    d. Abduction 50°, internal rotation 25°, flexion 10°

27. Which of the following is *not* true regarding osteoarthritis of the knee?
    a. It usually begins as a generalized phenomenon.
    b. It usually begins in one compartment.   **Ref. 8, 20:219, 1971**
    c. It can often be traced to derangement of a single meniscus.
    d. Pain arises from capsular stretching and not from erosion of cartilage.

28. With regard to manipulation, which one of the following is most accurate?
    a. Not indicated for the elbow
    b. More effective for the shoulder than for any   **Ref. 43, p. 1206** other joint
    c. Not needed following total joint replacement
    d. Never complicated by fractures
    e. All correct

29. Which one of the following is *not* a cause of extra-articular ankylosis of the knee in extension?
    a. Fibrosis of vastus intermedius
    b. Adhesions between patella and femur   **Ref. 43, p. 1213**
    c. Iatrogenic injections
    d. Septic arthritis

30. In manipulation of a frozen shoulder, which one of the following is usually *not* ruptured?
    a. Tendon of the long head of the biceps
    b. Subscapularis   Ref. 43, p. 1231
    c. Adhesions
    d. All of the above
31. Which of the following types of muscular dystrophy usually begins before age 10?
    a. Duchenne
    b. Limb girdle   Ref. 8, 19:82, 1970
    c. Fascioscapulo
    d. Myotonic
    e. More than one of the above
32. Which of the following statements pertains to formation of Brodie's abscess?
    a. Is a localized form of acute osteomyelitis
    b. Usually develops in diaphysis   Ref. 43, p. 1314
    c. Seen more frequently in debilitated patients
    d. May remain inactive for years
33. Which one of the following syndromes may be caused by a disc space infection in its early stages?
    a. Hip joint syndrome with signs of a septic joint
    b. Abdominal syndrome with suggestion of ap-   Ref. 43, p. 1319
       pendicitis
    c. Meningeal syndrome suggestive of tuberculosis
       or acute suppurative meningitis
    d. All of the above
34. Which of the following statements is correct with regard to osteoporosis?
    a. Osteoporosis in postmenopausal women is
       heritable.
    b. Osteoporosis is related to childbearing.   Ref. 8, 22:8, 1973
    c. The body height is a good measure of the
       progression of osteoporosis.
    d. Osteoporosis can be diagnosed before fracture.
35. Resection of which portion of the fibula should not be done because of residual instability?
    a. Proximal fourth
    b. Upper half   Ref. 43, p. 1320
    c. Middle two thirds
    d. Lower fourth
36. Which one of the following is *not* true regarding specific types of osteomyelitis?
    a. Brucellar osteomyelitis is most common in
       farmers and located most often in the
       lumbar spine.
    b. Coccidioidal osteomyelitis usually occurs in   Ref. 43, p. 1325
       multiple foci.

c. Actinomycotic osteomyelitis usually affects the femur.

d. Syphilitic osteomyelitis rarely requires surgery.

37. Which one of the following structures is commonly damaged by ischemic myositis of the upper extremity?
    a. Median and ulnar nerves
    b. Median and radial nerves   Ref. 43, p. 1459
    c. Flexor and extensor pollicis longus
    d. Flexor digitorum profundus and flexor carpi radialis longus

38. Which of the following statements does *not* apply to the anterior compartment syndrome?
    a. Sensation is usually lost first in the area between the first and second toes dorsally.
    b. Extensor hallucis longus function is usually   Ref. 43, p. 1462
       the first muscle to be lost.
    c. The dorsalis pedis pulse is usually absent.
    d. Cause is thought to be edema and small hemorrhages secondary to excessive activity in the unconditioned person.

39. In doing a shoulder arthrogram, the expected volume of the joint should be in the following range:
    a. 5 to 10 ml
    b. 15 to 20 ml   Ref. 43, p. 1478
    c. 20 to 30 ml
    d. 30 to 40 ml

40. Which of the following is *not* a component of a motor unit in EMG evaluations?
    a. Anterior horn cell
    b. Peripheral axon   Ref. 8, 21:25, 1972
    c. Lower motor neuron
    d. Innervated muscle fibers
    e. All of the above

41. Which of the following may indicate a need for surgery with regard to soft cervical disc herniation?
    a. Neurologic defect
    b. Intractable pain   Ref. 8, 21:123, 1972
    c. Failure to respond to conservative treatment
    d. Repeated attacks
    e. All of the above

42. A normal cervical disc holds how much saline solution under pressure?
    a. 0.2 ml
    b. 0.5 ml   Ref. 8, 21:124, 1972
    c. 0.8 ml
    d. 1.0 ml

43. Which of the following is *not* characteristic of the posterior interosseous nerve syndrome?
    a. May be caused by synovial proliferation

b. Patient unable to extend wrist   **Ref. 127, 55-A:753, 1973**

c. Can be confused with extensor tendon rupture

d. Can be confused with extensor tendon dislocation into intermetacarpal area

44. In patients with atlantoaxial subluxation secondary to rheumatoid arthritis, which of the following is *not* true?

a. It is seen in up to 25% of patients with rheumatoid arthritis.

b. Over half the patients show some neuro-   **Ref. 127, 55-A:458, 1973**
logic finding.

c. The degree of subluxation is proportional to the signs and symptoms.

d. Patients may show involvement of the trigeminal nerve.

45. Which of the following is *not* characteristic of pyogenic infections of the disc space.

a. Narrowing of disc space is the first change noted on x-ray examination.

b. Abscess formation is seen on x-ray exam-   **Ref. 127, 55-A:698, 1973**
ination.

c. *Staphylococcus aureus* is the most common organism.

d. A bone scan may show increased uptake in the infection.

46. With regard to classic hemophilia A, which of the following is *not* true?

a. It is due to a deficiency of factor VIII.

b. An AHG level above 4% usually prevents   **Ref. 8, 22:28-34, 1973**
hemorrhage.

c. Resorptive capacity of the synovium is limited by multiple hemorrhages.

d. The incidence of hemorrhage is not related to age.

e. Contractures are primarily extra-articular.

47. Which of the following is *not* a characteristic physical finding found in hysterical backache?

a. Abnormal movements such as astasia-abasia

b. Conversion symptoms that simulate physi-   **Ref. 8, 21:98, 1972**
cal illness

c. Dermatome neurologic defects

d. Severe disabling but vague, poorly localized pain

e. All of the above

48. Which of the following bursae is involved in weaver's bottom disease?

a. Subgluteal

b. Trochanteric   **Ref. 43, p. 1514**

c. Ischiogluteal

d. Iliopectineal

49. Which is the most commonly inflamed bursa?
    a. Trochanteric
    b. Subacromial   **Ref 43, p. 1515**
    c. Subscapular
    d. Olecranon

50. The most common cause for atlantoaxial subluxation is:
    a. Congenital absence of dens
    b. Atlantoaxial subluxation   **Ref. 127, 55-B:482, 1973**
    c. Fracture of the dens
    d. Rheumatoid arthritis

51. Which of the following is *not* true regarding proximal tibial fibular joint instability?
    a. Subluxation may compromise the peroneal nerve.
    b. Anterolateral dislocation is the most com-   **Ref. 127, 56-A:145, 1974**
       mon type.
    c. Superior dislocation is usually accompanied by fracture of the tibia.
    d. With chronic subluxation and arthritis, fusion of the joint is the treatment of choice.

52. With regard to a snapping scapula, which of the following is *not* true?
    a. Snapping of the shoulder more common
    b. May be caused by increased anterior in-   **Ref. 43, p. 1506**
       clination of the superior edge of the scapula
    c. Is frequently secondary to an osteochondroma
    d. May be caused by poor posture

53. With regard to prepatellar bursitis, which of the following is *not* applicable?
    a. It may be caused by acute or chronic trauma.
    b. In diagnosis it may be confused with   **Ref. 43, p. 1508**
       septic arthritis of the knee.
    c. Resecting the bursa following acute bursitis is easier than it is after chronic inflammation.
    d. A frequent complication following excision is a large hematoma.

54. Which of the following entities has *not* been implicated as a cause of tennis elbow?
    a. Inflammation of an adventitious bursa
    b. Calcification in the common extensor   **Ref. 43, p. 1496**
       origin
    c. Annular ligament
    d. Extensor carpi radialis brevis
    e. All of the above

55. With regard to displacement or subluxation of the peroneal tendons, which of the following is *not* true?
   a. It may be secondary to a congenitally shallow groove in the lateral malleolus.
   b. It may be repaired by reconstruction of a retinaculum from the Achilles tendon. **Ref. 43, p. 1495**
   c. It frequently follows skiing accidents.
   d. X-ray films are of no help in diagnosis.
   e. It may be secondary to paralytic calcaneo-valgus deformity.

56. Which of the following statements is *not* true regarding herniation of muscle through fascia?
   a. It occurs most commonly below the knee.
   b. It is usually not related to trauma. **Ref. 43, p. 1496**
   c. It is most common over the anterior tibial muscle.
   d. Repair of a defect in the fascia is the treatment of choice.
   e. Anterior tibial compartment syndrome may be iatrogenic.

57. Which of the following statements pertains to treatment of neglected patellar tendon ruptures?
   a. Skeletal traction through the patella is used preoperatively.
   b. Some type of tension-relieving suture is usually indicated. **Ref. 43, p. 1473**
   c. Quadricep exercises are begun as soon as possible.
   d. The semitendinosus tendon may be used to replace the patellar tendon.
   e. All of the above.

58. The most common serious complication of chemonucleolysis is:
   a. Disc space infection
   b. Increase of sciatic pain **Ref. 106, 99:68, 1974**
   c. Anaphylactic shock
   d. Spinal cord damage
   e. Meningitis

59. With regard to palindromic arthritis, which of the following statements is true?
   a. Hip and knee joints are predisposed.
   b. Attacks typically begin in the afternoon. **Ref. 105, p. 209**
   c. Anemia is a common constitutional effect.
   d. 75% have positive rheumatoid factor.

60. Which of the following is *not* true of ochronotic arthritis?
   a. It is inherited as Mendelian dominant.
   b. Cartilage is more brittle than normal. **Ref. 105, p. 86**
   c. Vitamin C in high doses tends to reduce excretion of homogentisic acid.
   d. No cure is known.

61. In complete traction injuries involving the whole brachial plexus, which is *not* true?
    a. C-6 to C-7 lesion is indicated by a positive Horner's syndrome.
    b. Useful recovery of the extensor muscle of the wrist is rarely seen.   Ref. 105, p. 535
    c. Useful recovery of the trapezius and seratus anterior is common.
    d. Sensory recovery is poor.
    e. All of the above.

62. Which of the following is *not* true of a bipartite patella?
    a. Usually bilateral
    b. Opposing margins smooth and dense   Ref. 105, p. 160
    c. Usually smaller fragment in upper inner quadrant
    d. Generally asymptomatic

63. The filum terminale syndrome is:
    a. Associated with the Arnold-Chiari syndrome
    b. Untreatable   Ref. 105, p. 245
    c. Seen most commonly between 7 and 10 years of age
    d. Not associated with scoliosis

64. Which of the following is *not* similar in gout and pseudojoint?
    a. Recurrent acute attack
    b. Precipitating factors, surgery, mercurial   Ref. 49, p. 785
       diuretics, trauma
    c. Duration of untreated attacks
    d. Radiograph of affected joints

65. Which is typical of Reiter's syndrome?
    a. Clinical features usually chronic
    b. Thought to be secondary to gonococcal   Ref. 49, p. 753
       infection
    c. Skin lesions rare
    d. May present in children following dysentery

66. Which of the following is *not* a cause of diaphysometaphyseal ischemia?
    a. Pancreatic disease
    b. Sickle cell anemia   Ref. 49, p. 1106
    c. Gaucher's disease
    d. Pheochromocytoma
    e. All may cause it

67. Which of the following is found radiographically in pigmented villo-nodular synovitis?
    a. Early joint narrowing
    b. Early stages that may mimic tuberculosis   Ref. 49, p. 827
       and rheumatoid arthritis   Ref. 127, 50-B:290, 1968
    c. Subchondral erosions, which are rarely seen early
    d. Nodular masses that frequently show calcification

68. The narrow lumbar canal syndrome:
    a. May cause claudication
    b. Presents symptoms rather acutely   Ref. 127, 50-B:595, 1968
    c. Cannot be diagnosed without help of
       myelography
    d. Is seen more frequently in thin people
69. With regard to osseous bridges of the lumbar spine, which is correct?
    a. Usually bilateral
    b. May have area of pseudarthrosis   Ref. 127, 50-A:513, 1968
    c. Rarely associated with scoliosis
    d. Usually spans more than two vertebras
70. Which of the following is *not* correct regarding complications of disc
    surgery?
    a. 50% of vascular accidents are not noted at
       the time of surgery.
    b. Typical infections of disc space occur   Ref. 127, 50A:382-428, 1968
       more often when the septic process is
       confined to the space than when an ob-
       vious wound infection is present.
    c. Patients with adequately repaired dural
       tears can be ambulated in a routine
       fashion postoperatively.
    d. There is aproximately 50% mortality in
       those patients sustaining vascular accidents.
    e. All are correct.

MULTIPLE CHOICE, MULTIPLE ANSWERS (answers on p. 273)

Select one or more answers that will best complete or answer each of the following statements or questions.

71. Which of the following are thought to be contraindicated in the treat-
    ment of anterior compartment syndrome?
    a. Fasciotomy of the crural fascia early
    b. Ice packs following surgery   Ref. 43, p. 1463
    c. Fasciotomy of crural fascia after fourth day
    d. Heat and elevation
    e. Tendon transfers in late stages of treatment
72. Which of the following statements are *not* true regarding the supra-
    spinatus syndrome?
    a. Pain is usually located in the region of
       greater tuberosity.
    b. Calcification seen by x-ray examination is   Ref. 43, p. 1475
       always symptomatic.
    c. The clinical diagnosis is less common than
       the number found at autopsy in those over
       60 years of age.
    d. Motion is usually not limited.
    e. Snapping is frequently noted.

73. In the treatment of rotator cuff lesions, which of the following are correct?
    a. Approximately 90% will recover without surgery.
    b. Abduction humeral splints are helpful. Ref. 43, p. 1480
    c. Physical therapy and manipulation under anesthesia may be helpful when adhesions have developed but may be complicated by fracture.
    d. Calcifications that appear dense, round, and circumscribed usually respond well to aspiration and steroid injection.
    e. A calcium deposit may form a mechanical block to motion.
74. The Hitchcock procedure is indicated in which of the following?
    a. Rupture of rotator cuff
    b. Tenosynovitis of the long head of biceps Ref. 43, p. 1489
    c. Rupture of the biceps insertion Ref. 105, p. 553
    d. Patient with positive Yergason's sign
75. In which of the following ways are palmar and plantar fibromatosis similar?
    a. Both begin on the medial side of an extremity.
    b. The cords are tender. Ref. 43, pp. 361, 1433, 1504
    c. Flexion contractures usually develop.
    d. May show mitoses microscopically and be confused with fibrosarcoma.
76. In a snapping hip which of the following are true?
    a. It rarely requires surgery.
    b. It is never confused with intra-articular pathology. Ref. 43, p. 1504
    c. It may be caused by an osteochondroma.
    d. It is always secondary to lesions about the greater trochanter.
    e. If surgical treatment is necessary, local anesthesia is preferable.
77. Which of the following are true regarding acute osteomyelitis of the sacroiliac joint?
    a. It may present as appendicitis.
    b. The patient usually has a history of trauma to the buttocks. Ref. 127, 55-A:630, 1973
    c. There is systemic temperature elevation.
    d. It may be misdiagnosed as a septic hip.
    e. Initial x-ray films are often of no help in diagnosis.
    f. All are true.

78. Which of the following are *not* typical of transient painful osteoporosis of the lower extremities?
    a. Ankle joint is most common.
    b. Symptoms usually arise spontaneously without a history of trauma.   **Ref. 127, 55-A:1188, 1973**
    c. Skin appears cold, clammy, and atrophic.
    d. Stiffness is noted to be increased in the morning.
    e. Symptoms are self-limited.
79. With respect to a popliteal cyst (Baker's cyst), which of the following are correct?
    a. It can be confused with a rheumatoid cyst.
    b. It does not communicate with the knee joint.   **Ref. 43, p. 1510**
    c. Intra-articular pathology has been found in about 50% of patients.
    d. It should be excised in the face of a torn meniscus.
    e. It may mimic acute thrombophlebitis.
80. Which of the following statements are correct regarding open reduction of clavicular fracture?
    a. Nonunion is more frequent following open reduction and internal fixation (ORIF) than in closed treatment.
    b. Pressure in the brachial plexus by one of fragments may be an indication for ORIF.   **Ref. 43, p. 631**
    c. Fracture of the distal clavicle and tearing of the coracoclavicular ligaments usually heals satisfactorily if properly immobilized.
    d. A surgical scar is always less unsightly than a bony prominence following fracture.
    e. Persistent wide separation of fragments may be an indication for ORIF.
81. In the diagnosis of a hysterical personality, which of the following are correct?
    a. The MMPI is often helpful.
    b. On the above test the typical result is the "conversion V of hysteria."   **Ref. 8, 21:100, 1972**
    c. The "conversion V of hysteria" is composed of the scores on the hysteria, depression, and hypochondriacal scales.
    d. The above test is of no help in diagnosis.
    e. The above diagnosis is purely a clinical impression.

82. Which of the following statements are applicable to fat embolism?
    a. 60% of patients showed symptoms in the first 24 hours after injury.
    b. Po₂ of less than 50 mm Hg on room air is an important diagnostic point.

    Ref. 8, 22:38-46, 1973

    c. Petechiae are the most classic physical findings and are related to prognosis.
    d. Petechiae are actually microscopic fat emboli and may appear in recurrent crops over 1 or 2 days.
    e. The histologic incidence of fat embolism is close to 100%, but the clinical incidence is only about 5% following a long bone fracture.

83. Which of the following are thought to be intrinsic predisposing causes of bunions?
    a. Ill-fitting shoes
    b. Pes planus

    Ref. 8, 22:220, 1973

    c. Comparatively long first toe
    d. Metatarsus primus varus
    e. Lateral, distal, and posterior slanting of the distal articular surface of the middle cuneiform

84. Which of the following are common physical findings of hallux rigidus?
    a. If an exostosis is present, it is usually located dorsally.
    b. The metatarsal phalangeal joint is enlarged circumferentially.

    Ref. 8, 22:240, 1973

    c. There is valgus deviation of the toe beyond normal.
    d. The greatest limitation of motion is in flexion.
    e. Both passive and active motion are painful.

85. With regard to a compression fracture in pathologic osteoporosis, which statements are correct?
    a. This is the only definitive diagnostic sign of pathologic osteoporosis.
    b. These usually occur in three sets.

    Ref. 8, 22:6, 1973

    c. These are usually quite painful.
    d. The total loss of height from these usually does not exceed 6 cm.
    e. A dowager's hump developing without warning pain in the sixth decade is almost diagnostic of osteoporosis.

86. In the x-ray diagnosis of rheumatoid arthritis, which of the following are true?
    a. A proximal interphalangeal joint is the first to show changes.

15

b. The spine may be involved with a rheu-   **Ref. 49, pp. 686-708**
matoid nodule.

c. The joint space is widened in early stages.

d. 85% of patients show changes through x-
ray examination within 6 months of the
onset of disease.

e. Cervical disc narrowing is commonly seen
with hypertrophic spurring.

87. Which of the following are typical of Jaccoud's arthritis?
   a. Results from multiple attacks of rheuma-
   toid arthritis
   b. Bony narrowing and erosion   **Ref. 49, p. 730**
   c. Fibrosis of tendons and periarticular soft
   tissues
   d. Radial deviation of metacarpal phalangeal
   joints
   e. Atrophy and flexion contracture

88. Which of the following are *not* typical of Sjögren's syndrome?
   a. Keratoconjunctivitis sicca
   b. Hypersecretion of lacrimal and salivary   **Ref. 49, p. 730**
   glands   **Ref. 109, pp. 1948-1949**
   c. Not associated with the collagen diseases
   d. Association with rheumatoid arthritis
   e. Commonly associated with chest disease

89. Which of the following are characteristic of ankylosing spondylitis?
   a. Positive rheumatoid factor
   b. Subcutaneous nodules   **Ref. 49, p. 733**
   c. More common in males   **Ref. 109, pp. 1955-1956**
   d. Hips and shoulders involved in 80% of
   cases
   e. Usually begins in the sacroiliac joints

90. Which of the following are correct statements regarding specific arthri-
tides?
   a. Calcaneal spur formation is common in
   Reiter's syndrome.
   b. Osteitis condensans ilii is a self-limited   **Ref. 49, pp. 753, 761, 762**
   disease commonly found in females of
   child-bearing age.
   c. Osteitis condensans ilii involves the sacroiliac joint.
   d. Destruction of the distal interphalangeal
   joints is uncommon in psoriatic arthritis,
   but nail changes are frequently seen.
   e. Periosteal reaction of the metatarsals and
   proximal phalanges is common in Reiter's
   syndrome.

91. Which of the following are contraindications to anterior disectomy and interbody fusion?
    a. Complete block on the myelogram
    b. Advanced spondylosis at a single level   **Ref. 8, 21:130, 1972**
    c. Disc fragment migration from level of interspace
    d. Severe osteoporosis
92. With regard to hematogenous osteomyelitis, which of the following are true?
    a. *Staphylococcus aureus* is no longer the most common cause.
    b. *Haemophilus influenzae* appears to be increasing, although the incidence of bacteremia has not really changed over the years.   **Ref. 8, 21:1, 1972**
    c. *Klebsiella* is usually not destructive of bone.
    d. Anaerobic bacteria are now more frequent because of improved methods of detecting them.
93. Which of the following statements are true regarding prosthetic femoral head replacement?
    a. The results are better in treatment of fractures and aseptic necrosis than in arthritic patients.
    b. The results of those patients with early and late infections are equally poor.   **Ref. 127, 55-A:516, 1973**
    c. Early dislocation, if treated properly, may not adversely affect the final result.
    d. Roughly as many improve as deteriorate in the long-term follow-up.
    e. All of the above.
94. Which of the following are correct in the relationship of ectopic bone formation and total hip replacement?
    a. Does not affect result unless ankylosis occurs
    b. Is found in 15% to 20% of cases by 6 months   **Ref. 127, 55-A:1629, 1973**
    c. Is not related to prior hip surgery
    d. Patients with prior prosthetic replacements more likely to have ectopic ossificacations but not necessarily a poor functional result
95. The amount of wear on the high-density polyethylene socket in the total hip replacement is:
    a. Related to the weight of the patient
    b. Greater than 3 mm per 10 years (average)   **Ref. 106, 95:19, 1973**
    c. Less than 3 mm per 10 years (average)

d. Greater than 5 mm per 10 years (average)

e. Not related to weight or activity

96. Which of the following are considered "first line" drugs for the treatment of tuberculosis of bone and joints?
    a. Rifampin
    b. Isoniazid   **Ref. 106, 97:6, 1973**
    c. Ethambutol
    d. Cycloserine
    e. Viomycin

97. Which of the following are common complaints of patients with Paget's disease?
    a. Headache
    b. Backache   **Ref. 105, p. 417**
    c. Bowing of thighs
    d. Kyphosis
    e. Muscle weakness and fatigue

SITUATION AND PROGRESSIVE THOUGHT (answers on p. 273)

Select the answer or answers that best apply in accordance with the information given in the following statements.

98. A 30-year-old man comes to your office complaining that on running in a lateral direction or cutting, he has a strange feeling that he loses control of his knee; otherwise his knee feels normal. Your initial impression would be:
    a. Osteochondritis dissecans
    b. Collateral ligament tear   **Ref. 127, 50-A:211, 1960**
    c. Loose body
    d. Rotatory instability
    e. Meniscal tear

99. The best way to test your impression would be:
    a. Test in full extension for valgus-varus laxity
    b. Arthrogram   **Ref. 127, 50-A:216, 1968**
    c. Standard x-ray examination of the knees
    d. Check anterior drawer sign in 90° flexion and 15° of external rotation
    e. Check anterior drawer sign with patient sitting, knee over the table at 90° flexion and neutral

100. The operation designed to correct this lesion is a change of:
    a. Primary flexor to collateral stabilizer
    b. Primary flexor to external rotator   **Ref. 127, 50-A:228, 1968**
    c. Primary flexor to internal rotator
    d. Patellar ligament to cruciate
    e. Patellar ligament to pull in a more medial direction

101. The results of this operation have been:
    a. Not tested with reference to biomechanical principles
    b. Based only on subjective analysis of patients
    c. Shown to be based on sound biomechanical principles
    d. Unable to be tested because of the complexity of the procedure

    Ref. 127, 55-A:1225, 1973

102. A 45-year-old man is found to have a L-4 to L-5 disc rupture, and surgery is performed to correct this lesion. The patient does well for six months until pain returns in the back and he begins having headaches and a stiff neck. On physical examination, which of the following would be a significant diagnostic finding?
    a. Pain on palpation of lower back
    b. Muscle spasm in the cervical paraspinal **Ref. 127, 50-A:208, 418, 1968** muscles
    c. Normal temperature and color of skin over operative area
    d. Questionable fluctuant mass in the area of prior surgery

103. Treatment at this time should be:
    a. Bedrest and antibiotics
    b. Cast immobilization and antibiotics
    c. Myelogram
    d. Observation at monthly intervals with decreased activity

    Ref. 127, 50-A:269, 1968

104. Following accurate diagnosis of the problem, treatment should be:
    a. Repeated aspiration
    b. Surgical repair of the pseudocyst by suture **Ref. 127, 50-A:275, 1968** of the defect
    c. Surgical repair of the pseudocyst by overlying muscle or gelfoam
    d. Intrathecal antibiotics

105. A 40-year-old white housewife who does a lot of gardening at home presents with an ulcer on the forearm. She states it began as a small nodule that gradually became reddened and subsequently broke down and drained pus. She has tried all her home remedies, but is unable to clear this lesion. Otherwise her general health is good. Your differential diagnosis would indicate:
    a. Tuberculosis
    b. Histoplasmosis
    c. Spirotrichosis
    d. Coccidioidomycosis
    e. All of the above

    Ref. 105, pp. 114-116

106. Skin tests, complement fixation tests, and agglutination tests are helpful in the diagnosis of all but:
    a. Tuberculosis
    b. Histoplasmosis   Ref. 105, pp. 114-116
    c. Spirotrichosis
    d. Coccidioidomycosis
    e. All of the above

107. The treatment of choice for the above answer is:
    a. Potassium iodide
    b. Penicillin   Ref. 105, pp. 114-116
    c. Isoniazid, PAS, streptomycin
    d. Amphotericin B
    e. Chloramphenicol

108. A 35-year-old man enters your office complaining of hip pain. X-ray films show that he has aseptic necrosis of the femoral head. Which of the following would *not* be a cause?
    a. Alcoholism
    b. Gout   Ref. 127, 55-A:1351, 1973
    c. Hemostatic alterations
    d. Steroid therapy
    e. All may be

109. The chances of eventually contracting the same condition in the other hip are:
    a. Rare
    b. 100%   Ref. 127, 55-A:1351, 1973
    c. 5% to 10%
    d. 25%
    e. 35% to 50%

110. The most likely time the patient would become symptomatic with this condition would be when:
    a. X-ray films show mottled areas of increased density
    b. X-ray films show an infarct demarcated by   Ref. 127, 55-A:1355, 1973
       a zone of increased density
    c. Osteochondral flap is present
    d. Crescent sign is present on x-ray films
    e. Loose osteochondral fragment is present

111. In treatment of the affected but asymptomatic hip:
    a. The results are not influenced by treatment of the symptomatic hip
    b. Position of bone graft is not as important   Ref. 127, 55-A:1365, 1973
       as timing of the operation
    c. The physician should not wait for even
       four months before treating one with bone
       grafting
    d. An uncooperative patient should not be
       bone grafted

112. A 25-year-old white man consults you regarding a painful hip. He has been in a neighborhood physical fitness group that has been running 2 to 3 miles a day for the past month. Which of the following would be significant?
    a. Negative x-ray examination
    b. Absence of pain over the greater tro-   Ref. 43, pp. 605-606
       chanter
    c. Pain on flexion and internal rotation
    d. Pain relieved after exercise, although stiff
       on awakening
113. Your treatment at this time would be:
    a. Continue exercises to see if it "works itself
       out"
    b. Crutches and x-ray reexamination in   Ref. 127, 48-A:1031, 1966
       2 to 3 weeks
    c. Phenylbutazone, 100 mg three times a day
    d. Steroid injection

TRUE OR FALSE (answers on p. 273)

114. Following an episode of acute traumatic synovitis of the knee in which an effusion is present, the pH changes from normal alkaline to acid.
    (T) (F)   Ref. 43, p. 906
115. The most common cause of loose bodies in the knee is osteochondritis dissecans, and it accounts for over 50% of them.   Ref. 43, p. 949
    (T) (F)
116. In Buerger's disease the lower extremities are involved in 95% of cases.
    (T) (F)   Ref. 105, p. 452
117. In Paget's disease, unlike polyostotic fibrous dysplasia, the bones of the hands and feet are seldom affected.   Ref. 105, p. 414
    (T) (F)
118. In the organic type of coccygodynia, surgery is usually indicated.
    (T) (F)   Ref. 43, p. 955
119. In a gonorrheal septic joint, surgical drainage should usually be performed.   Ref. 43, p. 963
    (T) (F)
120. There is an increased chance of infection postoperatively when a hematoma forms, but this can be reduced by preoperative antibiotics.
    (T) (F)   Ref. 127, 55-A:795, 1973
121. In causalgia the skin is initially cold, moist, and glossy, later turning warm and blotchy.   Ref. 105, p. 461
    (T) (F)
122. The most common cause of failure in synovectomy of a rheumatoid knee is preoperative degenerative changes of the joint.
    (T) (F)   Ref. 127, 55-A:539, 1973
123. In the fit of a femoral head prosthesis it is better if it is a little loose than too tight.   Ref. 43, p. 1014
    (T) (F)

124. The hypercalcemia of hyperparathyroidism can be differentiated from that of sarcoid and vitamin D intoxication by the administration of cortisone. **Ref. 105, p. 64**
(T) (F)

125. In sciatic scoliosis the patient will list away from the involved side when the disc protrusion is located medial to the root. **Ref. 105, p. 839**
(T) (F)

126. The first sign of a pyogenic disc space infection is narrowing of the disc space. **Ref. 105, p. 861**
(T) (F)

127. In shoulder fusions the degree of abduction is more critical than the degree of internal rotation. **Ref. 43, p. 1186**
(T) (F)

128. Hypophosphatasia is due to a lowered serum phosphorus. **Ref. 5, p. 418**
(T) (F)

129. In the spinal tumor syndrome associated with tuberculosis, the neurologic signs precede the radiograph of spinal tuberculosis.
(T) (F) **Ref. 43, p. 1114**

130. Extra-articular arthrodesis may occur independent of intra-articular arthrodesis, but not vice versa. **Ref. 43, p. 1206**
(T) (F)

131. Results of high tibial osteotomy for valgus deformity of the knee are less favorable than they are for a varus deformity.
(T) (F) **Ref. 127, 55-A:963, 1973**

132. The linings of true and adventitious bursae are the same.
(T) (F) **Ref. 43, p. 1507**

133. A tall person tolerates a hip fusion as well as a short person does.
(T) (F) **Ref. 43, p. 1256**

134. Tuberculosis of the tarsal navicular is treated by excision of the navicular. **Ref. 43, p. 1091**
(T) (F)

135. The lateral articular facet of the patella is the side of earliest and most severe changes in chondromalacia. **Ref. 43, p. 1076**
(T) (F)

136. Quadriplegia following cervical disc rupture is never seen without an associated fracture or fracture dislocation. **Ref. 43, p. 1051**
(T) (F)

137. The pain of a ruptured cervical disc may be differentiated from myocardial pain; the latter is usually medial arm pain and the former, lateral arm pain. **Ref. 43, p. 1048**
(T) (F)

138. In some cases brown tumors disappear following parathyroidectomy in primary hyperparathyroidism. **Ref. 105, p. 62**
(T) (F)

139. Extensive bone destruction is a contraindication to the use of methylmethacrylate in the treatment of pathologic fractures.
(T) (F) **Ref. 127, 56-A:40, 1974**

140. An adequate amount of cortical steroids counteracts gouty attacks; thus attacks may be precipitated by surgical trauma. **Ref. 105, p. 79**
(T) (F)

141. A normal person ingests about 1 gm of calcium a day, but the net absorption is only 250 mg. **Ref. 127, 56-A:103, 1974**
(T) (F)

142. 1,25-Dihydroxy vitamin D is a highly active form of vitamin D that is converted in the liver. **Ref. 127, 56-A:106, 1974**
(T) (F)

143. Looser's lines and milkman's pseudofractures are cardinal features of osteomalacia but are of no help in evaluation of treatment.
(T) (F) **Ref. 127, 56-A:114, 1974**

144. Serum values for inorganic phosphate are elevated in renal osteo-dystrophy because of inadequate filtration of phosphate through the glomerulus. **Ref. 127, 56-A:121, 1974**
(T) (F)

145. Instability of the pelvis may follow removal of the iliac bone for grafting purposes. **Ref. 127, 54-A:83, 1972**
(T) (F)

146. In those who are asymptomatic but overweight, hyperuricemia may be converted to a normal level with gradual weight reduction.
(T) (F) **Ref. 127, 54-A:365, 1972**

147. Renal insufficiency is the most common direct cause of death in primary gout. **Ref. 127, 54-A:370, 1972**
(T) (F)

148. The sensitized sheep cell agglutination test is less sensitive but more specific than the latex fixation test in detecting rheumatoid factor in the joint fluid of patients with rheumatoid arthritis.
(T) (F) **Ref. 127, 54-A:838, 1972**

149. Acute renal failure may follow the crush syndrome.
(T) (F) **Ref. 127, 54-A:1691, 1972**

150. Approximately 30% of patients with pathologic fractures from metastatic cancer live a year or more. **Ref. 127, 54-A:1665, 1972**
(T) (F)

151. In predicting a return to work of the back-injured patient, psychologic ratings by psychologists are superior to those of physicians.
(T) (F) **Ref. 127, 54-A:1610, 1972**

152. In patients taking levodopa, indications for replacement hip prosthesis are the same as for normal elderly patients. **Ref. 127, 54-A:1254, 1972**
(T) (F)

153. Anterior interbody spinal fusion has a poorer fusion rate than does a posterolateral fusion, but has equally good clinical results.
(T) (F) **Ref. 127, 54-A:1204, 1972**
  Ref. 127, 54-A:756, 1972

154. 90% of patients with popliteal cyst have a damaged meniscus.
(T) (F) **Ref. 127, 54-A:1058, 1972**

155. List eight causes of bursitis about the knee joint.   Ref. 105, p. 778
156. List four contraindications to simple exostectomy for removal of a bunion.   Ref. 43, p. 1824
157. List ten causes of metatarsalgia.   Ref. 105, p. 804
158. List three predisposing factors related to meniscal injuries.
     Ref. 43, p. 907
159. List four causes of locking in the knee.   Ref. 43, p. 910
160. List three maneuvers on physical examinations that point to a torn meniscus.   Ref. 43, p. 911
161. List the indications for partial meniscectomy and the advantages and disadvantages of this procedure.   Ref. 43, p. 913
162. List the three late radiographic changes Fairbank described in the knee joint following meniscectomy.   Ref. 43, p. 918
163. List five causes of acquired flatfoot.   Ref. 105, p. 813
164. List five causes of loose bodies in the knee joint.   Ref. 43, p. 949
165. List the typical x-ray findings in baseball pitcher's elbow. Ref. 43, p. 956
166. List the four radiographic criteria for diagnosis of primary protrusio acetabuli.   Ref. 106, 94:261
167. List the indications for proximal tibial osteotomy in osteoarthritis of the knee.   Ref. 43, p. 1006
168. List six signs of arteriovenous fistula found on physical examination.
     Ref. 105, p. 473
169. List five indications for operative treatment of sodium urate deposits in gout.   Ref. 43, p. 1054
170. List eight causes of Charcot joints.   Ref. 43, p. 1055
171. List six causes of torticollis.   Ref. 105, p. 516
172. List the four major causes of osteitis pubis.   Ref. 43, p. 1079
173. List the typical route of spontaneous drainage for tuberculosis infections of the cervical spine, lumbar spine, and hip.
     Ref. 43, pp. 1097, 1099, 1103
174. List four causes of periosteal reaction.   Ref. 105, p. 421
175. List five causes of extra-articular and intra-articular arthrodesis.
     Ref. 43, p. 1206
176. List the typical changes in order of progression in Charcot joints.
     Ref. 49, p. 817
177. List the five basic principles in treatment of acute hematogenous osteomyelitis in adults.   Ref. 43, p. 1305
178. List three indications for amputation in cases of osteomyelitis.
     Ref. 43, p. 1325
179. List five diagnostic points leading to diagnosis of the costoclavicular syndrome.   Ref. 105, p. 539
180. List six signs of a rotator cuff tear.   Ref. 43, p. 1486
181. List nine basic principles for the performance of a muscle transplantation operation.   Ref. 43, p. 1519
182. List the four classic x-ray findings in primary hyperparathyroidism.
     Ref. 49, p. 447

Anatomy

GEORGE R. SCHOEDINGER, III, B.S., M.D.

MULTIPLE CHOICE, SINGLE ANSWER (answers on p. 268)

Select the *one* answer that will best complete or answer each of the following statements or questions.

1. Where is Erb's point in the brachial plexus?
   a. The junction of the fifth and sixth cervical roots
   b. The junction of the anterior and posterior divisions of the superior and middle trunks   **Ref. 43, p. 1719**
   c. The junction of the posterior divisions of the superior, middle, and inferior trunks
   d. The junction of the medial and lateral cords
   e. The junction of the eighth cervical and first thoracic roots

2. In evaluating a patient with low back pain, it is noted that there is decreased sensation on the dorsum of the foot between the great and second toes. This area is supplied by the _____ nerve.
   a. Sural
   b. Saphenous   **Ref. 60, p. 1000**
   c. Medial plantar
   d. Superficial peroneal
   e. Deep peroneal

3. The "spring" ligament of the foot is virtually compressed between the:
   a. Talus and os calcis
   b. Talus and posterior tibial tendon   **Ref. 17, p. 410**
   c. Talus and anterior tibial tendon   **Ref. 20, p. 410**
   d. Talus and peroneus tendon
   e. Talus and long plantar ligament

4. The contents of the radial bursa include the _____ tendon.
   a. Flexor pollicis longus
   b. Abductor pollicis longus   **Ref. 60, p. 474**
   c. Flexor carpi radialis
   d. Palmaris longus
   e. Flexor digitorum sublimis to the second
      digit
5. In Bennett's fracture the fragments are displaced proximally by the unopposed pull of the _____ muscle.
   a. Extensor pollicis longus
   b. Flexor policis longus   **Ref. 43, p. 192**
   c. Flexor pollicis brevis
   d. Abductor pollicis longus
   e. Adductor pollicis
6. The so-called keystone of the foot is the _____ metatarsal.
   a. First
   b. Second   **Ref. 20, p. 413**
   c. Third
   d. Fourth
   e. Fifth
7. The tendon of the plantaris muscle inserts _____ to the tendo calcaneus.
   a. Medially
   b. Laterally   **Ref. 60, p. 507**
   c. Anteriorly
   d. Posteriorly
8. The nerve supply to the knee joint is from branches of the _____
   nerve.
   a. Obturator
   b. Femoral   **Ref. 60, p. 997**
   c. Tibial
   d. Peroneal
   e. All of the above
9. Anastomoses between the haversian canals and the marrow cavity occur
   through:
   a. Canaliculi
   b. Volkmann's canals   **Ref. 25, p. 226**
   c. Lacunae   **Ref. 63. p. 417**
   d. Sharpey's fibers
   e. Interstitial lamellae
10. A sarcomere is bounded by _____ discs.
    a. A
    b. H   **Ref. 25, p. 276**
    c. Z   **Ref. 63, p. 528**
    d. I
    e. M

11. Haversian canals are connected to lacunae by:
    a. Sharpey's fibers
    b. Cementing lines of von Ebner   Ref. 25, p. 225
    c. Canaliculi   Ref. 63, p. 417
    d. Volkmann's canals
    e. Lamellae

12. Hensen's or the H disc is located within the _____ disc.
    a. I
    b. Z   Ref. 25, p. 278
    c. A   Ref. 63, p. 529
    d. N
    e. M

13. Periosteum adheres densely to bone by virtue of connective tissue pro-
    longations called:
    a. Cement lines of von Ebner
    b. Interstitial lamellae   Ref. 25, p. 227
    c. Fibroblasts
    d. Sharpey's fibers
    e. Circumferential lamellae

14. The action of the quadratus plantae is to:
    a. Support the plantar fascia by muscle
       tension
    b. Aid in flexion of the toes by virtue of its   Ref. 60, p. 516
       insertion
    c. Work as a bowstring to maintain elevation
       of the medial longitudinal arch
    d. Aid in adduction of the great toe
    e. Stabilize the metatarsophalangeal joints in
       extension

15. From occiput to sacrum, the intervertebral discs contribute about what
    percentage of the total vertebral height?
    a. 10%
    b. 25%   Ref. 127, 47-A:212, 1965
    c. 40%
    d. 60%

16. The vertebral artery enters the vertebral column at the level of the
    _____ cervical vertebra.
    a. Second
    b. Fourth   Ref. 60, p. 602
    c. Fifth
    d. Sixth
    e. Seventh

17. By far the greatest percentage of rotation of the head occurs at the
    _____ joint.
    a. Atlantooccipital
    b. Atlantoaxial   Ref. 127, 46-A:1767, 1964
    c. Cervical intervertebral   Ref. 127, 47-A:211, 1965
    d. Thoracocervical

18. Unilateral fusion of the fifth lumbar vertebra to the sacrum occurs in about what percentage of persons?
    a. Less than 1%
    b. 5%   Ref. 127, 47-A:210, 1965
    c. 15%
    d. 20%
    e. 25%

19. Which of the following bones is occasionally pierced by a cutaneous nerve?
    a. Fibula
    b. Clavicle   Ref. 20, p. 103
    c. Humerus
    d. Ulna
    e. Radius

20. In the adult the angle formed by the long axis of the os calcis and the talus normally is about _____.
    a. 0° to 5°
    b. 5° to 10°   Ref. 114, 93:375, 1965
    c. 10° to 15°
    d. 15° to 30°
    e. 30° to 50°

21. Glenohumeral motion represents about _____ of total shoulder motion.
    a. 25%
    b. 33%   Ref. 20, p. 169
    c. 50%
    d. 66%
    e. 75%

22. When exposing the brachial artery, you generally would expect to find the median nerve _____ to the artery.
    a. Superficial
    b. Deep   Ref. 60, p. 614
    c. Lateral
    d. Medial

23. The autonomous area of sensation of the median nerve is the:
    a. Dorsum of the thumb
    b. Tip of the fifth digit   Ref. 17, p. 1064
    c. Tip of the second digit
    d. Hypothenar eminence
    e. Thenar eminence

24. The superior gluteal artery and nerve leave the pelvis lying superficial to the _____ muscle.
    a. Superior gemellus
    b. Inferior gemellus   Ref. 60, p. 649
    c. Quadratus femoris
    d. Piriformis
    e. Obturator internus

25. The carotid sheath contains which of the following?
    a. Carotid artery, phrenic nerve, and
       jugular vein
    b. Carotid artery and jugular vein   **Ref. 60, p. 395**
    c. Carotid artery, jugular vein, and vagus
       nerve
    d. Carotid artery, phrenic nerve, and vagus nerve
    e. Carotid artery and phrenic nerve
26. The artery of the ligamentum teres femoris arises from which artery?
    a. Femoral
    b. Obturator   **Ref. 60, p. 646**
    c. Middle sacral
    d. Inferior gluteal
    e. External iliac
27. The pes anserinus is formed by the insertion of which of the following?
    a. Semimembranosus, semitendinosus, and
       sartorius
    b. Semitendinosus, biceps femoris, and   **Ref. 98, p. 286**
       gracilus
    c. Gracilis, sartorius, and biceps femoris
    d. Sartorius, gracilis, and semitendinosus
    e. Semimembranosus, semitendinosus, and
       biceps femoris
28. When in the anatomic position, the boundaries of the anatomic snuff-
    box from the radial to the ulnar side are the:
    a. Extensor pollicis longus, extensor pollicis
       brevis, and extensor carpi radialis
    b. Abductor pollicis longus, extensor pollicis   **Ref. 20, p. 146**
       brevis, and extensor pollicis longus
    c. Extensor pollicis brevis, extensor pollicis
       longus, and abductor pollicis longus
    d. Abductor pollicis brevis, extensor pollicis
       longus, and extensor carpi radialis
    e. Extensor pollicis longus, extensor pollicis
       brevis, and extensor indicis proprius
29. The adductor canal contains which of the following structures?
    a. Femoral artery and vein, nerve to the
       vastus medialis, and saphenous nerve
    b. Femoral vein and nerve to the articularis   **Ref. 60, p. 657**
       genu
    c. Popliteal artery and saphenous nerve and
       vein
    d. Femoral artery and vein, nerve to the
       vastus medialis, and articularis genu
    e. Popliteal artery and vein and nerve to the
       vastus medialis

30. The rotator cuff is composed of which of the following?
    a. Supraspinatus, infraspinatus, teres major, and teres minor
    b. Supraspinatus, infraspinatus, teres minor, and subscapularis
    c. Supraspinatus, deltoid, and subscapularis
    d. Deltoid, latissimus dorsi, and serratus anterior
    e. Deltoid, trapezius, and teres major

    Ref. 36, p. 250
    Ref. 141, 75:443, 1942

31. The boundaries of the femoral triangle (Scarpa's triangle) are the:
    a. Inguinal ligament, pyramidalis, and external oblique
    b. Sartorius, inguinal ligament, and adductor longus
    c. Knee joint, sartorius, tensor faciae latae, and iliotibial band
    d. Sartorius, gracilis, and inguinal ligament
    e. Knee joint, rectus femoris, and sartorius

    Ref. 60, p. 656

32. The deep or fourth layer of the foot contains which muscles?
    a. Quadratus plantae and lumbricales
    b. Abductor hallucis, abductor digiti quinti, and flexor digitorum brevis
    c. Dorsal and plantar interossei
    d. Flexor hallucis brevis, flexor digiti quinti brevis and adductor hallucis
    e. Quadratus plantae, flexor hallucis brevis, and flexor digitorum brevis

    Ref. 60, p. 518

33. The boundaries of the lumbar triangle are the:
    a. Iliac crest, latissimus dorsi, and external oblique
    b. Musculotendinous junction of the latissimus dorsi, dorsal spinous processes, and inferior border of the trapezius
    c. Gluteus maximus, dorsal spinous processes, and inferior border of the trapezius
    d. Line between the posterior superior iliac spines and the musculotendinous junctions of the trapezius muscles
    e. Inferior border of the trapezius, lateral border of the serratus posterior, and superior border of the latissimus dorsi

    Ref. 60, p. 448

34. Rotation of the scapula, as in full abduction of the arm, is accomplished by the:
    a. Levator scapula and rhomboideus minor
    b. Deltoid and levator scapula
    c. Deltoid and rhomboideus major and minor
    d. Trapezius and serratus anterior
    e. Serratus anterior and deltoid

    Ref. 60, p. 454

35. The nutrient artery of the tibia enters the bone directly below what structure?
    a. Semimembranosus insertion
    b. Popliteal line   **Ref. 60, p. 249**
    c. Insertion of the ligamentum patellae
    d. Tibial tuberosity
    e. Pes anserinus
36. In exposing the posterior distal aspect of the humerus through a posterior midline incision after the triceps tendon has been divided, what artery comes into view crossing the supracondylar area?
    a. Superior ulner collateral
    b. Inferior ulnar collateral   **Ref. 60, p. 617**
    c. Radial collateral branch of the profunda
       brachii
    d. Middle collateral branch of the profunda
       brachii
    e. Posterior ulnar recurrent
37. The incision for a Bankart shoulder reconstruction lies along the deltopectoral groove and therefore exposes what vascular structure?
    a. Basilic vein
    b. Brachial vein   **Ref. 43, p. 458**
    c. Axillary vein   **Ref. 60, p. 700**
    d. Costoaxillary vein
    e. Cephalic vein
38. Which of the following make up the "cruciate anastomosis"?
    a. Superior and inferior gluteal arteries and
       medial and lateral femoral circumflex arteries
    b. Superior gluteal artery, medial and lateral   **Ref. 20, p. 358**
       femoral circumflex arteries, and second
       perforating branch of the profunda femoris
    c. Inferior gluteal artery, first perforating
       branch of the profunda femoris, and
       medial and lateral femoral circumflex arteries
    d. Superior gluteal artery, obturator artery,
       lateral femoral circumflex artery, and first
       perforating branch of the profunda femoris
    e. Inferior gluteal artery, lateral femoral circumflex artery, second perforating branch
       of the profunda femoris, and obturator
       artery
39. The boundaries of the quadrangular space in the axilla are the:
    a. Teres major, lateral head of the triceps,
       medial head of the triceps, and long head
       of the triceps

b. Teres major, teres minor, infraspinatus,   **Ref. 20, p. 83**
   and long head of the triceps
c. Inferior deltoid margin, lateral head of
   the triceps, lateral humeral margin, and
   teres minor
d. Teres major, teres minor, medial border of
   the humerus, and long head of the triceps
e. Teres minor, inferior deltoid margin,
   medial head of the triceps, and medial
   border of the humerus

40. The quadrangular space is important in that through it passes the:
   a. Radial nerve and profunda brachii
   b. Circumflex scapular artery   **Ref. 20, p. 83**
   c. Upper lateral cutaneous nerve of the arm
   d. Musculocutaneous nerve
   e. Axillary nerve and posterior humeral cir-
      cumflex artery

41. The optimum point for blocking the ilioinguinal and iliohypogastric
   nerves with a local anesthetic agent is:
   a. 1 to 2 cm medial to the anterior superior
      iliac spine
   b. Midway between the anterior superior   **Ref. 60, p. 986**
      iliac spine and the pubic tubercle
   c. 4 to 6 cm posterior to the anterior superior
      iliac spine at the iliac crest
   d. Equidistant between the anterior superior
      iliac spine, pubic tubercle, and greater
      trochanter
   e. Equidistant between the posterior superior
      iliac spine and the dorsal spinous process
      of L-4

42. Atrophy of the first dorsal interosseous muscle in the hand is usually
   found after damage to which of the following?
   a. Radial nerve
   b. Ulnar nerve   **Ref. 60, p. 486**
   c. Median nerve
   d. Musculocutaneous nerve
   e. Superficial branch of the radial nerve

43. The meniscofemoral ligaments insert on the:
   a. Medial aspect of the medial condyle
   b. Lateral aspect of the lateral condyle   **Ref. 60, p. 352**
   c. Medial aspect of the lateral condyle
   d. Lateral aspect of the medial condyle

44. The iliopsoas is a strong flexor at the hip and a moderately strong:
   a. Medial rotator
   b. Lateral rotator   **Ref. 60, p. 489**
   c. Both of the above
   d. Neither a nor b

45. With a sudden downward pull on the arm hanging at the subject's side, stability of the shoulder joint is maintained primarily by the:
    a. Deltoid
    b. Biceps brachii and long head of the triceps   Ref. 19, p. 198
    c. Infraspinatus and subscapularis
    d. Supraspinatus and superior capsule
    e. Pectoralis major

46. The hamstrings, relative to the gluteus maximus, are _____ active while walking or bending forward at the hip.
    a. More
    b. Less   Ref. 19, pp. 253-254
    c. Not
    d. Equally

47. The hip capsule is weakest:
    a. Inferiorly
    b. Posteriorly between the ischiofemoral   Ref. 17, p. 388
       (ischiocapsular) and the pubofemoral
       (pubocapsular) ligaments
    c. Posteriorly between the ischiofemoral
       (ischiocapsular) and the iliofemoral liga-
       ments
    d. Anteriorly between the iliofemoral and
       pubofemoral (pubocapsular) ligaments
       beneath the iliopectineal bursa

48. The meniscofemoral ligaments closely follow the course of the:
    a. Anterior cruciate ligament
    b. Posterior cruciate ligament   Ref. 60, p. 352
    c. Popliteus tendon   Ref. 127, 46-B:307, 1964
    d. Medial collateral ligament

49. Posteriorly, the talus is grooved in order to accept the tendon of which of the following?
    a. Flexor hallucis longus
    b. Flexor digitorum longus   Ref. 60, p. 260
    c. Tibialis posterior
    d. Peroneus longus
    e. Peroneus brevis

50. In whites the most distal vertebra with a bifid dorsal spinous process is:
    a. C-3
    b. C-4   Ref. 92, p. 99
    c. C-5
    d. C-6

51. The meniscofemoral ligaments originate from the:
    a. Anterior horn of the medial meniscus
    b. Posterior horn of the lateral meniscus   Ref. 60, p. 352
    c. Anterior horn of the lateral meniscus   Ref. 127, 46-B:307, 1964
    d. Posterior horn of the medial meniscus

52. A straight line through the body between the anterior superior iliac spine and the ischial tuberosity is known as _____ line.
   a. Poupart's
   b. Bull's   Ref. 93, p. 366
   c. Hilgenreiner's
   d. Perkin's
   e. Roser-Nélaton

53. When taut, the meniscofemoral ligaments pull the meniscus:
   a. Anteromedially
   b. Posteromedially   Ref. 127, 46-B:307, 1964
   c. Posterolaterally
   d. Anterolaterally

54. The talus best fits the ankle mortise in which of the following?
   a. All positions
   b. At no time   Ref. 93, p. 384
   c. Full dorsiflexion
   d. Full plantar flexion
   e. External rotation and inversion

55. In examining a patient with low back pain, an area of hypesthesia is noted over the dorsolateral aspect of the foot. This area is supplied by branches of the _____ nerve.
   a. Superficial peroneal
   b. Deep peroneal   Ref. 60, p. 1000
   c. Sural
   d. Lateral plantar
   e. Saphenous

56. This nerve (answer to 55) most commonly contains fibers from which spinal roots?
   a. L-2 and L-3
   b. L-3 and L-4   Ref. 60, p. 999
   c. L-4 and L-5
   d. L-5 and S-1
   e. S-1 and S-2

57. Lister's tubercle is a landmark on which bone?
   a. Navicular
   b. Capitate   Ref. 7, 16:54, 1959
   c. Hamate
   d. Radius
   e. Ulna

58. The dorsal radial tubercle forms a pulley for the _____ tendon.
   a. Extensor pollicis longus
   b. Extensor pollicis brevis   Ref. 110, p. 105
   c. Abductor pollicis longus
   d. Extensor carpi radialis longus
   e. Extensor indicus

59. Which of the following muscles has the greatest tendon excursion?
    a. Extensor carpi radialis longus
    b. Extensor digitorum communis   **Ref. 30, p. 15**
    c. Extensor pollicis longus
    d. Flexor digitorum sublimis
    e. Flexor digitorum profundus
60. Concerning normal articular cartilage, which of the following is *not* true?
    a. It lacks nerves.
    b. It is covered with a synovial membrane.   **Ref. 18, pp. 9, 25**
    c. It is devoid of blood vessels and lymphatics.
    d. It never ossifies.
    e. Mitotic figures are infrequent.
61. Normal hyaline cartilage proliferation occurs in the _____ stratum.
    a. Calcified cartilage
    b. Superficial or tangential   **Ref. 18, p. 13**
    c. Intermediate
    d. Radiate
62. Which of the following does not lie in the volar carpal canal?
    a. Palmaris longus tendon
    b. Median nerve   **Ref. 7, 16:57, 1959**
    c. Flexor digitorum sublimis tendons
    d. Flexor digitorum profundus tendons
    e. Flexor pollicis longus tendon
63. The periodicity of normal adult cartilage is _____ angstrom units.
    a. 690
    b. 300   **Ref. 18, p. 9**
    c. 410
    d. 220
    e. 815
64. Surgery in the area of the sternocleidomastoid muscle is complicated by the eleventh cranial nerve, which lies superficial to the _____ portion of the muscle.
    a. Cleidooccipital
    b. Superficial sternomastoid   **Ref. 125, 125:476, 1944**
    c. Deep sternomastoid
    d. Superficial sternooccipital
    e. Deep cleidomastoid
65. McRae's, Chamberlain's, and McGregor's lines form points of reference for evaluation of the:
    a. Base of the skull and upper cervical area
    b. Hip joint and proximal femur   **Ref. 105, p. 519**
    c. Subtalar joint
    d. Glenohumeral joint and scapulothoracic area
    e. Talotibial joint
66. Individual skeletal muscles are identifiable and well formed by the _____ week of fetal life.
    a. Fifth
    b. Tenth   **Ref. 4, p. 5**

c. Fifteenth
d. Twentieth
e. Twenty-fifth
67. The lateral dorsal cutaneous nerve of the foot is a terminal branch of the:
    a. Sural nerve
    b. Superficial peroneal nerve   **Ref. 60, p. 998**
    c. Deep peroneal nerve
    d. Lateral plantar nerve
68. After birth the normal increase in muscle mass is believed to be the result of:
    a. An increase in number of muscle fibers
       by division of existing myofibrils
    b. An increase in the size and length of   **Ref. 4, pp. 6, 7**
       existing muscle fibers
    c. An increase in the number of new muscle
       fibers from mesenchymal precursor cells
    d. An increase in both the number and size
       of the myofibrils
69. The deep peroneal nerve is expected to contain fibers from the _____
    nerve roots.
    a. L-2 and L-3
    b. L-3 and L-4   **Ref. 60, p. 999**
    c. L-4 and L-5
    d. L-5 and S-1
    e. S-1 and S-2
70. The tibialis posterior may help support the medial longitudinal arch by
    virtue of its insertions, the major one of which is on the:
    a. Navicular
    b. Three cuneiform bones   **Ref. 60, p. 509**
    c. Second, third, and fourth metatarsals
    d. Cuboid
    e. Os calcis
71. The mechanics of the subtalar joint are such that in the pronated foot
    the os calcis is displaced:
    a. Posteriorly
    b. Anteriorly   **Ref. 127, 34-A:927, 1952**
    c. Laterally
    d. Posterolaterally
    e. Anterolaterally
72. Chopart's joint is the:
    a. Distal radioulnar
    b. Radionavicular lunate   **Ref. 43, p. 849**
    c. Talonavicular and calcaneocuboid
    d. Navicular cuneiform
    e. Subtalar

73. In a long bone with two or more epiphyses the nutrient artery is directed
_____ the epiphysis, which is the first to unite with the shaft.
   a. Toward
   b. Away from   Ref. 17, p. 138
   c. Without known correlation to
   d. Neither toward nor away from
74. The hip joint is an example of a (an) _____ joint.
   a. Trochoidal
   b. Ginglymus   Ref. 17, p. 385
   c. Spheroid
   d. Ellipsoidal
   e. Spiral
75. The flexor hallucis longus is a _____ muscle.
   a. Unipennate
   b. Bipennate   Ref. 17, p. 593
   c. Multipennate
   d. Fusiform
   e. Hypersufficient
76. The lateral lip of the linea aspera is a downward continuation of the:
   a. Pectineal line
   b. Intertrochanteric line
   c. Intertrochanteric crest   Ref. 60, p. 240
   d. Gluteal tuberosity
   e. Lesser trochanter
77. The sternal angle occurs at the junction of the manubrium and the
sternum and is at the level of the _____ costal cartilage.
   a. First
   b. Second   Ref. 20, p. 422
   c. Third
   d. Fourth
   e. Fifth
78. Indicate the muscle that is the main abductor of the hip.
   a. Gluteus maximus
   b. Gluteus medius   Ref. 60, p. 497
   c. Gluteus minimus
   d. Tensor fasciae latae
   e. Iliopsoas
79. The tendo Achillis rotates about _____ on an axis between its origin and
its insertion.
   a. 30°
   b. 40°   Ref. 43, p. 1209
   c. 60°
   d. 75°
   e. 90°
80. The nutrient artery to the femur usually arises from a branch of the:
   a. Posterior circumflex femoral
   b. Second perforating artery   Ref. 60, p. 660

c. First perforating artery
d. Deep femoral artery
e. Obturator artery

MULTIPLE CHOICE, MULTIPLE ANSWERS (answers on pp. 268-269)

Select one or more answers that will best complete or answer each of the following statements or questions.

81. Which of the following attach to the coracoid process of the scapula?
    a. Biceps brachii (short head)
    b. Biceps brachii (long head)   **Ref. 60, p. 302**
    c. Coracobrachialis
    d. Pectoralis minor
    e. Pectoralis major

82. The median plantar nerve:
    a. Lies posterior to the tibial artery
    b. Lies deep to the quadratus plantae mus-   **Ref. 60, p. 998**
       cle
    c. Usually innervates only three muscles
    d. Supplies sensation to all of the plantar
       surface of the forefoot
    e. Lies deep to the abductor hallucis muscle

83. Fascia lata arises from the:
    a. Iliac crest
    b. Coccyx   **Ref. 60, p. 491**
    c. Sacrum   **Ref. 105, p. 286**
    d. Inguinal ligament
    e. Superior pubic ramus

84. The scapular notch allows passage of the:
    a. Suprascapular artery
    b. Dorsal scapular nerve   **Ref. 60, p. 201**
    c. Circumflex scapular nerve   **Ref. 110, p. 54**
    d. Suprascapular nerve
    e. Dorsal scapular artery

85. Anatomic shortening of the iliotibial band tends to produce:
    a. Abduction of the femur
    b. Hip flexion   **Ref. 105, p. 287**
    c. Internal rotation of the femur
    d. Flexion of the knee
    e. Genu valgum

86. The extensor carpi radialis brevis arises principally from the _____ and inserts on the base of the _____ metacarpal.
    a. Lateral epicondyle of the humerus
    b. Radial collateral ligament   **Ref. 60, p. 468**
    c. Intermuscular septum
    d. Second
    e. Third

87. If the radial nerve is divided 0.5 cm proximal to where it bifurcates into its superficial and deep branches, motor function will usually remain in the:
    a. Brachioradialis
    b. Extensor carpi radialis longus   Ref. 60, p. 976
    c. Extensor carpi radialis brevis
    d. Extensor pollicis longus
    e. Extensor digitorum longus
88. Fibrocartilage is found in the:
    a. Ventral ends of ribs
    b. Intervertebral discs   Ref. 25, p. 217
    c. Pinna of the ear
    d. Ligamentum teres femoris
    e. Symphysis pubis
89. Lateral rotators of the humerus include the:
    a. Teres major
    b. Teres minor   Ref. 60, p. 455
    c. Supraspinatus
    d. Posterior fibers of the deltoid
    e. Infraspinatus
90. The posterior cord of the brachial plexus gives rise to the:
    a. Ulnar nerve
    b. Median nerve   Ref. 60, p. 961
    c. Radial nerve
    d. Musculocutaneous nerve
    e. Axillary nerve
91. Which of the following arise from the fibula?
    a. Tibialis anterior
    b. Tibialis posterior   Ref. 60, pp. 504, 507, 509
    c. Gastrocnemius
    d. Soleus
    e. Extensor hallucis longus
92. Excision of the lateral meniscus is not infrequently complicated by injury to the:
    a. Anterior cruciate ligament
    b. Posterior cruciate ligament   Ref. 43, p. 917
    c. Biceps femoris tendon
    d. Lateral collateral ligament
    e. Popliteus tendon
93. A sarcomere contains which of the following discs?
    a. A
    b. I   Ref. 25, p. 276
    c. N
    d. H
    e. M

94. A median plantar neurectomy is expected to cause paralysis of the:
    a. Interossei
    b. Flexor hallucis brevis   Ref. 60, p. 998
    c. Adductor hallucis
    d. Flexor digitorum brevis
    e. Quadratus plantae

95. Indicate the muscle(s) that is (are) not likely to have dual innervation, that is, both preaxial and postaxial components.
    a. Pectineus
    b. Biceps femoris   Ref. 110, pp. 89, 541, 553, 555
    c. Adductor magnus
    d. Vastus medialis
    e. Brachialis

96. The peroneal division of the sciatic nerve passes through the piriformis muscle in about _____ of persons and above it in about _____ of persons.
    a. 34%
    b. 22%   Ref. 20, p. 353
    c. 12%
    d. 5%
    e. 0%

97. A crushing injury of the medial humeral epicondyle dividing the ulnar nerve would cause paralysis of the:
    a. Palmaris brevis
    b. Palmaris longus   Ref. 60, p. 972
    c. Interossei
    d. Adductor pollicis
    e. Adductor pollicis brevis

98. The pure flexors of the elbow are the:
    a. Biceps brachii
    b. Brachioradialis   Ref. 60, p. 460, 467
    c. Coracobrachialis
    d. Brachialis
    e. Flexor carpi radialis longus

99. Which of the following are innervated by the same terminal nerve?
    a. Flexor digitorum longus
    b. Peroneus longus   Ref. 60, pp. 492, 507, 511
    c. Peroneus brevis
    d. Peroneus tertius
    e. Quadriceps femoris

100. Arrange in order, from above downward, the insertions of the following muscles.
    a. Gemellus superior
    b. Gemellus inferior   Ref. 60, p. 499
    c. Obturator externus
    d. Obturator internus
    e. Piriformis

101. A median parapatellar incision frequently divides a branch of the:
    a. Obturator nerve
    b. Ilioinguinal nerve   **Ref. 60, p. 989**
    c. Medial femoral cutaneous nerve
    d. Intermediate femoral cutaneous nerve
    e. Saphenous nerve

102. Spondylolisthesis implies a defect in the bony structure of the vertebra in which area(s)?
    a. Lamina
    b. Pedicle   **Ref. 43, p. 2008**
    c. Pars interarticularis
    d. Superior articular facet
    e. Inferior articular facet

103. The posterior branch of the obturator nerve does not usually supply the:
    a. Adductor magnus muscle
    b. Obturator externus muscle   **Ref. 60, p. 987**
    c. Adductor brevis muscle   **Ref. 110, p. 553**
    d. Gracilis muscle
    e. Obturator internus muscle

104. The gluteus maximus is a strong _____ of the thigh.
    a. Extensor
    b. Abductor   **Ref. 60, p. 497**
    c. Lateral rotator
    d. Medial rotator

105. Distally, the radius is grooved to articulate with the:
    a. Scaphoid
    b. Hamate   **Ref. 60, p. 214**
    c. Lunate
    d. Greater multangular
    e. Capitate

106. Which of the following are unlikely to provide innervation to the hip joint?
    a. Terminal branches of the nerve to the rectus femoris
    b. Terminal branches of the nerve to the   **Ref. 110, pp. 553, 555** quadratus femoris
    c. Branches of the posterior division of the obturator nerve
    d. Branches of the anterior division of the obturator nerve
    e. Branches of the nerve to the adductor magnus

107. Which of the following lie between the brachialis and the brachioradialis muscles?
    a. Median nerve
    b. Radial nerve   **Ref. 60, p. 467**
    c. Dorsal interosseous branch of the radial nerve

d. The anastomosis between the radial collateral branch of the profunda brachii
artery and the radial recurrent
artery

e. Origin of the median antebrachial cutaneous nerve

108. The innervation of the shoulder joint is derived from branches of the:
a. Suprascapular nerve
b. Lateral cord   **Ref. 17, p. 360**
c. Dorsal scapular nerve
d. Axillary nerve
e. Subscapular nerves

109. In better than 50% of persons the abductor pollicis longus tendon is
divided into more than one part and when so divided may insert into
which of the following?
a. Base of the first metacarpal
b. Thenar fascia   **Ref. 7, 16:54, 1959**
c. Trapezium   **Ref. 43, p. 370**
d. Base of the first proximal phalanx
e. Trapezoid

110. Between the superficial and deep layers of the supinator muscle lie
the following important structure(s):
a. Median nerve
b. Deep branch of the radial nerve   **Ref. 60, p. 470**
c. Posterior interosseous artery
d. Nerve to the anconeus

SITUATION AND PROGRESSIVE THOUGHT (answers on p. 269)

Select the answer or answers that best apply in accordance with the information given in each of the following statements.

111. A patient is admitted having suffered a stab wound of the proximal
thigh immediately below the femoral triangle. After passing directly
posterior through the interval between the sartorius and rectus femoris,
the blade would next pierce the:
a. Nerve to the rectus femoris
b. Vastus intermedius   **Ref. 17, p. 573**
c. Profunda femoris artery
d. Obturator nerve
e. Vastus medialis

112. Directly deep to the structure indicated in 111 lies the:
a. Anterior division of the obturator nerve
b. Pectineus   **Ref. 17, p. 573**
c. Profunda femoris artery
d. Adductor brevis
e. Sciatic nerve

113. In the proximal area of the thigh, which of the following almost completely surrounds the femur and is closest to it?
    a. Rectus femoris
    b. Vastus lateralis   **Ref. 17, p. 573**
    c. Vastus medialis
    d. Vastus intermedius
    e. Adductor magnus

114. Assuming that the blade passed between the profunda femoris and femoral artery, what structure(s) would be immediately vulnerable?
    a. Posterior division of the obturator nerve
    b. Adductor brevis   **Ref. 17, p. 573**
    c. Sciatic nerve
    d. Gracilis
    e. Adductor longus

115. A foreign body is lodged in the plantar interossei between the second and third metatarsals at a midshaft level. The wound of entrance is on the plantar surface of the foot. How many potential spaces did this object traverse, assuming its present position?
    a. Zero
    b. Two   **Ref. 17, p. 601**
    c. Three
    d. Four
    e. Six

116. Which of the following did it last traverse in its migration upward?
    a. Quadratus plantae
    b. Transverse head of the adductor hallucis   **Ref. 17, p. 601**
    c. Oblique head of the adductor hallucis
    d. Flexor digitorum brevis
    e. Flexor hallucis

117. If an infection should start in the central fascial compartment of the foot, which of the following would be involved?
    a. Flexor hallucis longus
    b. Flexor hallucis brevis   **Ref. 17, p. 601**
    c. Flexor digitorum longus
    d. Oblique head of the adductor hallucis

118. A patient sustained a laceration of the volar surface of the forearm immediately proximal to the wrist joint. The pronator quadratus is divided partially. The exposed structure(s) immediately deep to it are the:
    a. Flexor pollicis longus
    b. Flexor carpi radialis   **Ref. 60, p. 479**
    c. Flexor digitorum profundus
    d. All of the above
    e. None of the above

119. Which of the following will lie between the flexor carpi ulnaris and the flexor pollicis longus?
    a. Ulnar nerve
    b. Flexor digitorum profundus   **Ref. 60, p. 479**

43

c. Radial artery

d. Flexor carpi radialis

e. Ulnar artery

120. In repair of the wound described in 118, from deep to superficial, the _____ should be reconstructed first.

a. Flexor pollicis longus

b. Median nerve   **Ref. 60, p. 479**

c. Palmaris longus

d. Flexor carpi radialis

121. A patient was struck in the midportion of the right arm by plate glass. There was a transverse fracture and a severance of major structures. The humerus was stabilized. The brachial artery and vein were anastomosed as well as the basilic vein. Between the latter two structures you would expect to see the:

a. Radial nerve

b. Median nerve   **Ref. 60, p. 459**

c. Ulnar nerve

d. Lateral antebrachial cutaneous nerve

e. Medial antebrachial cutaneous nerve

122. Anterior to the previously indicated structure would be the:

a. Radial nerve

b. Brachialis muscle   **Ref. 60, p. 459**

c. Biceps brachii muscle

d. Ulnar nerve

e. Medial head of the triceps muscle

123. The lateral antebrachial cutaneous nerve lies between the _____ and the _____.

a. Biceps brachii

b. Triceps brachii   **Ref. 60, p. 459**

c. Brachialis muscle

d. Brachial vein

e. Basilic vein

124. The radial nerve would be found between the _____ and the _____.

a. Biceps brachii muscle

b. Brachialis muscle   **Ref. 60, p. 459**

c. Triceps muscle

d. Brachial artery

e. Brachioradialis muscle

125. Posterior to the basilic vein lies the:

a. Radial nerve

b. Brachial artery   **Ref. 60, p. 459**

c. Ulnar nerve

d. Median nerve

e. Median antebrachial cutaneous nerve

126. The radial and ulnar bursae are found on the dorsal aspect of the wrist.
(T) (F)   **Ref. 60, p. 474**

127. In normal synovial lining there may be cartilage cells present.
(T) (F)   **Ref. 18, p. 29**

128. Osteoblasts, osteocytes, and osteoclasts are generally believed to develop from specific precursor cells, and transformation from one cell type to another is not seen.   **Ref. 25, p. 231**
(T) (F)   **Ref. 63, p. 398**

129. The obturator internus leaves the pelvis via the greater sciatic foramen, while the piriformis traverses the lesser sciatic foramen.   **Ref. 60, p. 500**
(T) (F)

130. It has been shown that the trunk of a nerve sending branches to a given muscle tends to supply branches to the joint moved by the muscle and to the area of skin over the insertion of the muscle.   **Ref. 93, p. 292**
(T) (F)

131. The nucleus pulposus is the remnant of the notochord.
(T) (F)   **Ref. 127, 47-A:209, 1965**

132. A venous cut down at the ankle most commonly utilizes the small saphenous vein or one of its branches.   **Ref. 60, p. 717**
(T) (F)

133. The H disc is usually seen best during relaxation of the myofibril.
(T) (F)   **Ref. 25, p. 279**
       Ref. 63, p. 532

134. Muscles are composed of both light and dark fibers, the former supposedly mediating quick movements.   **Ref. 93, p. 400**
(T) (F)

135. Methylene blue placed in the ring finger might be expected to be found in the supratrochlear nodes, since this is one finger drained by the superficial lymphatic system of the forearm.   **Ref. 60, p. 748**
(T) (F)

136. The major blood supply to the little, the ring, the long, and the ulnar side of the index fingers is from the deep palmar arterial arch.
(T) (F)   **Ref. 7, 16:58, 1959**

137. Knowledge of the two potential spaces on the dorsum of the hand is important, since both communicate with the palm and therefore may be a route for the spread of infection.   **Ref. 7, 16:55, 1959**
(T) (F)

138. Because of their insertion, it has been shown that the cruciate ligaments will allow 160° of internal rotation of the tibia on the femur if all other ligaments are divided.   **Ref. 127, 23:44, 1941**
(T) (F)

139. The tuber joint angle of the os calcis (Böhler's angle) normally measures 20° to 40°.   **Ref. 42, p. 1090**
(T) (F)

140. The cruciate ligaments seem to have more to do with resistance of varus and valgus forces than do the collateral ligaments since, when the cruciate ligaments are intact and the collateral ligaments are divided, there is instability of the knee; such instability does not occur when the reverse is true.   **Ref. 127, 23:44, 1941**

(T) (F)

LIST (answers on pp. 269-270)

141. List three types of "immovable" joints and describe the type of union in each.   **Ref. 93, p. 288**

142. List in order, from anterior to posterior, the structures encountered from the medial malleolus to the flexor hallucis longus tendon.

                                                      Ref. 60, p. 667

143. List six ligamentous structures that attach to the coracoid process of the scapula.   **Ref. 60, p. 319ff**

144. List in order, from medial to lateral, the structures crossing the ankle joint at the level of the transverse crural ligament.   **Ref. 60, p. 665**

145. List the nerve supply of the hip joint.   **Ref. 60, p. 344**

146. List the four major epiphyseal centers of the lower limb contributing to linear growth. Indicate the percentage of growth attributed to each.

                                            Ref. 127, 39-A:853, 1957
                                              Ref. 127, 45-A:1, 1963

147. List in order, from subchondral bone to joint cavity, the layers encountered in normal adult cartilage.   **Ref. 18, p. 10**

148. List four structures innervated by the axillary nerve.   **Ref. 60, p. 964**

149. List the muscles composing the floor of Scarpa's triangle.   **Ref. 60, p. 656**

150. List the vascular supply of the femoral head and indicate at what age each vessel or system of vessels is most important.   **Ref. 42, p. 750**

                                            Ref. 127, 35-B:442, 1953
                                            Ref. 127, 39-B:358, 1957

SECTION 3

Biomechanics

FLOYD G. GOODMAN, B.S., M.D.

MULTIPLE CHOICE, SINGLE ANSWER (answers on p. 270)

Select the *one* answer that will best complete or answer each of the following statements or questions.

1. Electrical current may be set up between two parts of the same metal if one part is exposed to a higher concentration of oxygen than the other. Corrosion will take place at the:
   a. Anode where there is a greater concentration of oxygen
   b. Anode where there is a lesser concentration of oxygen   **Ref. 127, 38-B:751, 1956**
   c. Cathode where there is a lesser concentration of oxygen
   d. Cathode where there is a greater concentration of oxygen

2. The 11 mm cloverleaf nail, when oriented to present its greatest resistance to bending forces, is approximately _____ stronger than the 9 mm size.
   a. 110%
   b. 80%   **Ref. 7, 11:93, 1954**
   c. 40%   **Ref. 106, 60:13, 20, 1968**
   d. 25%

3. The "swing phase" of the gait cycle:
   a. Is known as the high-energy phase
   b. Is initiated by action of the hip flexors, depends on pendulum action during "swing through," and terminates by deceleration action of the hamstrings in the "heel strike" position   **Ref. 15, p. 168**
   c. In contrast to the stance phase, is unaided by the pull of gravity
   d. Accounts for about 40% of the entire gait cycle and has its highest energy consumption at the "foot flat" position

47

4. The bullet from a .30-06 caliber sporting rifle weighing 150 grams, which has a velocity of 3,000 feet per second, would develop _____ the foot-pounds of energy as the same weight bullet traveling at 750 feet per second.
   a. Two times
   b. Four times
   c. Eight times
   d. Sixteen times

   Ref. KE $= \frac{1}{2}\, mv^2$

5. Those muscles that tend to elevate the arch of the foot as their sole effect on it are the:
   a. Tibialis anterior and peroneus brevis
   b. Tibialis posterior and peroneus longus
   c. Flexor hallucis and digitorum brevis, quadratus plantae, and abductor hallucis
   d. Extensor digitorum longus and brevis, and extensor hallucis longus and brevis

   Ref. 50, p. 183
   Ref. 106, 70:20, 122, 130, 1970

6. The primates differ from most other animals in that their center of gravity is:
   a. Midway between the shoulder and hip girdle at the second lumbar vertebra
   b. Above the level of the supporting joints
   c. Below the level of the supporting joints
   d. Relatively unimportant in the biome-chanical patterns of locomotion

   Ref. 127, 35-A:544, 1953

7. The stance phase of locomotion:
   a. Starts with the "foot flat" position, includes the "toe clearance" position, and ends with the "toe off" position
   b. Starts with the "knee bend" position, includes the "toe off" position, and ends with the "heel strike" position
   c. Starts with the "heel strike" position, includes the "foot flat" and "heel off" positions, and ends with the "toe clearance" position
   d. Starts with the "foot flat" position, includes approximately 60% of the gait cycle, and ends with the "toe clearance" position

   Ref. 15, p. 168

8. Stress may be defined as:
   a. The bend or deflection of the structure under load
   b. Intermolecular resistance within a body to the deforming action of force
   c. The maximum load-carrying capacity of a structure
   d. The bending or displacement of a structure under load

   Ref. 7, 9:257, 1952
   Ref. 7, 18:111, 1961
   Ref. 53, p. 40
   Ref. 56, pp. 33-38

9. During normal barefoot ambulation the major weight is found:
   a. On the first metatarsal head
   b. On the third metatarsal head   Ref. 127, 46-A:329, 1964
   c. On the fifth metatarsal head
   d. On the first toe and fifth metatarsal heads
10. The tibia rotates internally during the:
   a. First quarter of stance phase
   b. Second quarter of stance phase   Ref. 8, 19:63, 1970
   c. Third quarter of stance phase   Ref. 12, p. 203
   d. Fourth quarter of stance phase   Ref. 127, 46-A:364-365, 1964
11. A force acting upon a body (object) at a given point will create a moment about any other point in the body. This is best defined as:
   a. The perpendicular distance between the
      line of application of the force and the
      other point multipled by the magnitude of
      the force
   b. The magnitude of the force plus the   Ref. 53, pp. 13-20
      distance
   c. The magnitude of the force divided by the
      distance
   d. The magnitude of the force plus the dis-
      tance squared
12. The defect in the shaft of a tubular bone that will weaken the bone least per area of bone removed is a:
   a. Circle
   b. Triangle   Ref. 7, 9:261, 1952
   c. Rectangle   Ref. 106, 60:222, 1968
   d. Trapezoid
   e. Square
13. There are usually two components to a spiral fracture of long bones: a spiral component and a longitudinal component. The greatest stability to the fracture would be afforded by screw fixation perpendicular to the long axis of the bone and at:
   a. 30° on either side of the longitudinal com-
      ponent
   b. 45° on either side of the longitudinal com-   Ref. 7, 9:263, 1952
      ponent   Ref. 127, 52-A:507, 1970
   c. 60° on either side of the longitudinal com-
      ponent
   d. 90° to the longitudinal component
14. Fractures occurring in long bones as a result of torsion tend to follow a spiral course:
   a. 30° from the long axis
   b. 45° from the long axis   Ref. 7, 9:268, 1952
   c. 60° from the long axis   Ref. 127, 52-A:507, 1970
   d. 90° from the long axis

15. When the force vectors set up in Russell's traction are perpendicular to each other, the longitudinal force, discounting friction, will be:
    a. Twice the vertical force
    b. One half the vertical force   Ref. 106, 66:144, 1969
    c. One fourth the vertical force   Ref. 127, 17:175, 1935
    d. The same as the vertical force

16. A subject stands on one leg with the pelvis level. The pressure occurring on the femoral head will be approximately:
    a. The body weight minus the weight of the
       leg
    b. Two and one-half times the body weight   Ref. 53, pp. 26-27
    c. Four times the body weight   Ref. 127, 29:618, 1947
    d. Eight times the body weight

17. A child standing on the toes of one foot weighs 100 pounds. The distance from the ankle joint to the area of toe contact with the floor is two times the distance from the ankle joint to the Achilles tendon. The total weight-bearing force across the ankle joint is:
    a. 100 pounds
    b. 200 pounds   Ref. 7, 9:258, 1952
    c. 300 pounds
    d. 400 pounds

18. The lumbar vertebrae of normal young men are known to withstand compressive forces of over:
    a. 400 pounds
    b. 600 pounds   Ref. 11, p. 1
    c. 800 pounds   Ref. 113, 31(Fasc. 2):135, 1961
    d. 1,000 pounds   Ref. 127, 43-A:328, 1961

19. The change in the linear dimensions of a body as the result of the application of force best defines:
    a. Strain
    b. Stress   Ref. 7, 9:257, 1952
    c. Modulus of elasticity   Ref. 7, 18:111, 1961
    d. Work   Ref. 56, pp. 38-47

20. The successive joints within a limb enabling precision movement are termed the "kinetic chain." The freedoms of motion in the upper extremity chain from the shoulder to the fingertip would be:
    a. Three
    b. Five   Ref. 100, p. 63
    c. Seven
    d. Eleven

21. The maximum amount of force that you should expect the strongest bony component of the posterior spinal elements to tolerate, according to Harrington, is approximately:
    a. 50 pounds
    b. 100 pounds   Ref. 127, 44-A:597, 1962
    c. 300 pounds
    d. 500 pounds

22. When standing on tiptoe, the force of the Achilles tendon acting across the ankle joint represents a:
    a. First-class lever system
    b. Second-class lever system   Ref. 56, pp. 402-406
    c. Third-class lever system   Ref. 91, p. 106
    d. Fourth-class lever system   Ref. 100, p. 68
23. The resistance of a material to deformation or bending expressed as stress divided by strain best defines:
    a. Strength
    b. Modulus of elasticity   Ref. 7, 9:257, 1952
    c. Toughness   Ref. 7, 18:111, 1961
    d. Elastic bend
24. Fracture of long bones occurs most frequently as a result of excessive:
    a. Tensile stress
    b. Shear   Ref. 7, 9:268, 1952
    c. Compressive stress   Ref. 56, pp. 386-389
    d. Stiffness
25. The removal of a longitudinal bone graft, creating a slotted defect in a tubular bone, is estimated to reduce the resistance of that bone to torsion by:
    a. 12 times
    b. 100 times   Ref. 7, 9:261, 1952
    c. 200 times   Ref. 106, 60:223, 1968
    d. 1,200 times
26. The superior structural configuration for the resistance to torsion and bending forces per cross-sectional area of material used is the:
    a. Solid rod
    b. I beam   Ref. 7, 9:259, 1952
    c. Flat beam   Ref. 106, 60:15, 221, 1968
    d. Cylinder
27. Five ⅛-inch pins or a Smith-Petersen nail takes up approximately the same cross-sectional area of the femoral neck. This is about _____ of the cross-sectional area.
    a. 2%
    b. 5%   Ref. 45, 13:282, 1959
    c. 10%
    d. 25%
28. The proper drill size when screw fixation is to be used in bone is reported to be the:
    a. Root diameter (screw diameter minus the thread depth on both sides of the screw)
    b. Root diameter plus one third of the   Ref. 106, 72:283, 1970
       thread depths   Ref. 119, 64:347, 1952
    c. Root diameter plus one half of the thread depths
    d. Root diameter plus two thirds of the thread depths

29. As the child adapts from embryonic life to the erect position, the spine develops two countercurves. The first of these to develop is:
    a. Cervical lordosis
    b. Dorsal kyphosis   **Ref. 100, p. 127·**
    c. Lumbar lordosis
    d. Sacral kyphosis
30. A young adult man lifts a 200-pound weight from the floor during weight lifting. Intra-abdominal and intrathoracic pressure would be expected to:
    a. Shift to a negative value
    b. Maintain a constant gradient throughout   **Ref. 11, p. 1**
       the lifting period to ensure uniform car-   **Ref. 119, 107:418-433, 1973**
       diorespiratory function   **Ref. 127, 43-A:334, 1961**
    c. Increase to as high as 50 to 100 mm Hg,
       with the intrathoracic pressure exceeding
       the intra-abdominal pressure
    d. Increase to as high as 50 to 100 mm Hg,
       with the intra-abdominal pressure exceed-
       ing the intrathoracic pressure

MULTIPLE CHOICE, MULTIPLE ANSWERS (answers on pp. 270-271)

Select one or more answers that will best complete or answer each of the following statements or questions.

31. The major stability of the trunk under heavy loading is believed to be provided by the:
    a. Vertebrae, discs, and interspinous ligaments
    b. Deep back and paraspinous muscles   **Ref. 11, p. 1**
    c. Intercostal muscles   **Ref. 119, 107:418-423, 1973**
    d. Abdominal and thoracic cavities   **Ref. 127, 43-A:327, 347, 1961**
32. The primary support and maintenance of the arch of the foot is by the:
    a. Peroneus longus and tibialis posterior
    b. Intrinsic muscles of the foot   **Ref. 106, 70:20, 122, 130, 1970**
    c. Ligamentous structures of the foot   **Ref. 127, 46-A:480, 492, 1964**
    d. Tibialis anterior and peroneus brevis   **Ref. 127, 45-A:1189, 1963**
33. During the walking-gait cycle, the knee reaches maximum flexion of approximately _____ during _____ phase.
    a. 45°
    b. 65°   **Ref. 12, pp. 105-110**
    c. Stance   **Ref. 119, 107:406-410, 1973**
    d. Swing   **Ref. 120, 6(2):18, 1962**
34. The joint(s) having 2° freedom of motion is (are) the:
    a. Proximal interphalangeal joint
    b. Radiohumeral joint   **Ref. 100, p. 62**
    c. Hip joint
    d. Knee joint

35. The myoelectric prosthesis:
    a. Depends on electrical stimulus
       from normally functioning muscles
       for control
    b. Derives its name from utilizing   Ref. 127, 47-B:411, 416, 421, 1965
       electrical motors as a substitute for
       muscle power
    c. Ideally is designed with a feedback
       mechanism that gives a sense of
       tactile or pressure sensation
    d. Depends on electrical stimulus
       from normally functioning muscles
       to provide its power supply
36. Acrylic cement used in the placing of femoral head prostheses:
    a. Gives a permanent bony bond between
       the bone, the cement, and the prosthesis
    b. Is reported to effectively distribute the   Ref. 106, 62:156, 1969
       weight load more evenly throughout the   Ref. 106, 72:145, 239, 1970
       upper femur   Ref. 127, 47-B:361, 1965
    c. Is reported to effectively reduce bone   Ref. 127, 50-B:822, 1968
       reabsorption and migration of the pros-
       thesis
    d. Is replaced by cortical bone within twelve
       to eighteen months
37. The strongest anatomic sites for the placement of the distraction hooks
    used in Harrington rod internal fixation are:
    a. Bases of transverse processes
    b. Tips of transverse processes   Ref. 127, 44-A:597, 1962
    c. Articular processes
    d. Laminae
38. During lifting, with the knees straight, muscle activity in the erector
    spinae muscle occurs when the back is in:
    a. Full flexion
    b. Midflexion   Ref. 19, pp. 183, 297-300
    c. Extension
    d. All of the above
39. The proper and strongest reliable method of securing the ends of wire
    is reported to be:
    a. A square knot
    b. A double twist   Ref. 21, p. 154
    c. Securing all ends together when more than
       one strand is utilized
    d. Securing the two ends separately when
       more than one strand is utilized
40. The resistance of stainless steel implants to corrosion is at least in part
    dependent on:
    a. The presence of from 2% to 4% molyb-
       denum within the composition of the metal

b. A thin invisible protective film of ferrous oxide

Ref. 106, 72:233, 1970
Ref. 127, 38-B:749, 1956

c. A thin invisible film of ferrous sulfide
d. A thin invisible film of chromium oxide

41. Stability is afforded the hip joint by the iliofemoral ligaments that become tight when the femur is in:
   a. Full extension
   b. Full flexion and external rotation   **Ref. 100, pp. 273, 274**
   c. Full flexion and internal rotation
   d. Adduction

42. Electromyographic studies have demonstrated the relative unimportance of which of the following muscle(s) in maintaining the erect position during stance?
   a. Gluteus maximus
   b. Hamstrings   **Ref. 19, pp. 248-249**
   c. Iliopsoas
   d. Quadriceps femoris

43. In the so-called antalgic gait common to patients with painful hip disease:
   a. The center of gravity is shifted away from the painful hip joint to relieve pain
   b. The center of gravity is shifted over the painful hip joint to relieve pain   **Ref. 106, 58:153, 1968**
       Ref. 127, 29:619, 1947
   c. There is increased abduction of the femur
   d. The gait pattern is nearly the same as that seen in abductor weakness

44. Which of the following are biomechanical factors not considered valid in a subject standing on one leg?
   a. The pressure applied to the femoral head is in a vertical plane.
   b. Severance of the fascia lata in a normal individual would not alter the biomechanics of the hip joint.   **Ref. 100, pp. 269, 285, 287**
       Ref. 106, 58:153, 1968
       Ref. 106, 72:15, 1970
   c. The gluteus minimus, because of its angle of force, becomes the prime stabilizer of the hip joint in the adducted position.   **Ref. 127, 29:608, 617, 1947**
   d. A shift of the center of gravity over the supporting foot is necessary to maintain balance in spite of increased tension in the abductors.

45. Vertical loading of the proximal femur will show the earliest cracking of the "stress coat":
   a. Along the superior margin of the neck
   b. Along the inferior margin of the neck   **Ref. 127, 33-A:489, 1951**
   c. Along the lateral aspect of the greater trochanter
   d. Along the intertrochanteric line

46. A criterion of 800 pounds has been set up as the minimum desirable standard for fracture fixation devices of the femoral neck and intertrochanteric areas. Which of the following meet this criterion?
    a. Jewett nail
    b. Holt nail   Ref. 45, 13:281, 1959
    c. Deyerle plate, with five ⅛-inch pins   Ref. 127, 38-A:832, 1956
    d. Thornton plate, with a Smith-Petersen nail   Ref. 127, 45-A:694, 1963
47. Biomechanical studies of the hip joint have shown that pressure on the femoral head in one-leg stance:
    a. Occurs at an angle of 165° to 170° to the vertical
    b. Occurs at an angle of 140° to 150° to the vertical   Ref. 53, pp. 26-28
                           Ref. 106, 72:15, 1970
    c. Is decreased with a shift of the center of   Ref. 127, 29:617-618, 1947
    gravity over the hip joint
    d. Requires a force of 1.5 to 1.9 times the body weight in the abductors to keep the pelvis level
48. Parham bands placed circumferentially around a long bone:
    a. Set up an in vivo battery within the ring and cause electrolytic dissolution and grooving of the bone within 3 weeks, even when present-day accepted metals for surgical implants are used
    b. Are considered a mechanically and surgically sound type of fixation when indicated   Ref. 21, p. 155
    c. Will cut off the periosteal blood supply to the underlying bone within one month
    d. Were originally made of brass and intended for removal after fracture healing
49. Among those who are known to have contributed greatly to biologic engineering and metallurgic principles are:
    a. Venable and Stuck
    b. Bechtol, Ferguson, and Laing   Ref. 21, pp. 1-16
    c. Key
    d. Blunt, Hudack, and Murray
50. Electromyographic studies have shown that the popliteus muscle apparently acts:
    a. As a medial rotator of the tibia
    b. In early flexion to unlock the knee   Ref. 19, p. 140
    c. During standing to prevent knee buckling
    d. During crouching to prevent forward slipping of the femur on the tibia in conjunction with the posterior cruciate ligament

51. During running gait, which of the following is (are) true?
    a. The hip and knee reach maximum exten-
       sion during "follow-through."
    b. The knee reaches maximum extension   Ref. 12, pp. 105-110
       during "foot descent."
    c. Knee flexion is maximum during "forward
       swing" and is well in excess of 90°.
    d. The velocity of the foot is 0 in its most for-
       ward and in the trailing position.
52. The clavicle would be expected to move through a range of motion up to
    _____ when the shoulder is moved from adduction and internal
    rotation to full abduction and external rotation.
    a. 50° of rotation
    b. 30° in a vertical (forward and backward)   Ref. 106, 58:21, 1968
       axis   Ref. 119, 107:425-432, 1973
    c. 50° in a horizontal axis
    d. No greater than 25° on any single axis
53. Repeated pressure gauge studies of the above-knee (AK) socket during
    ambulation have shown:
    a. Maximum socket pressures usually develop
       at the brim
    b. Maximum socket pressures usually develop   Ref. 122, 10-8:20-55, 1967
       at the distal stump
    c. Pressures developed during walking are
       markedly higher than those experienced
       during stance
    d. Local pressure rarely exceeds 25 psi
54. The axis of vertebral rotation:
    a. Throughout the thoracic level tends to be
       at the center of the spinal cord
    b. Throughout the thoracic level tends to be   Ref. 122, 10-8:66-75, 1967
       at the center of the disc space
    c. Throughout the lumbar level tends to be
       centered between the facets
    d. At the L-5 level tends to be posterior to
       the facets
55. Torsional load applied to long bones would be expected to:
    a. Produce a transverse fracture
    b. Produce a transverse fracture if a drill   Ref. 53, pp. 90-91
       hole were present   Ref. 127, 52-A:507, 1970
    c. Result in spiral fractures along planes of
       maximum tensile stress
    d. Result in fracture through the region of
       the drill hole
56. Biomechanical studies on pes anserine transfers in reconstruction of the
    knee suggest:
    a. The rotatory efficiency is increased by
       nearly 100%

b. The flexor efficiency is increased by   **Ref. 127, 55-A:1225-1241, 1973**
nearly 100%
c. The transplantation is based on sound
biomechanical principles
d. All of the above
57. Synovial fluid:
a. Demonstrates a nonnewtonian behavior
b. Tends to decrease viscosity with increased   **Ref. 56, pp. 252-256**
rate of joint motion, i.e., with increased
shear rate
c. Viscosity is related to the size of the hyaluronic acid molecules and is variable
d. Provides nutrition as a carrier to articular
cartilage
58. The viability and integrity of the skin depend on its nutrition, i.e., blood
supply. Which of the following factors are accurate?
a. Normal skin can easily withstand prolonged pressures of 5 to 7 psi, although
this is above the capillary fill level.
b. The major difference contributing to   **Ref. 56, pp. 263-268**
breakdown of the skin of the buttocks of
a paraplegic patient and a normal individual is protective sensation.
c. Skin repair is scar. It reaches its maximum
strength and maturity at about 6 weeks.
d. The harmful effects of pressure arise from
interference of the blood supply to the
skin.
59. When measured with strain gauges, compression applied to living cortical bone through the use of bone plates and screws would be expected
to show:
a. A decrease to immeasurable levels rapidly
over the first 5 to 7 days.
b. A decrease rapidly by about 20%, then   **Ref. 113, Supp. 125, pp. 5-41**
continue to slowly decrease, showing re-
sidual compressive forces up to 4 months.
c. Decreased compressive forces due primarily to bone necrosis.
d. Decreased compressive forces due primarily to bone remodeling.
60. A force (vector) is a push or pull and will have which of the following
defining characteristics?
a. Magnitude
b. Direction   **Ref. 53, pp. 13-20**
c. Point of application
d. Shear stress

Select the answer or answers that best apply in accordance with the information given in each of the following statements.

61. As a newly appointed team physician to a small college, you find what seems to be an unusual number of knee injuries. On physical examination, nearly 70% of the athletes are judged to have abnormal mechanical knee instability. A likely cause for this would be:
    a. Excessive deep squatting exercises
    b. Excessive progressive resistance exercises to the hamstrings
    c. Excessive progressive resistance exercises to the quadriceps carried out improperly
    d. Excessive lateral bending exercises causing unguarded stress to the medial and lateral collateral ligaments of the knee

    Ref. 12, p. 178
    Ref. 127, 44-A:1192, 1962

62. The pathology incriminated in the mechanical instability from the aforementioned cause is:
    a. Overstretching and relaxation of the quadriceps mechanism
    b. Overpulled hamstrings, with laxity of the pes anserinus
    c. Laxity of the posterior cruciate ligament
    d. Laxity of the medial and lateral collateral and the anterior cruciate ligaments

    Ref. 127, 44-A:1192, 1962

63. While watching the team undergo strenuous conditioning exercises, you find your suspicions were correct. In instituting corrective measures, the greatest protective stability to the knee would be afforded by specific resistance extension exercises between:
    a. 0° and 10° flexion
    b. 20° and 30° flexion
    c. 30° and 45° flexion
    d. 45° and 90° flexion

    Ref. 127, 44-A:1182, 1962

64. This exercise would be primarily directed at strengthening the:
    a. Articularis genu
    b. Vastus intermedius
    c. Relaxed structures contributing to the mechanical instability
    d. Vastus medialis

    Ref. 127, 44-A:1182, 1962

65. The trainer seeks your advice on ankle taping. You would advise him that stress tests have shown over 60% of the initial support given the athlete by ankle taping would be maintained up to _____ during heavy exercise.
    a. 10 minutes
    b. 30 minutes
    c. 1 hour
    d. 2 hours

    Ref. 127, 44-A:1189, 1961

66. The maximum support of the ankle by taping will be given the athlete by:
   a. Standard basket-weave pattern
   b. Standard basket-weave and stirrup pattern   Ref. 127, 44-A:1187, 1962
   c. Standard basket-weave and heel-lock pattern
   d. Standard basket-weave and combination stirrup and heel-lock pattern

67. A 35-year-old white man has a transverse fracture of the midshaft of the femur. Internal fixation is elected by the attending surgeon. If two longitudinal plates and screw fixation are used, the greatest resistance to bending and torsion will be obtained if they are placed at:
   a. 45° to each other
   b. 90° to each other   Ref. 7, 9:263, 1952
   c. 135° to each other   Ref. 53, p. 177
   d. 180° to each other

68. When three screws are used on either side of the fracture site, which screws must withstand the greatest force to maintain fixation?
   a. Those farthest from the fracture line
   b. Those closest to the fracture line   Ref. 7, 11:263, 1952
   c. Those midway between the fracture line and the end of the plate
   d. Theoretically, equal distribution between all six screws

69. If intramedullary fixation is used, the superior structural configuration for the resistance of torsion and bending would be a:
   a. Solid round rod
   b. Diamond-shaped nail   Ref. 7, 11:93, 1954
   c. Triangular-shaped nail   Ref. 106, 60:13-19, 1968
   d. Cloverleaf nail

70. A cloverleaf nail is finally chosen by the surgeon. It will present its greatest resistance to bending when the open side is:
   a. Toward the concave side of the bend
   b. Away from the concave side of the bend   Ref. 7, 11:99, 1954
   c. At 90° to the concave side of the bend   Ref. 45, 2:66-74, 1953
   d. At 45° to the concave side of the bend

TRUE OR FALSE (answers on p. 271)

71. A painless range of hip motion after arthroplasty of flexion 120°, abduction 20°, and external rotation 20° should adequately accommodate the common activities of daily living.   Ref. 106, 72:205, 1970
   (T)   (F)

72. Mechanical properties of bone exhibit increased ability of cancellous bone to absorb energy over cortical bone.   Ref. 106, 58:249, 1968
   (T)   (F)

73. A drill hole in bone causes local stress concentration when the bone is subjected to loading forces. **Ref. 106, 60:222, 1969**
(T) (F)

74. Absence of loss of function of the vastus medialis would be expected to preclude the last 15° of knee extension. **Ref. 127, 50-A:1594, 1968**
(T) (F)

75. Rotary motion of the vertebrae at the lumbosacral junction in the normal adult is expected to be nearly 15° but can be effectively controlled with the use of the chairback brace. **Ref. 127, 50-A:1591, 1968**
(T) (F)

76. The high-heel shoe tends to throw the weight in the forefoot toward the fourth and fifth metatarsal heads. **Ref. 127, 46-A:333, 1964**
(T) (F)

77. Force-plate studies have shown that at "heel strike" and "heel off" positions the forces applied to the weight-bearing surface normally rise as high as 120% of body weight. **Ref. 15, p. 178**
(T) (F)

78. The bullet of a .38 caliber special handgun may attain a muzzle velocity up to 1,350 feet per second. This would be considered a high-velocity missile. **Ref. 7, 10:193, 1954**
(T) (F)

79. Crystalline structure as well as chemical composition may affect the stability of a metallic implant. **Ref. 106, 72:233, 1970**
(T) (F) **Ref. 127, 38-B:750, 1956**

80. When testing microhardness of cortical bone by the Vicker's indenter, it has been shown that hardness is more closely related to the mineral content than to the water content of the bone. **Ref. 50, p. 46**
(T) (F)

81. Stress-coat techniques have proved useful in measuring both stress and strain production in bone. **Ref. 7, 9:265-268, 1952**
(T) (F)

82. Dorsiflexion of the toes tends to increase the arch of the foot.
(T) (F) **Ref. 50, p. 176**

83. Plasticity may be defined as the physical property that allows a body to return to its original shape after having been deformed by force.
(T) (F) **Ref. 7, 18:111, 1961**

84. When lifting a 200-pound weight, increased intra-abdominal and intra-thoracic pressures may reduce the load on the lumbar spine by nearly 30%. **Ref. 56, pp. 333-338**
(T) (F) **Ref. 119, 107:418-423, 1973**
Ref. 127, 43-A:344-345, 1961

85. The stability of the spine depends primarily on the ligamentous structures binding the bony parts. **Ref. 11, p. 1**
(T) (F) **Ref. 56, pp. 333-338**
Ref. 119, 107:418-423, 1973
Ref. 127, 43-A:347, 1961

86. List the six basic determinants of gait.   Ref. 15, pp. 171-173
                                                       Ref. 106, 72:205, 1970
                                                       Ref. 127, 35-A:546, 1953

87. List four processes or means that may allow movement of metallic screws placed in bone.   Ref. 127, 38-B:745, 1956

88. List three structural mechanisms contributing to the weight-bearing function of the foot.   Ref. 50, p. 161

89. List five factors that may influence the corrosion of metallic implants.
                                                       Ref. 56, pp. 138-143
                                                       Ref. 106, 72:233, 1970
                                                       Ref. 127, 38-B:748, 1956

90. List six cavitary defects occurring in the normal basic structure of lamellar bone.   Ref. 55, p. 6

91. A load is defined as an outside force applied to a structure. List five basic types or classes of mechanical loads.   Ref. 56, pp. 116-117

92. List four methods of measuring or detecting strain.   Ref. 56, pp. 45-48

93. List and define six parameters or descriptive properties of solids.
                                                       Ref. 56, pp. 49-56

94. The femoral neck may fracture from absorption of some 60 kg/cm of energy. A 50 kg woman develops up to 2,700 kg/cm of kinetic energy during a fall. List the means of energy absorption that prevent fracture during each fall.   Ref. 53, p. 83

95. List five causes of orthopaedic implant failure.   Ref. 56, pp. 409-448

Children's orthopaedics

VIRGINIA M. BADGER, M.D.

MULTIPLE CHOICE, SINGLE ANSWER (answers on pp. 272-273)

Select the *one* answer that will best complete or answer each of the following statements or questions.

1. The most important nonoperative use of the Milwaukee brace is:
    a. Prevention of the worsening of small curves
    b. Correction of a thoracic curve from 50° to 40°　　**Ref. 132, 3-1:11, 1972**
    c. Prevention of the progression of double curves of less than 25°
    d. One of the above
    e. Two of the above

2. A useful guide indicating completion of vertebral growth is:
    a. Fusion of the proximal tibial epiphysis
    b. Fusion of the proximal humeral epiphysis　　**Ref. 45, 11:111, 1958**
    c. Progression of the iliac epiphysis to the　　**Ref. 71a, p. 135**
       posterior inferior iliac spine
    d. Ossification of the carpal bones
    e. Closure of the vertebral ring apophysis

3. Failure of the development of normal acetabular slope in the child may indicate:
    a. Cretinism
    b. Congenital anterior dislocation of the hip　　**Ref. 34, p. 1002**
    c. Congenital syphilis
    d. Arthrogryposis
    e. Achondroplasia

4. The bone most frequently involved in hematogenous osteomyelitis of the prepubertal age group is the:
    a. Femur
    b. Humerus　　**Ref. 5, p. 281**
    c. Tibia　　**Ref. 132, 3-1:227, 1972**
    d. Ulna
    e. Dorsal vertebra

5. The incidence of bilaterality in Legg-Perthes disease affecting males is usually reported to be:
   a. 5%
   b. 10%
   c. 15%
   d. 20%
   e. 25%

   Ref. 34, p. 1150

6. The modified Caldwell procedure to improve quadriceps function implies transfer of the tendon(s) of the:
   a. Semimembranosus
   b. Sartorius
   c. Adductor magnus
   d. Gracilis
   e. Semitendinosus and biceps femoris

   Ref. 43, pp. 1559-1560
   Ref. 103, p. 967

7. The complete classification of the congenital anomaly absence of the fibula is:
   a. Terminal, transverse, incomplete paraxial hemimelia fibula
   b. Intercalary, transverse, complete paraxial phocomelia fibula
   c. Congenital limb deficiency, L/R fibula, total
   d. Terminal, longitudinal, complete acheiria
   e. Terminal, longitudinal, incomplete paraxial hemimelia fibula

   Ref. 94, p. 119
   Ref. 127, 43-A:1203, 1961
   Ref. 127a, 1:11, 1976
   Ref. 132, 3-1:187, 1972

8. In an adolescent girl with a rigid scoliotic (R) thoracolumbar curve of about 70° the treatment of choice is:
   a. Hold in the Milwaukee brace until skeletal maturity
   b. Place in a series of Risser localizer casts until skeletal maturity
   c. Immediate correction and spinal fusion
   d. Halo-femoral traction for 3 weeks followed by spinal fusion
   e. Watchful waiting

   Ref. 132, 3-1:11, 1972

9. Which of the following is *not* true regarding osteochondritis of the tibial tubercle (Osgood-Schlatter disease)?
   a. It is twice as common unilaterally as bilaterally.
   b. It usually runs a self-limited two- to three-year course.
   c. It is more common in males than in females.
   d. Swelling of the tendon shadow at its bony insertion is an inconstant finding on x-ray examination in the active phase.
   e. Rapid growth usually has preceded the symptoms.

   Ref. 94, p. 398

10. Which of the following is *not* true with regard to tuberculosis affecting a joint?
    a. The synovial membrane is usually involved first.
    b. The synovial fluid sugar is usually less than 20% of the blood sugar level drawn at the same time.   Ref. 51, p. 102   Ref. 94, pp. 812, 832
    c. Pain is a common presenting complaint.
    d. So-called kissing sequestra are the late result of subchondral bone involvement.
    e. There is an increase of the lymphocyte to monocyte ratio, although the total white blood count may not be markedly elevated.

11. The earliest manifestation of slipped capital femoral epiphysis is:
    a. Widening of the epiphyseal line and irregular demineralization of the adjacent metaphysis upon x-ray examination
    b. Narrowing of the joint line, with irregular   Ref. 127, 31-A:734, 1949 calcification within it
    c. Decrease in the *C-E* angle of Wiberg
    d. Increased density of the femoral head, with irregular loss of trabecular pattern
    e. The appearance of radiolucent areas in the epiphysis, with an increase in trabeculation

12. Marked ability to internally rotate an otherwise normal hip is usually due to:
    a. Valgus of the neck
    b. Varus of the neck   Ref. 51, p. 125
    c. Anteversion of the neck
    d. Posterior inferior slip of the capital femoral epiphysis
    e. Anterior medial slip of the capital femoral epiphysis

13. Synovitis affecting the hip is believed by some authorities to be premonitory to:
    a. Slipped capital femoral epiphysis
    b. Legg-Perthes disease   Ref. 51, p. 170
    c. Coxa vara
    d. Coxa valga
    e. Epiphyseal dysplasia

14. Involvement of the hip accounts for about what percent of bone or joint tuberculosis in children under 10 years?
    a. 5%
    b. 10%   Ref. 94, p. 832
    c. 20%
    d. 50%

15. Which portion of the capital femoral epiphysis has the most abundant vascular supply?
    a. Anterior medial
    b. Anterior lateral   Ref. 127, 39-B:358, 1957
    c. Central
    d. Posterior
    e. All about the same

16. In the erect position, weight is borne by what portion of the femoral head?
    a. Anterior lateral
    b. Anterior medial   Ref. 51, p. 177
    c. Central   Ref. 127, 29:608, 617, 1947
    d. Posterior lateral
    e. Posterior medial

17. In idiopathic scoliosis the primary curve is usually:
    a. Thoracic
    b. High thoracic   Ref. 127, 52-A:1512
    c. Lumbar
    d. Cervicothoracic
    e. Thoracic

18. In a patient with known tuberculosis of the spine the most constant sign of imminent paraplegia due to pressure on the cord is:
    a. Depressed deep tendon reflexes
    b. Hyperactive deep tendon reflexes   Ref. 127, 32-A:87, 1950
    c. Babinski's sign   Ref. 127, 35-A:735, 1953
    d. Sensory change
    e. Clonus

19. In the Klippel-Feil syndrome the primary defect is generally believed to be:
    a. Soft tissue webs
    b. Failure of neurologic development in the   Ref. 51, p. 275
       neck muscles   Ref. 89, p. 54
    c. Absence of the normal atlantooccipital
       joint
    d. Failure of cervical vertebral segmentation
    e. Cervical spina bifida with asymptomatic
       meningocele

20. The omovertebral bone is associated with which of the following?
    a. Congenital hemivertebra
    b. Klippel-Feil syndrome   Ref. 51, p. 276
    c. Ellis–van Creveld syndrome   Ref. 89, p. 53
    d. Sprengel's deformity
    e. Ribbing's disease

21. Muscular torticollis is frequently associated with which of the following?
    a. Placenta previa
    b. Abruptio placentae   Ref. 89, p. 401

c. Breech presentation   **Ref. 125, 125:476, 1944**
d. Premature delivery   **Ref. 127, 30-A:556, 1948**
e. Premature rupture of the membranes   **Ref. 127, 51-B:432, 1969**

22. Which of the following is most frequently congenitally absent?
    a. Sternomastoid
    b. Trapezius   **Ref. 51, p. 282**
    c. Pectoralis major or minor
    d. Serratus anterior
    e. Biceps brachii

23. In a 2-year-old child who is walking and who has bilateral, supple pronated feet and internal tibial torsion, what should you do?
    a. Do not treat the child, since he will outgrow both defects.
    b. Do not treat the child, since the foot deformity is merely the result of the tibial torsion.   **Ref. 51, p. 62**
                                      Ref. 127, 51-B:263, 1969
    c. Plan for bilateral Grice procedures and tibial derotational osteotomies.
    d. Treat the pronation defect with corrective shoes and forget the torsion of the tibia.
    e. Treat the torsion with twisters or a Denis Browne splint and the feet with fully corrected shoes.

24. The biceps brachii is frequently absent in patients with no radius; however, when present, the site of its insertion is usually the:
    a. Trochlea
    b. Capitellum   **Ref. 7, 15:172, 1958**
    c. Coronoid process of the ulna   **Ref. 51, p. 295**
    d. Lacertus fibrosus
    e. Brachialis fascia

25. The carpal bone most frequently found to be congenitally absent is the:
    a. Navicular
    b. Lunate   **Ref. 51, p. 295**
    c. Capitate
    d. Pisiform
    e. Greater multangular

26. The mother of a patient 18 months old is worried because her son uses his left hand more than he uses his right. All members of her husband's family are right-handed. What should you do?
    a. Do not worry, since there is a 50-50 chance of developing left-handedness.
    b. Consider the possibility of marital infidelity.   **Ref. 51, p. 5**
    c. Realize this as increased motor development of the right side of the brain.

d. Reassure the mother that this is just a
   passing phase in his life.
e. Consider the possibility of underlying
   neural damage.

27. Considering a patient in whom the limit of dorsiflexion of the ankle is 10° of plantar flexion with the knee flexed or extended and who otherwise is normal, the surgical procedure of choice is:
    a. Strayer release
    b. Vulpius procedure   Ref. 43, p. 1693
    c. Soleus neurectomy   Ref. 94, p. 569
    d. Heel cord lengthening   Ref. 127, 54-B:272, 1972
    e. Silfverskiöld procedure

28. Which type of cerebral palsy improves most with age?
    a. Spastic
    b. Ataxic   Ref. 43, p. 1687
    c. Athetoid   Ref. 94, p. 529
    d. Rigid

29. Differentiating rickets from achondroplasia is usually possible by which of the following?
    a. Decreased length of long bones, with
       widening of the transverse diameter
    b. Prominent frontal bossae of the skull   Ref. 86, p. 34
    c. Bowlegs   Ref. 89, p. 77
    d. Capping of the epiphyses, with fraying of
       their margins
    e. Scoliosis

30. The omovertebral bone is usually connected between the fifth or sixth cervical vertebra and the:
    a. Scapular spine
    b. Occiput   Ref. 86, p. 95
    c. Inferior angle of the scapula
    d. Medial border of the scapula

31. Corneal opacities, hepatosplenomegaly, and mental retardation are associated with:
    a. Ollier's disease
    b. Maffucci's syndrome   Ref. 86, p. 42
    c. Hurler's syndrome
    d. Morquio's disease
    e. Achondroplasia

32. A patient with increased prominence of the cheeks and facial changes consistent with leontiasis ossea most likely has:
    a. Fibrous dysplasia
    b. Pyle's disease   Ref. 86, p. 54
    c. Achondroplasia
    d. Rickets
    e. Engelmann's disease

33. Concerning rheumatoid arthritis of the spine, which of the following is *not* true?
    a. Like peripheral rheumatoid arthritis, it occurs more frequently in females than in males.
    b. The sacroiliac joints are usually affected first.　　　　　　　　　　Ref. 126, p. 1218
    c. Ossification of the annulus fibrosus gradually occurs
    d. Subcutaneous nodules are not seen unless the peripheral form of the disease is present also.
    e. Ocular involvement is commonly seen.
34. In a patient with hemarthrosis due to hemophilia and mild trauma you should control the hemophilia and then:
    a. Leave the joint alone
    b. Aspirate the joint and start guided motion　　Ref. 51, p. 525
    after the acute phase subsides　　　　　　　　Ref. 89, p. 158
    c. Instill antibiotics as a prophylactic measure against infection
    d. Surgically drain the joint and do a lavage with plasma solution
    e. Aspirate the joint and immobilize in a plaster cast to prevent contracture or reinjury
35. Myelophthisic anemia is found in which diseases?
    a. Letterer-Siwe disease
    b. Gaucher's disease　　　　　　　　　　Ref. 5, p. 222
    c. Albers-Schönberg disease　　　　　　　Ref. 51, p. 535
    d. Niemann-Pick disease　　　　Ref. 109, pp. 1626, 1674
    e. All of the above
36. Acquired hip dislocation in myelomeningocele is most frequently due to:
    a. Acetabular incompetence
    b. Muscle imbalance between hip flexor-ad-　　Ref. 103, p. 905
    ductors and hip extensor-abductors
    c. Congenital coxa vara
    d. Flail lower limb musculature
37. The so-called Erlenmeyer-flask deformity of the metaphyses of long bones is sometimes seen in:
    a. Metaphyseal dysplasia
    b. Gaucher's disease　　　　　　　　Ref. 5, pp. 171, 245
    c. Albers-Schönberg disease　　　　Ref. 86, pp. 46, 49, 222
    d. All of the above
    e. None of the above
38. In a brachial plexus injury with associated Horner's syndrome you would expect an injury to which root?
    a. C-5
    b. C-6　　　　　　　　　　　　　　Ref. 51, p. 408

c. C-7

d. C-8

e. T-1

39. Unilateral chondrodysplasia (Ollier's disease) seems to represent one end of a spectrum of disease, at the other end of which is:

a. Diaphyseal aclasis

b. Achondroplasia   **Ref. 51, p. 426**

c. Hurler's syndrome

d. Morquio's disease

e. Maffucci's syndrome

40. In ulnar clubhand the digits most often absent are:

a. None

b. Second, third, fourth, and fifth   **Ref. 51, p. 293**

c. Second, third, and fourth

d. Third, fourth, and fifth

e. Fifth

41. Regarding primary anterior congenital dislocation of the hip, which is *not* true?

a. Lumbar lordosis is increased.

b. Trendelenburg's sign is positive.   **Ref. 7, 4:125, 1948**

c. The greater trochanter is always above Nélaton's line.

d. There is usually a prominence in the femoral triangle.

e. The femoral head is anterior to the axis of weight bearing.

42. The incidence of primary anterior congenital dislocation of the hip in infancy is usually reported as _____.

a. 12%

b. 18%   **Ref. 127, 21:648, 1939**

c. 23%

d. 28%

e. 35%

43. A 12-year-old girl is admitted with a history of gradually developing paralysis of both lower limbs over the past few months. An older brother has the same problem, as did her father. Physical examination reveals flail lower limbs below the knee and absent ankle jerk. Quadriceps, biceps, and triceps reflexes are 2+. Sensation is intact; however, there is decreased position and vibratory sense. Although there is marked atrophy, the muscles are not tender. There is no ataxia. The most likely diagnosis is:

a. Friedreich's disease   **Ref. 83, p. 1301**

b. Chronic polyneuritis

c. Poliomyelitis

d. Charcot-Marie-Tooth disease

e. Werdnig-Hoffmann disease

44. Hauser's procedure for treatment of a recurrent patellar dislocation is:
    a. Transplantation of the tibial tubercle medially and of the semitendinosus tendon to the patella
    b. Inferior medial transplantation of the insertion of the ligamentum patella   **Ref. 43, pp. 451, 1955**
    c. A checkrein procedure using medial joint capsule
    d. Medial transfer of the lateral half of the ligamentum patella
    e. Patellectomy and plastic repair of the ligamentum patella

45. Greater than half of all patients with cerebral palsy may be classified in which general group?
    a. Hemiplegic
    b. Paraplegic   **Ref. 89, p. 170**
    c. Monoplegic
    d. Quadriplegic
    e. Diplegic

46. In hereditary multiple osteocartilaginous exostosis the classic triad of features is (1) osteochondromas, (2) shortening of the radius and fibula, and (3) _____.
    a. Widening of the epiphysis
    b. Widening of the metaphysis   **Ref. 5, p. 114**
    c. Widening of the diaphysis
    d. All of the above
    e. None of the above

47. Which of the following is not usually associated with neurofibromatosis?
    a. Skeletal and soft tissue hypertrophy
    b. Scoliosis   **Ref. 5, p. 192**
    c. Congenital pseudarthrosis   **Ref. 51, p. 633**
    d. Phakomas   **Ref. 94, p. 91**
    e. Osteochondritis   **Ref. 127, 32-A:601, 1950**

48. In scurvy, pseudoparalysis is usually seen in which age group, as compared to patients with congenital syphilis?
    a. Older
    b. Younger   **Ref. 51, p. 519**
    c. Same
    d. Is not seen in scurvy

49. The monostotic form of fibrous dysplasia comprises about _____ of reported cases of this disease.
    a. 5%
    b. 10%   **Ref. 51, p. 532**
    c. 20%   **Ref. 94, p. 86**
    d. 30%

50. Dense transverse lines in the area of the metaphysis are frequently noted in which of the following?
    a. Melorheostosis
    b. Osteopathia striata   **Ref. 51, p. 538**

c. Osteopoikilosis

d. Osteopetrosis

e. Neurofibromatosis

51. Manifestations of Ehlers-Danlos syndrome include in addition to hyper-elasticity of the skin:

    a. Fragility of blood vessels

    b. Subcutaneous tumors   Ref. 51, p. 552

    c. A Raynaud-like phenomenon   Ref. 127, 40-A:663, 1958

    d. All of the above

    e. None of the above

52. Which of the following is not usually seen in patients with congenital absence of the fibula?

    a. Leg length discrepancy

    b. Equinovarus position of the foot   Ref. 94, p. 119

    c. Anterior bowing of the tibia   Ref. 127, 34-A:941, 1952

    d. Absence of one or more metatarsal rays   Ref. 127, 39-A:1229, 1957

    e. A heavy fibrous band attached to the in-terosseous membrane

53. Concerning Milroy's disease, which of the following is *not* true?

    a. Unilateral cases are common.

    b. The ankle is usually affected first.   Ref. 51, p. 567

    c. It usually starts during puberty.

    d. It is a hereditary condition.

    e. It is rapidly progressive.

54. Congenital radioulnar synostosis usually occurs at the:

    a. Distal radioulnar joint

    b. Elbow joint involving the humerus   Ref. 43, p. 2032

    c. Midshaft area   Ref. 94, p. 136

    d. Proximal end of the forearm

55. The most frequent congenitally absent long bone is the _____.

    a. Tibia

    b. Fibula   Ref. 43, p. 1928

    c. Radius

    d. Ulna

56. The second most common type of cerebral palsy is:

    a. Spastic

    b. Athetotic   Ref. 43, p. 1685

    c. Rigid type

    d. Ataxic

    e. Mixed type

57. In the ataxic type of cerebral palsy the neurologic lesion is generally believed to be in the:

    a. Motor cortex

    b. Thalamus   Ref. 43, p. 1685

    c. Cerebellum

    d. Globus pallidus

    e. Medulla and pons

58. In a patient with residual muscle weakness and paralysis due to polio-myelitis, the tibialis anterior muscle will cause motion of the foot against gravity, but not against resistance. This muscle should therefore be graded as:
    a. Trace
    b. Poor   **Ref. 51, p. 603**
    c. Fair
    d. Good
59. Contractures develop most commonly in which type of cerebral palsy?
    a. Athetoid
    b. Ataxic   **Ref. 51, p. 587**
    c. Spastic
    d. Rigid
    e. Flaccid
60. A dorsal bunion may be seen:
    a. In imbalance between the tibialis anterior and the peroneus longus
    b. In imbalance between the dorsiflexors of   **Ref. 43, p. 1544**
       the foot and the triceps surae group and
       long toe flexors
    c. In conjunction with hallux rigidus
    d. In a congenital flatfoot with a rocker-bottom deformity
    e. All of the above
61. Madelung's deformity may be caused or imitated by which of the following?
    a. Aberration of radial epiphyseal growth
    b. Epiphyseal injury   **Ref. 30, p. 281**
    c. Infection
    d. Rickets
    e. All of the above
62. In a slipping capital femoral epiphysis the proximal portion usually moves:
    a. Posteroinferiorly
    b. Laterally   **Ref. 51, p. 163**
    c. Anteroinferiorly   **Ref. 94, p. 190**
    d. Medially
    e. Anterolaterally
63. In a child 3 years of age, periosteal new bone formation primarily involving the metaphysis of long bones, with a corner sign, lateral spur of Pelkan, and Wimberger's line, is diagnostic of:
    a. Lead intoxication
    b. Scurvy   **Ref. 5, p. 373**
    c. Caffey's disease   **Ref. 62, p. 363**
    d. Hypervitaminosis A   **Ref. 105, p. 78**
    e. Battered-child syndrome

64. In the scoliotic curve of 35° to 40° the Milwaukee brace is *most* efficient in providing which of the following forces?
   a. Side-to-side lateral support
   b. Distraction from chin to pelvic girdle   Ref. 27, p. 21
   c. Three-point medial holding force of the
      pads
   d. Distraction from occipital pads to pelvic
      girdle

65. Central nervous system involvement in children with congenital syphilis occurs in about _____.
   a. Less than 10%
   b. 25%   Ref. 105, p. 108
   c. 50%
   d. 70%
   e. Almost 100%

66. A patient was treated with a cast for a congenital clubfoot and associated tibial torsion. The clubfoot was nicely corrected; however, the internal tibial torsion persisted. This should be corrected if it exceeds:
   a. 5°
   b. 10°   Ref. 94, p. 237
   c. 15°   Ref. 127, 31-A:511, 1949
   d. 20°

67. In patients with hemophilia the joint most commonly subject to hemarthroses is the:
   a. Ankle
   b. Hip   Ref. 45, 82:92, 1972
   c. Knee   Ref. 127, 30-A:589, 1948
   d. Wrist
   e. Elbow

68. Changes resembling those seen in coxa plana are frequently seen in all but:
   a. Morquio's disease
   b. Achondroplasia   Ref. 51, p. 414
   c. Rickets   Ref. 127, 30-A:603, 1948
   d. Melorheostosis
   e. Ollier's disease

69. In rheumatoid spondylitis the earliest clinical sign is:
   a. Skin eruption
   b. Decrease in chest expansion   Ref. 126, p. 15
   c. Interphalangeal joint pain
   d. Sacroiliac pain
   e. Knee effusion

70. The epiphyseal injury most commonly needing open reduction is the:
   a. Salter type I
   b. Salter type II   Ref. 127:45-A:611, 1963
   c. Salter type III
   d. Salter type IV
   e. Salter type V

71. In osteomyelitis associated with sickle cell disease, the organism most often isolated is:
    a. *Pseudomonas*
    b. *Streptococcus*   Ref. 5, p. 292
    c. *Salmonella*   Ref. 127, 53-A:1, 1971
    d. *Proteus*
    e. Colibacillus

72. After hamstring transfer to combat quadriceps weakness, recurvatum is generally minimized if:
    a. The triceps surae is adequate
    b. The knee is not immobilized in hyper-   Ref. 43, p. 1581
       extension and braces cause no recurvatum
    c. Any talipes equinus is corrected before
       weight bearing is started
    d. Physical therapy initiates active knee
       flexion
    e. All of the above

73. An infant is being evaluated for the x-ray finding of "osteopetrosis." The hospital course reveals generalized muscular weakness and hypotonia, anorexia, vomiting, and an increased serum calcium. A tentative diagnosis is:
    a. Leri's melorheostosis
    b. Albers-Schönberg disease   Ref. 86, p. 248
    c. Idiopathic hypercalcemia
    d. Rickets
    e. Fanconi syndrome

74. The Campbell bone block procedure and the Lambrinudi arthrodesis ablate which function in the foot?
    a. Dorsiflexion
    b. Plantar flexion   Ref. 43, pp. 1547, 1553
    c. Inversion
    d. Eversion

75. A positive Trendelenburg sign may be due to weakness or paralysis of the:
    a. Gluteus maximus
    b. Gluteus medius   Ref. 51, p. 136
    c. Rectus femoris
    d. Adductor magnus
    e. Iliopsoas

76. Intersection of a line drawn from the hard palate through the posterior border of the foramen magnum and one drawn through the body of the first cervical vertebra should lead you to suspect:
    a. Arnold-Chiari malformation
    b. Platybasia   Ref. 109, p. 1850
    c. Porencephalic cyst
    d. Rachischisis

77. In children with myelomeningocele what neuro-osseous defect frequently occurs in addition to the lower spinal abnormality?
    a. Platybasia
    b. Porencephalic cyst   Ref. 51, p. 623
    c. Diastematomyelia   Ref. 109, p. 1850
    d. Arnold-Chiari malformation
78. Congenital coxa vara is believed to be due to a disturbance in ossification and growth originating in the _____ portion of the epiphyseal plate.
    a. Anterior
    b. Posterior   Ref. 113, 30:48, 1960
    c. Medial   Ref. 127, 51-B:106, 1969
    d. Lateral
    e. All of the above
79. Congenital coxa vera at birth is:
    a. More common than in later childhood
    b. Less common than in later childhood   Ref. 43, p. 1999
    c. Equally as common as in later childhood   Ref. 127, 51-B:106, 1969
    d. Without known relation to later childhood
80. A 15-year-old boy has gradually developing muscle weakness accompanied by muscular pain on movement. There are associated erythematous skin eruptions and diplopia. This suggests:
    a. Pseudohypertrophic muscular dystrophy
    b. Syringomyelia   Ref. 51, p. 639
    c. Dermatomyositis   Ref. 109, p. 1922
    d. Myasthenia gravis   Ref. 130, 273:537, 1965
    e. Progressive muscular atrophy

MULTIPLE CHOICE, MULTIPLE ANSWERS (answers on p. 273)

Select one or more answers that will best complete or answer each of the following statements or questions.

81. Osteomyelitis caused by *Streptococcus* is to be expected most frequently in which of the following age groups?
    a. Under 1 year
    b. 5 to 10 years   Ref. 6, p. 1634
    c. 10 to 20 years   Ref. 45, 27:189, 1963
    d. 20 to 50 years   Ref. 45, 96:152, 1973
    e. Over 50 years   Ref. 119, 32:462, 1936
82. List in the order of their appearance the various ossification centers about the elbow.
    a. Capitellum
    b. Olecranon   Ref. 86, pp. 19, 20
    c. Radial head
    d. Lateral epicondyle
    e. Medial epicondyle
    f. Trochlea

83. Which of the following have been associated with peroneal spastic flat feet?
    a. Rheumatoid arthritis of the subtalar joint   **Ref. 45, 70:73, 1970**
    b. Tuberculosis of the tarsal joints   **Ref. 127, 30-B:624, 1948**
    c. Bony anomalies such as calcaneonavicular bar or talocalcaneal bridge
    d. Osteoid osteoma of the foot
    e. Congenital vertical talus
84. Which of the following will tend to produce a rocker-bottom foot?
    a. Dorsiflexing the forefoot in exercises to stretch the heel cord   **Ref. 45, 70:10, 1970**
    b. Walking on a foot with an uncorrected equinus deformity   **Ref. 51, p. 72**
    c. Attempting correction of forefoot equinus before correction of hindfoot equinus
    d. Too rapid correction of forefoot varus
    e. Slipping of the foot up in the corrective cast, with subsequent overdorsiflexion of the forefoot
85. Excessively small calf size in a patient with clubfeet is frequently seen in which of the following?
    a. Arthrogryposis congenita multiplex
    b. Charcot-Marie-Tooth disease   **Ref. 51, p. 66**
    c. Pseudohypertrophic muscular dystrophy
    d. Phenylketonuria
    e. Congenital syphilis
86. After the age of 1 year, the etiologic agent in aseptic arthritis is most likely _____, whereas before that age the organism most commonly isolated is _____. In both age groups the route of infection is usually _____.
    a. *Streptococcus*   **Ref. 45, 96:152, 1973**
    b. *Staphylococcus*   **Ref. 51, p. 101**
    c. Direct contamination
    d. Hematogenous
    e. Lymphogenous
87. Slipped capital femoral epiphysis occurs mainly in which of the following?
    a. Very tall, very thin children
    b. Thin children with precocious puberty   **Ref. 89, p. 343**
    c. Heavily muscled children
    d. Obese children with underdeveloped sexual characters
    e. Normal children without a previous history of somatic complaints
88. The Heyman procedure associated with treatment of slipped capital femoral epiphysis refers to:
    a. A type of transcervical osteotomy
    b. A type of subtrochanteric osteotomy   **Ref. 127, 36-A:539, 1954**

c. Removal of bony deformity of the femoral   **Ref. 127, 39-A:293, 1957**
neck
d. Metallic fixation of the capital femoral
epiphysis
e. A bone grafting operation across the
epiphyseal plate

89. Which of the following should be included in the differential diagnosis
of coxa vara?
a. Rickets
b. Osteomalacia   **Ref. 127, 30-B:161, 595, 1948**
c. Melorheostosis   **Ref. 127, 51-B:106, 1969**
d. Tuberculosis
e. Legg-Calvé-Perthes disease

90. Which of the following should occur before allowing the patient with
Legg-Perthes disease to start weight bearing on the affected side?
a. Complete remineralization of the femoral
head
b. Evidence of advancing bony reconstruc-   **Ref. 51, p. 182**
tion at the surface of the epiphysis   **Ref. 127, 53-B:54, 1971**
c. No new dense area formation over the
past two or three months
d. Full range of motion at the hip
e. None of the above

91. Congenital kyphosis is frequently seen in:
a. Hurler's syndrome
b. Morquio's disease   **Ref. 51, p. 199**
c. Cretinism   **Ref. 127, 55-A:223, 1973**
d. Oppenheim's disease
e. Werdnig-Hoffmann disease

92. Idiopathic scoliosis is most commonly seen in _____, and in this
type the convexity usually is toward the _____.
a. Males
b. Females   **Ref. 43, p. 1839**
c. Right   **Ref. 51, p. 237**
d. Left   **Ref. 89, p. 293**

93. In a child who has torticollis, the differential diagnosis might include:
a. Tuberculosis of the cervical spine
b. Cervical osteomyelitis   **Ref. 51, p. 285**
c. Acute myositis   **Ref. 89, pp. 401-404**
d. Tonsillitis with lymphadenopathy
e. Congenital anomalies of the cervical spine

94. In juvenile rheumatoid arthritis, which of the following may frequently
be within normal limits?
a. Erythrocyte sedimentation rate
b. ASO titers   **Ref. 51, p. 527**
c. Latex fixation   **Ref. 126, p. 1214**
d. Bentonite flocculation   **Ref. 135, 50:940, 1972**
e. Leukocyte count

95. In a radial clubhand with the thumb and first metacarpal present, which muscles are usually present?
    a. Extensor pollicis longus
    b. Extensor pollicis brevis   **Ref. 51, p. 295**
    c. Adductor pollicis brevis   **Ref. 127, 52-A:966, 1970**
    d. Adductor pollicis
    e. Opponens pollicis
96. Which of the following osteochondritides are more frequently seen in males than in females?
    a. Legg-Calvé-Perthes disease
    b. Osgood-Schlatter disease   **Ref. 45, 14:7, 1959**
    c. Haglund's disease
    d. Freiberg's disease
    e. Scheuermann's disease
97. The upper plexus type of obstetric paralysis occurs about _____ times as often as that including the whole arm, and both types occur far _____ commonly than the lower plexus form.
    a. Two
    b. Four   **Ref. 43, p. 1719**
    c. Six
    d. More
    e. Less
98. Which of the following x-ray findings are commonly found in vitamin C deficiency?
    a. Ringing of the epiphyses
    b. "White line" corresponding to the zone of   **Ref. 86, p. 109**
       provisional calcification
    c. Rarefaction in the metaphysis
    d. Coarse and irregular appearance of the
       metaphyseal ends
    e. Subperiosteal new bone formation
99. Which of the following may be included in the differential diagnosis of infantile cortical hyperostosis?
    a. Hypervitaminosis A
    b. Engelmann's disease   **Ref. 5, p. 502**
    c. Trauma
    d. Scurvy
    e. Hypervitaminosis D
100. In Volkmann's ischemic contracture of the forearm, which two muscles are usually affected more severely than any other?
    a. Flexor pollicis longus
    b. Flexor digitorum sublimis   **Ref. 43, p. 1459**
    c. Fexor digitorum profundus
    d. Flexor carpi ulnaris
    e. Flexor carpi radialis
101. In congenital pseudarthrosis of the tibia the bowing deformity points:
    a. Anteriorly
    b. Posteriorly   **Ref. 43, p. 1946**

    c. Medially

    d. Anterolaterally

    e. Posteromedially

102. A 10-year-old girl with a previously untreated unilateral congenitally dislocated hip is seen. Which of the following are justifiable?

    a. Arthrodesis of the hip

    b. Traction followed by acetabuloplasty and   **Ref. 7, 4:125, 1948**
       derotational osteotomy

    c. Prosthetic replacement of the femoral head

    d. Cup arthroplasty

    e. Osteotomy

103. Which of these measurements are related to the same clinical entity?

    a. The Y coordinate of Ponseti

    b. Hilgenreiner's D line   **Ref. 43, p. 1962**

    c. Hilgenreiner's H line

    d. Perkin's line

    e. Poupart's line

104. An increased incidence of café au lait spots seen in neurofibromatosis may also be seen in:

    a. Fibrous dysplasia

    b. Acromegaly   **Ref. 5, p. 193**

    c. Hyperparathyroidism

    d. Gout

    e. Pseudarthrosis of the tibia

105. An arthrogram is stated to be of value in the treatment of congenital dysplasia and dislocation of the hip. Allegedly it will do which of the following?

    a. Demonstrate the degree of dysplasia

    b. Allow you to see if the acetabulum contains   **Ref. 43, p. 1962**
       much soft tissue

    c. Show the size of the femoral head

    d. Make possible more accurate measurement
       of the alpha angle of Hilgenreiner

    e. Demonstrate the status of the acetabular
       labrum

106. A valgus deformity of the knee is usually not seen in which of the following?

    a. Morquio's disease

    b. Familial metaphyseal dysplasia   **Ref. 51, p. 453**

    c. Achondroplasia   **Ref. 89, pp. 61, 82**

    d. Postpoliomyelitis

    e. Scurvy

107. An increased incidence of mental deficiency would not be expected in:

    a. Hurler's syndrome

    b. Morquio's disease   **Ref. 51, p. 447**

    c. Ellis–van Creveld syndrome   **Ref. 89, pp. 58, 69**

    d. Pleonosteosis

    e. Achondroplasia

108. Which of the following have been suggested as the cause of adolescent kyphosis (Scheuermann's disease)?
   a. Osteochondritis of the vertebral epiphysis
   b. Excessively tight hamstring muscles   **Ref. 127, 38-A:149, 1956**
   c. Deficient growth of the vertebral body   **Ref. 141, 72:798, 1941**
      anteriorly, with herniation of the disc
      (Schmorl's nodes)
   d. Viral infection of the disc space
   e. Persistent anterior vascular grooves

109. The Steindler flexorplasty at the elbow transfers the muscles arising from the medial epicondyle of the humerus to a position more proximal on the shaft. A good result usually depends on good muscle strength, particularly in which of the following?
   a. Palmaris longus
   b. Flexor digitorum sublimis   **Ref. 127, 36-A:775, 1954**
   c. Pronator teres
   d. Flexor carpi ulnaris
   e. Flexor carpi radialis

110. Ideally, what muscles must be strong before an iliopsoas tendon transfer to the greater trochanter (Mustard's procedure) should be considered?
   a. Gluteus maximus
   b. Gluteus minimus   **Ref. 127, 41-B:289, 1950**
   c. Adductor magnus   **Ref. 127, 34-A:647, 1952**
   d. Sartorius   **Ref. 127, 52-A:1364, 1970**
   e. Quadriceps

111. In a patient with vitamin D–deficiency rickets the renal excretion of which of the following will be high?
   a. Citric acid
   b. Amino acid   **Ref. 51, p. 512**
   c. Ca^{++} **Ref. 94, p. 695**
   d. PO_4
   e. Alkaline phosphatase

112. Which of the following are early findings in a patient with hyperparathyroidism?
   a. Polyuria and polydipsia
   b. Anorexia   **Ref. 51, p. 516**
   c. Irritability
   d. Flaccidity of muscles
   e. Nausea

113. Tenderness over the end of the long bone in a patient with scurvy is usually due to:
   a. Subperiosteal hemorrhage
   b. Cortical infractions   **Ref. 51, p. 519**
   c. Epiphysitis
   d. Epiphyseal separation
   e. Secondary synovitis

114. Which of the following are the most commonly involved bones in mono-stotic fibrous dysplasia?
   a. Humerus
   b. Femur   **Ref. 51, p. 532**
   c. Clavicle
   d. Skull
   e. Tibia

115. Congenital constricting bands are most often seen in the _____ extremity and occur most frequently _____ the elbow or knee.
   a. Upper
   b. Lower   **Ref. 43, p. 1894**
   c. Above   **Ref. 51, p. 560**
   d. Below

116. Lesions of the motor cortex may cause which types of cerebral palsy?
   a. Spastic
   b. Athetotic   **Ref. 43, p. 1685**
   c. Ataxic
   d. Rigid
   e. Flaccid

117. Which of the following are known to contribute to paralytic dislocation of the hip?
   a. Absence of abductor force
   b. Coxa valga deformity   **Ref. 43, p. 1614**
   c. Tightness of adductors
   d. Poorly formed acetabulum
   e. Redundant hip capsule

118. Congenital clubfoot occurs about _____ per thousand births, and is _____ in boys than in girls.
   a. Once
   b. Five times   **Ref. 51, p. 65**
   c. Ten times
   d. More common
   e. Less common

119. Recurrent dislocation of the patella is _____ common in males and _____ tend to be familial.
   a. More
   b. Less   **Ref. 51, p. 110**
   c. Does   **Ref. 89, p. 367**
   d. Does not

120. Recurrent dislocation of the patella is usually _____ and the dislocation generally is:
   a. Unilateral
   b. Bilateral   **Ref. 51, p. 110**
   c. Medial   **Ref. 89, p. 367**
   d. Lateral

121. The femoral neck at birth forms an angle of about _____ with the shaft of the femur; however, this angle changes with growth and weight bearing to about _____.
    a. 160°
    b. 150°   **Ref. 52, p. 313**
    c. 135°   **Ref. 60, p. 239**
    d. 125°   **Ref. 127, 53-A:1007, 1971**
    e. 110°

122. Anteversion of the femoral neck at birth approximates _____, but with normal development it changes to about _____.
    a. 35°
    b. 25°   **Ref. 51, p. 125**
    c. 15°   **Ref. 127, 53-A:1007, 1971**
    d. 10°
    e. 5°

123. Osteomyelitis in a patient with sickle cell disease occurs:
    a. Most often in children
    b. Most often in adults   **Ref. 5, p. 292**
    c. In the epiphysis   **Ref. 127, 53-A:1007, 1971**
    d. In the metaphysis
    e. In the diaphysis

124. Madelung's deformity is most commonly seen in _____ and is bilateral in _____ of persons.
    a. Males
    b. Females   **Ref. 30, p. 281**
    c. 33%
    d. 66%
    e. 75%

125. Which of the children's fractures listed below should be treated by open means to gain anatomic reduction?
    a. Femoral neck
    b. Lateral epicondyle of the elbow   **Ref. 26, pp. 27, 43, 57, 147, 171**
    c. Displaced fracture of the radial head
    d. Supracondylar fracture of the humerus
    e. Transverse fracture of the patella

126. Hutchinson's triad in congenital syphilis includes:
    a. Deformity of the secondary incisor teeth
    b. Saber shins   **Ref. 105, p. 110**
    c. Interstitial keratitis
    d. Eighth nerve deafness
    e. Charcot joint

127. In the spastic cerebral palsy child the muscles of the lower extremity that generally demonstrate the greatest degree of spasticity are the:
    a. Hip abductors
    b. Hip flexors   **Ref. 132, 3-1:113, 1972**
    c. Hip external rotators
    d. Knee flexors
    e. Knee extensors

128. In congenital pes valgus, which of the following deformities are a part of the pathologic anatomy?
    a. The navicular articulates with the dorsal aspect of the neck of the talus.
    b. The talus rocks laterally out of the ankle mortice.   Ref. 132, 3-1:132, 1972
    c. The sustentaculum tali is blunted.
    d. The cuboid is malrotated in relation to the navicular.
    e. The tibionavicular ligament is contracted.

129. Legg-Perthes disease has been found in association with which of the following?
    a. Hurler's syndrome
    b. Gaucher's disease   Ref. 34, p. 1150
    c. Engelmann's disease
    d. Congenital dislocation of the hip
    e. Achondroplasia

130. The tumorlike osseous lesions seen in patients with hemophilia are thought to be due to:
    a. Benign neoplasms
    b. Subperiosteal hemorrhages   Ref. 127, 30-A:589, 1948
    c. Hemarthrosis   Ref. 127, 47-A:517, 1965
    d. Vascular abnormalities within the bone with hemorrhage   Ref. 127, 51-B:614, 1969
    e. Abnormalities of calcium and phosphorus balance

SITUATION AND PROGRESSIVE THOUGHT (answers on p. 273)

Select the answer or answers that best apply in accordance with the information given in the following statements.

131. A 13-year-old boy with a history of hip pain for several weeks is admitted with a history of a fall with sudden acute hip pain and inability to bear weight. The most likely diagnosis is:
    a. Legg-Calvé-Perthes disease
    b. Scheuermann's disease   Ref. 51, p. 160
    c. Slipped capital femoral epiphysis   Ref. 89, pp. 343, 345
    d. Fracture of the hip

132. The best treatment of this patient would be:
    a. Nonweight bearing, with a Snyder-Fort sling on the affected side
    b. Reduction and internal fixation with multiple pins or a Smith-Petersen nail   Ref. 51, p. 160
    c. Bed rest, with subsequent use of an ischial weight-bearing brace   Ref. 89, p. 345
    d. Aspiration of the hip joint, culture, and antibiotic therapy
    e. Bed rest until immediate tenderness is gone and then physical therapy in conjunction with steroids

133. A patient with bilateral clubhands, with absent first rays, is being pre-
     pared for surgery when it is noted that he is anemic and thrombocy-
     topenic. The mother states that another member of the family has had
     similar troubles. The most likely diagnosis is:
     a. Gaucher's disease
     b. Tay-Sachs disease   **Ref. 109, p. 1629**
     c. Hand-Schüller-Christian disease
     d. Fanconi syndrome
     e. Albright's syndrome
134. You might also expect to find:
     a. Hemangiomas
     b. Café au lait spots   **Ref. 109, p. 1629**
     c. Generalized olive-brown pigmentation
     d. Excessively fair skin
     e. Vitiligo
135. In a mentally retarded child with congenital glaucoma who is chron-
     ically acidotic due to kidney dysfunction related to failure of the renal
     tubules to reabsorb glucose, amino acids, etc., and who has abnormally
     wide epiphyses, the serum chemistries would probably be:
     a. High Ca, low P, and high alkaline phos-
        phatase
     b. Low Ca, low P, and high alkaline phos-   **Ref. 5, p. 410**
        phatase   **Ref. 89, p. 81**
     c. High Ca, high P, and low alkaline phos-
        phatase
     d. Low Ca, high P, and low alkaline
        phosphatase
     e. High Ca. low P, and normal alkaline phos-
        phatase
136. This child most likely has:
     a. Rickets
     b. Melorheostosis leri   **Ref. 5, p. 410**
     c. Scurvy   **Ref. 89, p. 81**
     d. Gaucher's disease
     e. Fanconi syndrome
137. A 2-year-old white girl is seen because, according to the mother, she
     "stands and walks funny." Physical examination demonstrates a 2.5 cm
     shortening of the right lower extremity, with an extra thigh fold and
     equivocal decrease in the ability to abduct the right hip. The minimum
     x-ray views that should be obtained for adequate diagnosis and treat-
     ment are:
     a. Anteroposterior
     b. Frog-leg lateral   **Ref. 7, 18:207, 1961**
     c. Cross-table lateral   **Ref. 43, p. 1964**
     d. Anteroposterior in full internal rotation   **Ref. 127, 21-A:648, 1939**
     e. All of the above   **Ref. 127, 51-A:601, 1969**

138. Following diagnosis, the patient should be:
    a. Started on a course of physical therapy
    b. Placed in an ischial weight-bearing brace   Ref. 43, p. 1964
       on the right
    c. Placed in a skeletal traction on the right
    d. Evaluated for neurofibromatosis
    e. Scheduled for a Syme or Chopart amputa-
       tion on the right
139. The next step in therapy should include:
    a. Closed or open reduction and immobiliza
       tion in a spica cast
    b. Femoral shortening on the left   Ref. 43, p. 1964
    c. Removal of the hypertrophic area on the
       left by local incision
    d. Arthroplasty in later childhood or early
       teens
    e. Prosthesis fitting after amputation
140. A 14-year-old boy is brought to you for evaluation of muscle weakness
    that is said to have begun about six or eight months before. Physical
    examination reveals a retarded muscle relaxation time, especially in the
    hand; atrophy of the muscles of the face and neck with expressionless
    facies; and monotonic speech. You might expect to find:
    a. Excessive hair growth
    b. Typical senile cataracts   Ref. 7, 9:171, 1952
    c. Testicular enlargement   Ref. 109, p. 1930
    d. Blepharoconjunctivitis
    e. All of the above
141. Which of the following have been shown to be of some value in the
    treatment of this disease?
    a. Neostigmine
    b. Thyroid hormone   Ref. 7, 9:171, 1952
    c. Quinine   Ref. 109, p. 1321
    d. Ephedrine
    e. Potassium chloride
142. A 10-year-old girl comes to you for treatment of a "curve in the back."
    This has progressed over the past year and is associated with back pain
    after exercise and at the end of the day. There is no history suggestive
    of neuromuscular disease. Physical examination, except for a compen-
    sated dextroscoliosis, is within normal limits. X-ray films reveal a thoracic
    scoliosis between T-6 and L-1, with the apex at the disc space between
    T-9 and T-10, that measures 36°. Anteroposterior x-ray views of the
    pelvis reveal open iliac epiphysis. Acceptable treatment would include:
    a. Spinal fusion and Harrington rod instru-
       mentation
    b. Milwaukee brace   Ref. 127, 44-A:591, 1962
    c. Risser jacket   Ref. 132, 3-1:10, 1972
    d. Hyperextension and hyperflexion exercises

143. Assuming that the patient is treated with Harrington rods and spinal fusion, the distraction force should be on the _____ side of the vertebral column and the proximal hook placed at the level of _____.
    a. Right
    b. Left   Ref. 127, 44-A:600, 1962
    c. T-6   Ref. 132, 3-1:44, 1972
    d. T-7
    e. T-8
144. Compression forces should be placed on the _____ side of the vertebral column, with the distal hook implanted in the _____ of L-1.
    a. Right
    b. Left   Ref. 127, 44-A:603, 1962
    c. Pedicle   Ref. 132, 3-1:42, 1972
    d. Facet joint
    e. Transverse process
145. A secondary supplementary force is sometimes necessary if the sacral triangle is _____, and when this requires use of a universal hook, there should be an overlap of the tips of the instruments of at least _____ vertebral segments.
    a. Isosceles
    b. Obtuse   Ref. 127, 44-A:605, 1962
    c. Two   Ref. 132, 3-1:52, 1972
    d. Four
    e. Six

TRUE OR FALSE (answers on pp. 273-274)

146. The predisposition to osteomyelitis in the metaphysis of a long bone is indirectly related to the rate of growth and size of the bone.
    (T) (F)   Ref. 105, p. 90
147. Differentiation on physical examination of a congenital vertical talus from the simple calcaneovalgus foot is not possible, since in both the os calcis is usually reducible into normal relationship with the talus.
    (T) (F)   Ref. 51, p. 49
                                               Ref. 127, 45-A:413, 1963
148. Differentiation of aseptic necrosis of the tarsal navicular (Köhler's disease) from normally occurring multiple ossification centers is possible, since the former is usually seen in a much younger age group.
    (T) (F)   Ref. 51, p. 79
149. The knock-knee deformity associated with rickets disappears with flexion of the knee because the posterior portions of the femoral condyles are normal, while anteriorly the medial femoral condyle is of abnormal length.   Ref. 89, p. 377
    (T) (F)
150. Coxa plana is considered by many authorities to be a soft tissue disease, since one of the earliest changes found is a bulging of the capsule and joint space widening.   Ref. 45, 4:180, 1954
    (T) (F)   Ref. 127, 53-B:37, 1971

151. A primary focus of epiphyseal involvement is common in tuberculosis.
(T) (F) Ref. 51, p. 190

152. Subchondral cortical bone is denser in the posterior portion of the femoral head than in the anterior. Ref. 51, p. 177
(T) (F)

153. The hip joint is more commonly affected by tuberculosis than is any other single joint. Ref. 51, p. 189
(T) (F)

154. Vertebral plana (Calvé's disease) initially was believed to be due to aseptic necrosis but recently has been linked to eosinophilic granuloma. Ref. 127, 36-A:969, 1954
(T) (F) Ref. 127, 53-B:37, 1971

155. In cerebral palsy the defect is in the lower motor neurons.
(T) (F) Ref. 89, p. 170

156. Because of their more supple musculature, reconstructive surgical procedures in athetoid cerebral palsy patients are usually most successful.
(T) (F) Ref. 125, 150:1396, 1952
Ref. 125, 161:781, 1956
Ref. 125, 174:1266, 1960

157. One common difference between psoriatic arthropathy and rheumatoid arthritis is that early in the former the distal interphalangeal joints are involved, whereas in the latter the reverse is true.
(T) (F) Ref. 126, pp. 1213, 1686

158. "Trigger thumb" is seen in children as well as adults; however, in children it is more frequently bilateral. Ref. 43, p. 374
(T) (F) Ref. 51, p. 301

159. The development of contractures in athetotic cerebral palsy is more common than in any other type. Ref. 43, p. 1690
(T) (F)

160. In "upper arm" or Erb-Duchenne palsy there is usually profound sensory loss over the area of the involved roots. Ref. 105, p. 540
(T) (F)

161. In cerebral palsy, damage of the motor cortex, that is, hemorrhage, always causes the spastic type. Ref. 43, p. 1685
(T) (F)

162. In children, back pain is usually not associated with any serious clinical condition. Ref. 51, p. 199
(T) (F)

163. The ossification center of the femoral head is usually present at birth.
(T) (F) Ref. 86, pp. 19, 20

164. Osteogenesis imperfecta is a form of osteomalacia.
(T) (F) Ref. 86, p. 45

165. It has been shown experimentally that venous obstruction as well as arterial occlusion or spasm will cause Volkmann's ischemic contracture. Ref. 51, p. 368
(T) (F) Ref. 132, 3-1:175, 1972

166. The muscle imbalance that causes the initial deformities seen in rheumatoid arthritis is believed to be caused by reflex muscle spasm due to joint irritation. Ref. 127, 33-A:849, 1951
(T) (F) Ref. 127, 37-A:759, 1955
Ref. 135, 50-6:940, 1972

167. In rheumatoid arthritis, hand deformities usually fall into two groups, the "claw" type and the "pill-roller" type, with the latter being the more common of the two. Ref. 51, p. 362
(T) (F)

168. In a patient 5 years old with a solitary bone cyst, surgical ablation and bone grafting would be expected to result in complete cure.
(T) (F) Ref. 127, 36-A:267, 1954

169. Radiologic examination of an area thought to be involved by osteomyelitis is of no value during the first 7 to 10 days after onset of the disease. Ref. 51, p. 472
(T) (F)

170. Patients with renal phosphate–losing rickets may often be differentiated from patients with rickets due to other renal defects by the fact that in the former the BUN and NPN are usually elevated. Ref. 51, p. 514
(T) (F) Ref. 132, 3-1:243, 1972

171. In a 13-month-old patient with low serum calcium and phosphorous values and a high serum alkaline phosphatase, vitamin D–deficiency rickets can be differentiated from vitamin D–resistant rickets only by the patient's response to vitamin D therapy. Ref. 51, p. 516
(T) (F) Ref. 132, 3-1:243, 1972

172. The response of a patient to vitamin D therapy is useful in differentiating between the rickets due to defects in renal function and the inherited vitamin D–resistant variety. Ref. 51, p. 516
(T) (F) Ref. 132, 3-1:244, 1972

173. Rather rapid extension of lesions in the polyostotic form of fibrous dysplasia is uncommon. Ref. 51, p. 533
(T) (F)

174. Both sexes are afflicted with precocious puberty in polyostotic fibrous dysplasia. Ref. 51, p. 532
(T) (F)

175. Otosclerosis is most common in the prenatal form of osteogenesis imperfecta. Ref. 51, p. 539
(T) (F) Ref. 138, 40:145, 1943

176. Treatment of radioulnar synostosis by resection of the involved portion of the radius has generally yielded poor results in the past.
(T) (F) Ref. 43, p. 2032
Ref. 94, p. 136
Ref. 127:404, 1932

177. Anterior bowing of the leg in congenital absence of the tibia is *not* a prominent feature, as in congenital absence of the fibula.
(T) (F) Ref. 43, p. 1929
Ref. 127, 34-A:941, 1952
Ref. 132, 3-1:187, 1972

178. Constricting bands need be excised for cosmesis only, since they rarely interfere with limb function.   **Ref. 43, p. 1894**
    (T) (F)   **Ref. 51, p. 560**
179. Prompt treatment of congenital dislocation of the radial head by its surgical excision is generally recommended.   **Ref. 43, p. 2032**
    (T) (F)
180. The Egger's procedure (transplantation of the hamstring tendons to the distal femur) was devised primarily for patients with poliomyelitis to reinforce weak hip extension.   **Ref. 51, p. 591**
    (T) (F)

LIST (answers on pp. 274-275)

181. List the basic elements of the congenital clubfoot and the joint where the deformity occurs.   **Ref. 51, p. 65**
182. List the conditions that should alert you to the presence of a cavus deformity.   **Ref. 51, p. 75**
183. List five causes reported in the literature that possibly contribute to the formation of spondylolisthesis.   **Ref. 127, 44-A:539, 1962**
184. List three operative procedures that have been described to maintain reduction of a vertical talus.   **Ref. 43, p. 1562**
           Ref. 127, 32-A:344, 1950
           Ref. 127, 38-B:334, 1956
185. List six operative procedures that have been recommended for the treatment of paralytic dislocation of the hip.   **Ref. 43, p. 1614**
           Ref. 127, 46-B:426, 1964
186. List five operative procedures that have been recommended for stabilizing the paralytic foot.   **Ref. 43, pp. 1550, 1569**
187. List two operations that are used to treat metatarsus varus.   **Ref. 43, p. 1903**
188. List five causes of cerebral palsy.   **Ref. 43, p. 1685**
189. List six surgical procedures that have been devised to restore elbow flexion after paralysis of the elbow flexors.   **Ref. 43, p. 1640**
190. List five causes of unilateral hypertrophy of a limb.   **Ref. 43, p. 1892**
191. List five methods of operatively treating talipes equinus.   **Ref. 43, pp. 1550, 1569**
192. List in order of increasing severity the five reticuloendothelioses.   **Ref. 5, p. 222**
193. List the areas where tuberculous abscesses involving (a) cervical, (b) dorsal, and (c) lumbar vertebral areas tend to point or drain.   **Ref. 51, p. 210**
194. List the five generally accepted types of cerebral palsy. **Ref. 43, p. 1685**
195. List five pathologic diseases or entities in which there is a known increase of scoliosis.   **Ref. 51, p. 224**
196. List five conditions (other than idiopathic) that can contribute to genu valgum.   **Ref. 51, p. 108**
           Ref. 89, p. 377

197. List six conditions in which periosteal new bone formation may be seen in the infant and toddler age group.   **Ref. 5, pp. 272, 286, 371, 500, 510**
198. List five implicated causes of lateral dislocation of the patella.

Ref. 43, p. 448

Ref. 127, 27:446, 1945

199. List five entities that should be included in a differential diagnosis of a cystic mass in the popliteal fossa.   **Ref. 43, p. 1510**
200. List four indications for removal of an osteochondroma.

Ref. 105, p. 325

SECTION 5

Hand surgery

FLOYD G. GOODMAN, B.S., M.D.

MULTIPLE CHOICE, SINGLE ANSWER (answers on pp. 275-276)

Select the *one* answer that will best complete or answer each of the following statements or questions.

1. Extensor tendons in advanced rheumatoid arthritis of the hand tend to rupture most frequently at the:
   a. Distal interphalangeal joint level   Ref. 43, pp. 341-342
   b. Proximal interphalangeal joint level   Ref. 127, 51-A:15, 1969
   c. Dorsal carpal ligament level   Ref. 132, 2-3:643, 663, 1971
   d. Carpometacarpophalangeal level   Ref. 132, 5-2:432-436, 1974
2. The extensor hood of the digits is formed by which of the following?
   a. Long extensor tendon
   b. Dorsal interosseous muscle insertion   Ref. 7, 16:66, 1959
   c. Volar interosseous muscle insertion
   d. Insertion of the lumbrical
   e. All of the above
3. The excursion of an extensor tendon to a finger is approximately:
   a. 1.5 cm
   b. 3 cm   Ref. 30, p. 15
   c. 4 cm   Ref. 31, p. 412
   d. 5 cm
4. Flexor tendons after suture anastomosis usually should be immobilized for:
   a. 3 weeks
   b. 4 weeks   Ref. 43, p. 162
   c. 5 weeks   Ref. 132, 1-2:369, 1970
   d. 6 weeks
5. The most common cause of Volkmann's ischemic contracture is:
   a. Severance of the brachial artery
   b. Fracture of both bones of the forearm   Ref. 30, p. 245
   c. Supracondylar fracture of the humerus   Ref. 132, 4-4:983-986, 1973
   d. Spiral fracture of the midshaft of the humerus

91

6. Arthrodesis of the metacarpophalangeal joints in the hand, although rarely indicated, is recommended at:
   a. 0°
   b. 10° to 20°   Ref. 43, p. 234
   c. 20° to 30°
   d. 30° to 40°
7. The long extensor tendon of the thumb in advanced rheumatoid arthritis of the hand is most likely to rupture at the area of:
   a. Insertion   Ref. 43, p. 342
   b. Metacarpophalangeal joint   Ref. 127, 51-A:15, 1969
   c. Carpometacarpal joint   Ref. 132, 2-3:643, 1971
   d. Lister's tubercle   Ref. 132, 5-2:432-436, 1974
8. When the sublimis tendon only is severed just distal to the metacarpophalangeal joint in a child, it should be:
   a. Excised as allowed without increasing the
      incision   Ref. 31, pp. 552-557
   b. Repaired primarily   Ref. 41, p. 1659
   c. Repaired secondarily at a later date   Ref. 43, p. 179
   d. Excised at a later date with a tendon graft   Ref. 132, 1-2:363, 1970
9. Surgically improved function of cerebral palsy of the hand would be most likely in the _____ type.
   a. Ataxic   Ref. 38, p. 319
   b. Rigid   Ref. 113, 41:439-445, 1972
   c. Spastic   Ref. 127, 52-A:907-920, 1970
   d. Athetotic   Ref. 127, 56-A:466-472, 1974
10. A 32-year-old laborer suffered a gunshot wound to his left hand, The middle ray is missing to the base of the metacarpal. There is a scarred cleft present the full depth of the missing ray. The other digits, although somewhat stiff, function well. The procedure that would probably give the best functional and cosmetic result is:
   a. Excision of the scar and filling of the defect with abdominal pedicle graft
   b. Maintaining the width of the palm with a   Ref. 30, pp. 270, 276
      bone graft between the metacarpal heads to the index and ring fingers, followed by an abdominal pedicle graft to cover the defect
   c. Transposition of the base of the metacarpal to the ring finger radially to fill the defect, excision of the scar, and closure primarily
   d. Transposition of the base of the metacarpal to the index finger ulnarly to fill the defect, excision of the scar, and closure primarily

11. The most important aspect of treatment recommended in early Volk-
    mann's ischemia after removal of the constricting dressings is:
    a. Incision of the skin to allow swelling
    b. Division of the brachial artery in the ante-   Ref. 30, p. 253
       cubital space to break up arterial spasm   Ref. 132, 4-4:983-986, 1973
    c. Stellate ganglion block
    d. Fasciotomy of the flexor compartment of
       the forearm
12. Extensor tendons should be immobilized approximately _____ after
    suturing.
    a. 2 weeks
    b. 4 weeks   Ref. 43, p. 162
    c. 6 weeks   Ref. 132, 1-2:337, 1970
    d. 8 weeks   Ref. 141, 128:1269, 1969
13. Absence of the hands is correctly termed:
    a. Phocomelia
    b. Ectromelia   Ref. 30, p. 55
    c. Acheiria
    d. Perochiria
14. Syndactylia is noted in a newborn infant. There is no evidence of bony
    involvement, and function appears to be good. Repair would probably
    be best carried out:
    a. Before 6 months
    b. About 3 years   Ref. 30, p. 90
    c. About 6 years
    d. About 10 years
15. During surgery of the hand, which one of the following is frequently
    seen?
    a. Meissner's corpuscle
    b. Ruffini's nerve ending   Ref. 30, p. 19
    c. Pacinian corpuscle
    d. Merkel-Ranvier nerve ending
16. The least motion normally occurs at the carpometacarpal joints of the:
    a. Thumb
    b. Index and long fingers   Ref. 30, p. 20
    c. Long and ring fingers
    d. Little fingers
17. In what percent of cases does the sole blood supply to the carpal navic-
    ular bone enter distal to its waist?
    a. Less than 1%
    b. 7%   Ref. 127, 20:424, 1938
    c. 13%   Ref. 127, 48-A:1125, 1966
    d. 19%
    e. 27%
18. The collateral ligaments of the interphalangeal joints of the fingers are
    the tightest when the joint is:
    a. Fully flexed
    b. Extended   Ref. 7, 16:57, 1959

c. Hyperextended   Ref. 127, 49-A:306, 1967
d. Flexed to 45°

19. During embryonic development the finger buds grow out from the web space beginning about the:
   a. Fifth week
   b. Seventh week   Ref. 26, p. 81
   c. Ninth week   Ref. 31, pp. 54-55
   d. Twelfth week

20. Spontaneous rupture of flexor tendons in the hand most frequently involves the:
   a. Profundus
   b. Sublimis   Ref. 31, p. 436
   c. Pollicis longus   Ref. 43, p. 188
   d. Carpi ulnaris   Ref. 132, 5-2:437-440, 1974

21. Nonunion of the metacarpals is most frequently due to:
   a. Traction and distraction of the fracture fragments
   b. Bone loss at the fracture sight   Ref. 43, p. 225
   c. Interposing tissue
   d. Malalignment

22. Arthrodesis of the distal interphalangeal joints of the fingers is recommended at:
   a. 0° flexion
   b. 15° to 20° flexion   Ref. 43, p. 234
   c. 30° to 40° flexion
   d. 40° to 50° flexion

23. Spontaneous flexor tendon rupture usually occurs at the:
   a. Site of insertion   Ref. 31, p. 436
   b. Level of the metacarpophalangeal joint   Ref. 43, p. 188
   c. Midpalm   Ref. 132, 5-2:437-440, 1974
   d. Proximal interphalangeal joint   Ref. 137, 56:260-264, 1972

24. Nonunion of the phalanges in treated fractures is most frequently due to:
   a. Traction and distraction of the fracture fragments
   b. Infection   Ref. 43, p. 225
   c. Malalignment
   d. Interposing soft tissue

25. The most common destructive bone tumor occurring in the hand is:
   a. Enchondroma   Ref. 1, pp. 1032, 1042
   b. Aneurysmal bone cyst   Ref. 5, p. 528
   c. Chondrosarcoma   Ref. 43, p. 379
   d. Epidermal inclusion cyst of bone   Ref. 127, 50-A:365, 1968

26. Incision and drainage of a "collar-button" abscess is usually best accomplished:
   a. Through a palmar incision
   b. Through a dorsal incision   Ref. 30, p. 672

   c. Through a web space incision opening   **Ref. 43, p. 393**
       deep between the metacarpal heads   **Ref. 71, p. 184**
   d. Through both palmar and dorsal incisions

27. When the profundus tendon is cleanly severed distal to the proximal interphalangeal joint, it should be:
   a. Repaired primarily
   b. Repaired secondarily   **Ref. 31, pp. 552-557**
   c. Excised primarily and repaired with a   **Ref. 43, p. 179**
       tendon graft   **Ref. 132, 1-2:360-372, 1970**
   d. None of the above   **Ref. 132, 4-4:865-876, 1973**

28. A midpalmar space abscess:
   a. Occurs superficially to the flexor tendon sheaths
   b. Is usually best drained through dorsal   **Ref. 30, p. 672**
       longitudinal incisions   **Ref. 43, p. 394**
   c. Nearly always involves the wrist joint   **Ref. 71, pp. 35, 78, 397-406**
   d. Occurs deep to the flexor tendon sheaths and usually does not extend above the wrist

29. The usually accepted treatment of glomus tumor is:
   a. Drilling of the nail bed to relieve pressure
   b. X-ray therapy   **Ref. 30, p. 749**
   c. Surgical excision   **Ref. 137, 47:345-346, 1971**
   d. Aspiration and injection with a cortisone derivative

30. The most common malignant tumor of the hand is:
   a. Metastatic carcinoma
   b. Squamous cell carcinoma   **Ref. 30, p. 721**
   c. Fibrosarcoma
   d. Chondrosarcoma

31. A 60-year-old white man is seen with a lesion of the right thumb, which has been present for three to four months. He reports hitting the thumb with a hammer and that it initially got better. Since then, a fungating mass has made its appearance along the margin of the nail. The mass has a granular appearance and is bordered by a narrow pigmented band. The most likely diagnosis is:
   a. Carcinoma of the nail
   b. Subungual melanoma   **Ref. 30, p. 765**
   c. Glomus tumor   **Ref. 127, 48-A:92, 1966**
   d. Fibroma

32. Restoration of intrinsic muscle function is best when:
   a. A tenodesis effect is created
   b. The tendon transfers pass to the volar   **Ref. 43, pp. 304, 305**
       side of the deep transverse carpal ligament   **Ref. 112, pp. 23-50**
   c. The tendon transfers insert on the   **Ref. 127, 52-A:868, 1970**
       ulnar aspects of the extensor hoods   **Ref. 127, 55-A:1675-1677, 1973**
   d. The tendon transfers insert on the base of the proximal phalanx

33. The sublimis tendon to a finger is presumed to be severed when:
    a. The finger assumes a hyperextended posi-
       tion
    b. The distal interphalangeal joint cannot be   Ref. 43, pp. 167-168
       flexed while stabilizing the proximal inter-
       phalangeal joint
    c. The proximal interphalangeal joint cannot
       be flexed independently when the two
       adjacent fingers are held in extension
    d. The metacarpophalangeal joints cannot
       be independently flexed
34. X-ray films of a 32-year-old woman were presented at a conference. No
    history was given other than that the patient was not paralyzed. The
    hands showed atrophy of the soft tissues, especially the fingers. There
    was generalized demineralization of the bone and erosion of the tufts
    of many distal phalanges. Soft tissue calcification was noted within the
    pulp of several digits. The most likely diagnosis is:
    a. Gout   Ref. 22, p. 812
    b. Diabetic neuropathy   Ref. 30, p. 344
    c. Scleredema   Ref. 95, pp. 122, 188
    d. Hyperparathyroidism   Ref. 125, 215:1113-1116, 1971
35. The greatest functional intrinsic muscle loss to the thumb in median
    nerve palsy is the:
    a. Abductor pollicis brevis
    b. Opponens pollicis   Ref. 43, p. 308
    c. Flexor pollicis brevis   Ref. 127, 49-A:653, 1967
    d. Adductor pollicis
36. Which of the following has the strongest synergistic action and should
    not be used for transfer to an antagonistic action when another selection
    is available?
    a. Flexor carpi ulnaris
    b. Flexor carpi radialis   Ref. 30, p. 443
    c. Flexor digitorum sublimis   Ref. 31, pp. 411, 413
    d. Pronator teres
37. Finkelstein's test is associated with:
    a. Dupuytren's contracture
    b. Carpal tunnel syndrome   Ref. 43, p. 371
    c. de Quervain's disease
    d. Synovial fluid examination in rheumatoid
       arthritis
38. A thenar space infection is:
    a. Limited ulnarly by a fascial membrane
       arising from the third metacarpal
    b. Limited ulnarly by a fascial membrane   Ref. 30, p. 672
       arising from the second meta-
       carpal   Ref. 43, p. 395

c. Usually best drained through the dorsum of the hand to prevent scarring of the palm

d. Usually deep to the abductor pollicis muscle

Ref. 71, p. 407

39. A 40-year-old Jewish man has had a one-month history of increasing severe pain in the end of his ring finger. The pain is stabbing and burning in character and radiates up the arm. It is helped with aspirin. On physical examination a bluish discoloration is noted under the nail. X-ray examination reveals minimal bone erosion of the dorsal surface of the distal phalanx. The probable diagnosis is:
    a. Epidermal inclusion cyst
    b. Subungual melanoma
    c. Glomus tumor
    d. Terminal arterial aneurysm

Ref. 30, p. 748

40. Brachial plexus exploration, when indicated, is best carried out through:
    a. Axillary approach
    b. Infraclavicular approach
    c. Supraclavicular approach
    d. Transclavicular approach

Ref. 127, 55-A:1159-1176, 1973

41. Instability with subluxation of the wrist joint secondary to rheumatoid arthritis is best treated by:
    a. Arthrodesis
    b. Dorsal wrist stabilization (ligamentous reconstruction)
    c. Palmar shelf arthroplasty
    d. Darrach procedure

Ref. 127, 47-A:741, 1965
Ref. 127, 51-A:1, 1969
Ref. 127, 52-A:896, 1970
Ref. 132, 2-3:649-661, 1971

42. A 22-year-old mechanic was referred for care of an impacted right fifth metacarpal neck fracture, 18 days after injury. X-ray films showed 40° of angulation. There was residual discoloration, swelling, and restriction of motion. No rotational deformity was noted. The treatment of choice would be:
    a. Closed reduction under ulnar nerve block
    b. Attempted closed reduction with the patient under general anesthesia; if this fails, then open reduction or osteotomy of the healing fragments and pin fixation
    c. Cast or splint until healing is complete, then carry out correctional osteotomy
    d. Accept the present deformity and encourage immediate active range of motion and light work

Ref. 127, 52-A:1159, 1970

43. A 30-year-old male shopworker suffered a stab wound over the dorsum of his long finger, middle phalanx, right hand. After healing of the skin a hard mass was present, which after six months continued to be tender and nonmovable and elevated the skin into a mound. Loss of flexion of the digit was noted. The most likely diagnosis would be:
    a. Epidermal inclusion cyst
    b. Osteogenic sarcoma

Ref. 127, 48-A:105, 1966

c. Foreign body reaction

d. Turret exostosis

44. The wrist flexion (Phalen's) test would be expected to be positive in a patient suffering from:

    a. Dupuytren's contracture

    b. Carpal tunnel syndrome   **Ref. 127, 48-A:211, 1966**

    c. de Quervain's disease

    d. Scleroderma

45. After injury or reconstructive surgery to the hand, stiff joints can best be mobilized by:

    a. Daily treatment with microwave diathermy or ultrasound

    b. Biweekly passive stretching of the in-   **Ref. 31, pp. 431-433**
       volved joints   **Ref. 132, 2-3:623-628, 1971**

    c. Frequent whirlpool baths with tempera- **Ref. 132, 5-2:445-449, 1974**
       tures similar to hot bath water to increase circulation

    d. Frequent instruction and encouragement by the surgeon or a "knowledgeable" therapist on active range of motion and muscle strengthening exercises only

46. Displaced proximal phalangeal finger fractures should:

    a. Be treated with fingers splinted or casted in full extension until healed at approximately 8 weeks

    b. Be casted or splinted with fingers in   **Ref. 127, 55-A:1651, 1973**
       flexion for 8 weeks to control rotation   **Ref. 132, 1-2:261-273, 1970**

    c. Be expected to do well with closed or open reduction with cross-pin fixation and simple side-to-side finger splinting allowing immediate early motion

    d. Be treated with complete immobilization of the joints proximal and distal to the fracture until the fracture lines appear healed on x-ray evaluation, to avoid malunion or nonunion

47. An interosseous ganglion of the distal radius would be expected to have which of the following characteristics?

    a. Irregular poorly defined osseous margins by x-ray evaluation

    b. Epiphyseal in position but may cross the **Ref. 111, pp. 325-328, 1973**
       old epiphyseal line

    c. Containing thin serous fluid and synonymous with a unicameral bone cyst

    d. May be multilocular, filled with blood, and expanding the cortex; synonymous with an aneurysmal bone cyst

48. Following a crush injury, a hand is noted to be markedly swollen throughout, with loss of intrinsic muscle function and pain when straightening the fingers. The highest priority of consideration would be:
    a. Ulnar nerve decompression
    b. Compressive dressings, elevation, and ice   Ref. 119, 106:826-828, 1973
    c. Intrinsic muscle decompression   Ref. 137, 50:341-349, 1972
    d. Arteriography

49. A patient presents with symptoms compatible with carpal tunnel compression but also reports gradual weight gain, overall joint pain, and mild effusion of both knees with pretibial edema. A most likely diagnosis would be:
    a. Rheumatoid arthritis
    b. Congestive heart failure   Ref. 127, 55-A:78-82, 1973
    c. Hypothyroidism   Ref. 111, pp. 336-337, 1972
    d. Degenerative arthritis with congestive heart failure

50. The painful thumb carpometacarpal joint:
    a. Occurs most frequently in men
    b. Is due primarily to degenerative   Ref. 127, 55-A:1655-1666, 1973
    articular changes without significant   Ref. 132, 4-2:331-347, 1973
    capsular loosening or pathology
    c. Results primarily from increasing capsular laxity, which results in subluxation and degenerative changes
    d. Requires prosthetic replacement of the trapezium even before advanced articular destruction has occurred

MULTIPLE CHOICE, MULTIPLE ANSWERS (answers on p. 276)

Select one or more answers that will best complete or answer each of the following statements or questions.

51. When an infant presents with a congenital defect of the radius, which of the following conditions would you expect?
    a. Absence of the first and second metacarpals would be expected in 85% of such cases.
    b. The segment most likely to be present   Ref. 30, p. 68
    would be the radial head.   Ref. 127, 51-B:399, 1969
    c. Absence of the scaphoid and trapezium would be expected on a statistical basis.
    d. Early conservative treatment by casting manipulation and bracing has proved unhelpful. The treatment of choice, therefore, is waiting patiently until the child is old enough for definitive surgery, usually at 4 to 6 years of age.

52. Dupuytren's contracture has been shown to have association with:
    a. Peyronie's disease
    b. Epilepsy   Ref. 30, p. 231
    c. Plantar fascitis   Ref. 66, pp. 12-21
    d. Trauma
    e. Sex
53. The superficial volar arterial arch lies beneath which of the following?
    a. Palmar aponeurosis
    b. Palmaris brevis   Ref. 60, p. 624
    c. Transverse carpal ligament
    d. Flexor digiti quinti brevis
    e. Divisions of the ulnar and median nerves
54. Concerning the deep palmar arterial arch, which of the following are true?
    a. It lies on the proximal portions of the metacarpals.
    b. It is covered by the flexor tendons of the fingers.   Ref. 60, pp. 619-621
    c. In 60% of cases it is superficial to the ulnar nerve.
    d. It anastomoses with the deep volar branch of the ulnar artery.
    e. The adductor pollicis lies deep to it.
55. Subungual melanoma:
    a. Most frequently presents early as a black spot underneath the thumbnail
    b. May split the nail, protruding as a fungus-like growth   Ref. 30, pp. 763-765
    c. Usually ulcerates and weeps a thin brown fluid
    d. Should be treated with amputation and regional lymph node dissection
56. Ganglions tend to occur frequently over the:
    a. Dorsum of the wrist, arising from the scaphoid lunate ligament
    b. Dorsum of the wrist, arising from the capitohamate ligament   Ref. 30, p. 722
                                            Ref. 127, 53-A:299-302, 1971
    c. Volar ulnar aspect of the wrist, arising from the pisohamate ligament
    d. Volar aspect of the metacarpophalangeal joints, arising from the flexor tendon fibro-osseous canal
57. Vasomotor conditions occasionally warrant sympathetic block. The ganglia that have greatest effect on the arm and hand is (are):
    a. Stellate
    b. T-2   Ref. 30, p. 712
    c. T-3   Ref. 132, 1-2:255-259, 1970
    d. T-4

58. Giant cell tumor of the tendon sheath:
    a. Occurs most frequently in the hand
    b. Is associated with xanthelasma   Ref. 30, pp. 275, 276
    c. Usually presents as a painful nodular
       lesion
    d. Commonly involves joints and erodes bone
59. Lateral to the pisiform bone there is a hiatus between the volar carpal
    ligament and the transverse carpal ligament that allows passage of
    the:
    a. Palmaris longus
    b. Median nerve   Ref. 7, 16:88, 1959
    c. Ulnar artery   Ref. 127, 51-A:1095, 1969
    d. Ulnar nerve   Ref. 127, 51-B:471, 1969
    e. Flexor carpi ulnaris
60. The content(s) of the ulnar bursa is (are) the:
    a. Flexor digitorum sublimis
    b. Flexor digitorum profundus   Ref. 60, p. 474
    c. Flexor carpi radialis
    d. Palmaris longus
    e. Median nerve
61. In advanced rheumatoid arthritis the hand usually takes on the appear-
    ance of:
    a. Intrinsic minus
    b. Intrinsic plus   Ref. 43, pp. 329, 340, 343
    c. Ulnar deviation of the fingers   Ref. 112, p. 102
    d. Radial deviation of the wrist   Ref. 132, 4-4:1039-1056, 1973
62. Regarding the extensor digiti quinti, which of the following is (are) *not*
    true?
    a. Its innervation differs from that of the
       extensor indicis proprius.
    b. It is inserted principally into the extensor   Ref. 7, 16:54, 1959
       hood of the fifth digit.
    c. It lies to the ulnar side of the nearest
       common extensor tendon
    d. It does not share a compartment at the
       wrist.
    e. It commonly is divided into two
       tendinous slips.
63. When multiple tissues must be reconstructed in the hand, attention
    should be given in what order?
    a. Tendons
    b. Skin   Ref. 43, p. 213
    c. Nerves
    d. Bone
    e. Joints

64. In dislocations of the metacarpophalangeal joint of the thumb the meta-carpal head usually protrudes _____, and closed reduction often is impossible because the head is usually trapped by fibers of the _____ muscle.
   a. Volarly
   b. Dorsally
   c. Opponens pollicis
   d. Abductor pollicis longus
   e. Flexor pollicis brevis

Ref. 30, p. 662
Ref. 38, p. 118
Ref. 43, p. 183

65. de Quervain's disease:
   a. Involves the synovial sheaths of the extensor pollicis longus and abductor pollicis brevis
   b. Is more common in women than men
   c. Is most painful when the thumb is extended and the wrist is deviated radially
   d. Is often associated with aberrant tendons within the involved sheath

Ref. 30, p. 472
Ref. 31, p. 445
Ref. 43, pp. 371-372

66. Trigger finger or thumb:
   a. Is not known to be present at birth
   b. Is frequently associated with trauma
   c. Results from stricture of the fibro-osseous canal at the level of the proximal interphalangeal joint
   d. Usually demonstrates microscopic involvement of both the tendon and the fibro-osseous canal

Ref. 30, p. 474
Ref. 31, p. 447
Ref. 113, 41:419-432, 1970

67. An infected radial bursa:
   a. Will communicate with the ulnar bursa in over 50% of cases
   b. Is usually satisfactorily drained by a single appropriately placed incision along the lateral aspect of the thumb
   c. Is best drained by two incisions, one above the wrist and a second along the lateral aspect of the thumb
   d. Involves only the tendon sheath of the flexor pollicis longus by definition

Ref. 43, p. 395
Ref. 71, p. 351

68. The Littler release is designed to:
   a. Preserve the transverse fibers of the extensor hood to avoid hyperextension of the metacarpophalangeal joint
   b. Release the insertion of the oblique fibers into the extensor tendon
   c. Permit flexion of the interphalangeal joints in the intrinsic minus hand
   d. Rehabilitate the intrinsic plus hand

Ref. 43, p. 344

69. Which of the following have been found to be associated with rheumatoid arthritis?
    a. de Quervain's disease
    b. Carpal tunnel syndrome   Ref. 30, p. 363
    c. Trigger finger   Ref. 43, p. 329
    d. Mucous cyst
70. Epidermal inclusion cysts in the hand:
    a. Are believed to result from implantation
       of epithelium due to injury
    b. May present as an expansile destructive   Ref. 30, pp. 727-729
       lesion of bone   Ref. 127, 50-A:365, 1968
    c. Occur less frequently than do sebaceous
       cysts
    d. Should be treated with radiation as the
       procedure of choice
71. Silicone rubber implants have proved useful as:
    a. Finger-joint prostheses
    b. Tendon replacement prostheses   Ref. 111, pp. 315-319, 1972
    c. Molds to form gliding surfaces for flexor Ref. 127, 53-A:829-838, 1971
       tendon grafts   Ref. 137, 47:576-579, 1971
    d. A nonreactive substance well tolerated by   Ref. 142, 48:1113, 1968
       the body in most instances
72. Monteggia's fracture usually:
    a. Demands open reduction in children
    b. Involves fracture of the proximal one third   Ref. 106, 66:94, 1969
       of the ulna
    c. Requires internal fixation of the ulna to
       prevent malunion in adults
    d. Requires fascial loop reconstruction of the
       annular ligament
73. Indications for surgery after injury to the finger joints would include:
    a. Volar plate injuries allowing hyperexten-
       sion of the proximal interphalangeal joint
    b. Acute collateral ligament injuries with   Ref. 127, 52-A:937, 1970
       instability   Ref. 132, 1-2:261-273, 1971
    c. Fractures disrupting the articular surfaces
    d. Boutonnière deformity
74. Dupuytren's contracture:
    a. Is virtually confined to people of Euro-
       pean descent
    b. Is always directly or indirectly relatable to   Ref. 31, pp. 226-239
       incidents of trauma   Ref. 66, pp. 12-50
    c. Is a disease of the palmar aponeurosis   Ref. 111, pp. 296-299, 1972
       and the tissues deep to it
    d. Usually requires release of the sublimis
       tendons for correction of contracture of
       the ring and small fingers

75. Island pedicle grafts to a denervated area of the hand can be expected to:
    a. Retain heat and cold sensation
    b. Retain normal two-point discrimination over long-term follow-up   Ref. 31, p. 382
             Ref. 127, 51-A:1257-68, 1969
    c. Readily convert to accurate localizing of stimulus to the new area of coverage   Ref. 127, 52-A:1181, 1970
    d. Provide protective sensation as a major objective
76. A low radial nerve palsy usually spares the:
    a. Extensor carpi ulnaris muscle
    b. Extensor digitorum longus muscle   Ref. 43, p. 306
    c. Abductor pollicis longus muscle
    d. Brachioradialis muscle
77. Which of the following are synergistic muscles?
    a. Flexor carpi ulnaris and flexor digitorum sublimus
    b. Flexor carpi radialis and extensor digitorum communis   Ref. 30, p. 443
             Ref. 31, pp. 411-413
    c. Extensor carpi radialis longus and flexor digitorum profundus
    d. Extensor carpi ulnaris and palmaris longus
78. The tendon "T" operation is designed to restore:
    a. Adduction to the thumb
    b. Abduction to the index fingers   Ref. 30, p. 513
    c. Opposition to the thumb
    d. The metacarpal arch
79. Indicate the procedure(s) most likely to be necessary in a high ulnar nerve palsy in the presence of normal median nerve function.
    a. Restoration of sublimis function to the ring and small fingers
    b. Restoration in intrinsic function to the ring and small fingers   Ref. 43, p. 309
    c. Restoration of profundus function to all fingers
    d. Restoration of abduction to the index finger and adduction to the thumb
80. Commonly recommended restoration procedures for high median nerve palsy would include:
    a. Restoration of profundus function to the index and long fingers by attachment to the profundus tendons of the ring and small fingers
    b. Restoration of the intrinsic muscle function to the index and long fingers by the Brand or Fowler technique   Ref. 30, p. 450
             Ref. 43, p. 312
             Ref. 127, 49-A:653, 1967

c. Restoration of opposition of the thumb
by use of the sublimis to the ring fingers

d. Restoration of flexion of the thumb by
transfer of the extensor carpi radialis or
brachioradialis

81. Early treatment of frostbitten extremities would include:
a. Rapid rewarming to 40° C
b. Elevation of limbs to lessen edema   **Ref. 132, 1-2:321-323, 1970**
c. Tetanus prophylaxis and antibiotics
d. Low molecular dextran
e. Drainage of tissue blisters

82. Repair of a lacerated flexor tendon in the distal forearm, wrist, or palm
should:
a. Include resection of adjacent overlying
palmar and antibrachial fascia
b. Under no circumstances include repair of   **Ref. 132, 1-2:357-367, 1970**
both sublimis and profundus tendons
within the same wound
c. Be carried out primarily after adequate
wound toilet in otherwise clean wounds
less than 6 hours old
d. Never sacrifice an intact sublimis for a
profundus repair to the same digit

83. Ulnar nerve compression at the elbow may be differentiated in what
way from compression at the wrist?
a. In the former, flexor carpi ulnaris and
profundus strength to the small finger
would tend to be decreased.
b. In the latter, Allen's test for ulnar artery   **Ref. 128, 38:780-785, 1973**
patency may be positive.
c. Nerve conduction studies can be expected
to accurately reflect the level of pathology
in most cases.
d.. Intrinsic atrophy and weakness do not occur with compression at the elbow but
are prominent features when there is
pathology at the wrist.

84. Epithelioid sarcoma of the hand and forearm:
a. Is rare among soft tissue malignancies in
this region
b. Usually presents as a nodule or group   **Ref. 127, 56-A:458-465, 1974**
of nodules along fascial or tendinous
structures
c. Rarely if ever metastasizes
d. Frequently involves skin and warrants
amputation of the involved part as the
treatment of choice

85. Dorsal tenosynovectomy at the wrists in active rheumatoid synovitis:
   a. May reduce incidents of future tendon rupture
   b. Rarely is successful in preventing rapid return of proliferative synovium in dorsal tendon sheath   Ref. 111, pp. 370-374, 1972
   Ref. 127, 56-A:601-610, 1974
   c. Is indicated immediately should tendon rupture occur
   d. Should not be combined with tendon repair

SITUATION AND PROGRESSIVE THOUGHT (answers on p. 276)

Select the answer or answers that best apply in accordance with the information given in each of the following statements.

86. A 47-year-old white woman has crippling arthritis of the hands. The deformities are severe, with x-ray and clinical evidence of dislocation and overriding of the metacarpophalangeal joints of the right hand. The articular surfaces are eroded. There is thinning of the cortex. It is believed that the patient may be helped operatively. Indicate the procedure(s) that is (are) most frequently recommended.
   a. Insertion of a Flatt prosthesis
   b. Fusion of the metacarpophalangeal joints   Ref. 30, p. 338
   c. Synovectomy   Ref. 43, pp. 333-335
   d. Resection of the metacarpal heads and repositioning of the soft tissue structures or a silicone rubber prosthetic arthroplasty replacement   Ref. 45, 15:127, 1959
   Ref. 112, p. 64
   Ref. 127, 50-A:609, 1968
   Ref. 132, 4-2:349-371, 1972
   Ref. 142, 48:1113, 1968
87. In reconstructing a hand affected by rheumatoid arthritis, the least desirable arthrodesis and one to be avoided when possible is the:
   a. Wrist joint
   b. Proximal interphalangeal joints of the fingers   Ref. 30, p. 338
   Ref. 127, 50-A:609, 1968
   c. Distal interphalangeal joints of the fingers   Ref. 127, 51-A:1, 1969
   d. Metacarpophalangeal joints of the fingers
88. On the left there is marked ulnar drift, with subluxation of the extensor tendons. None of the metacarpophalangeal joints is dislocated. They cannot, however, be fully extended and assume increased ulnar deviation when this is attempted. The joints are puffed and boggy. Which of the following operative procedures are frequently recommended as helpful at the metacarpophalangeal level?
   a. Incision of the extensor hood on the ulnar side of the long extensor tendon, synovectomy and release of the collateral ligaments, and repositioning of the extensor hood
   b. Tenotomy of the lumbrical muscles at their insertion into the extensor hood   Ref. 30, p. 374
   Ref. 43, p. 331

c. Tenotomy of the first volar interosseous, the third and fourth dorsal interosseous, and the abductor digiti quinti

Ref. 45, 36:62, 1964
Ref. 111, pp. 370-372, 1972
Ref. 112, p. 64

d. Transfer of the extensor indicis proprius and proprius quinti into the extensor hood on the radial side of the index and small fingers

89. A 16-year-old white boy has a radial nerve palsy of eight years' duration. He has a history of a fracture of the midshaft of the humerus that was fixed by internal fixation. The loss would be expected to include:
   a. Paralysis of the long head of the triceps
   b. Supination of the forearm   **Ref. 43, pp. 306, 307**
   c. Wrist and finger extension
   d. Paralysis of the abductor pollicis longus and brevis

90. The boy is able to weakly extend the distal phalanx of the thumb. This is most likely due to the:
   a. Aberrant insertion of the extensor pollicis brevis
   b. Action of the opponens pollicis, which   **Ref. 30, p. 511** frequently inserts into the extensor head
   c. Action of the abductor pollicis longus on the extensor hood
   d. Abductor pollicis brevis and the adductor pollicis muscles

91. The most acceptable procedure(s) for restoring thumb function would be:
   a. Transfer of the palmaris longus to the rerouted extensor pollicis brevis
   b. Transfer of the palmaris longus to the   **Ref. 43, pp. 306-307** rerouted extensor pollicis longus
   c. Transfer of the flexor carpi radialis to the extensor pollicis brevis and abductor pollicis longus and transfer of the flexor digitorum sublimis of the ring finger to the extensor indicis proprius and extensor pollicis longus
   d. Fusion of the metacarpophalangeal joint of the thumb in the position of function and transfer of either the flexor carpi radialis or the palmaris longus to the rerouted extensor pollicis longus

92. The best method of restoring function to the entire hand, according to Riordan, is:
   a. Fusion of the wrist, with transfer of the flexor carpi ulnaris to the extensor digitorum communis, transfer of the palmaris longus to the extensor pollicis longus, and

transfer of the flexor carpi radialis to the abductor pollicis longus and extensor pollicis brevis

b. Transfer of the sublimis of the long and ring fingers to the common digital extensors and transfers of the indicis proprius and extensor pollicis longus, respectively, with the pronator teres, to the extensor digitorum longus and brevis

Ref. 7, 16:89, 1959
Ref. 31, p. 411
Ref. 43, pp. 285, 306-307

c. Fusion of the wrist, with transfer of the flexor carpi ulnaris to the common digital extensors, transfer of the flexor carpi radialis to the extensor pollicis longus, and transfer of the palmaris longus to the abductor pollicis longus

d. Transfer of the flexor carpi ulnaris to the common digital extensors, transfer of the palmaris longus to the rerouted long extensor of the thumb, and transfer of the pronator teres to the extensor carpi radialis longus and brevis

93. A 22-year-old man is seen in the emergency room with a painful deformed right hand. Clinical and x-ray examinations show the metacarpophalangeal joint of the index finger to be dislocated, with the head displaced volarly. It is resistant to closed reduction. According to Kaplan, the proper incision for open reduction is the:

a. Midlateral approach
b. Dorsal approach
c. Palmar approach
Ref. 43, pp. 186, 187
Ref. 127, 39-A:1081, 1957
d. Web space approach between the index and long fingers

94. The restricting structures that are most frequently found to prevent closed reduction include the:

a. Flexor tendons slipped to the radial side and the lumbrical muscle slipped to the ulnar side, entrapping the metacarpal head

b. Natatory and anterior fibrocartilaginous plate distally and the superficial transverse metacarpal ligament proximally
Ref. 43, p. 187
Ref. 127, 39-A:108, 1957

c. Deep transverse carpal ligament proximally

d. Lumbrical muscle slipped to the radial side of the metacarpal head

95. A 39-year-old woman has suffered a C-6 cord lesion in an automobile accident. Functional loss would not be expected to include:
    a. Extension of the index fingers and thumb
    b. Flexion of the fingers   Ref. 30, pp. 253-255
    c. Extension of the wrist   Ref. 43, p. 314
    d. Abduction of the thumb   Ref. 112, pp. 155-169

96. Assume that in this or a similar patient with quadriplegia the following muscles are available for transfer: extensor carpi radialis longus and brevis, fair to good; brachioradialis, fair. The operative procedure usually recommended for rehabilitating the hand is:
    a. Fusion of the wrist in 20° of extension and transfer of the extensor carpi radialis brevis to the extensor digitorum communis, extensor carpi radialis longus to the flexor profundus of the fingers, and brachioradial is to the flexor pollicis longus
    b. Fusion of the wrist in 20° of extension;   Ref. 30, p. 453
    fusion of the thumb in position of func-   Ref. 43, p. 314
    tion; transfer of the extensor carpi radi-   Ref. 112, pp. 155-169
    alis brevis to the common digital ex-   Ref. 127, 56-A:951-959, 1974
    tensors, brachioradialis to the flexor digitorium profundus of the fingers, and extensor carpi radialis longus to the extensor indicis proprius
    c. Transfer of the brachioradialis for thumb opposition and transfer of the extensor carpi radialis longus to the profundus of the index and long fingers
    d. Tenodesis of the flexor digitorum profundus and flexor pollicis longus to the radius; tenodesis of the rerouted extensor pollicis brevis to the ulna to give opposition; transfer of the brachioradialis to the profundus tendons beyond tenodesis if desired

97. When a cord lesion is one segment lower, several other muscles become available for transfer. The reconstruction for this type of lesion has been outlined by Riordan and modified by Lipscomb, Elkins, and Henderson. They recommend _____ operations, one of which _____ entail arthrodesis of the wrist.
    a. Two
    b. Three   Ref. 30, p. 453
    c. Does   Ref. 43, pp. 314-315
    d. Does not   Ref. 112, pp. 155-169
                                          Ref. 127, 56-A:951, 1974

98. A 40-year-old housewife has a firm erythematous nodule over the dorso-radial surface of her long finger at the distal interphalangeal joint. The nodule measures 0.5 cm in diameter. The skin over the nodule is tense and shiny. There is no increased heat or other periarticular swelling. Other joints do not appear to be involved. The most likely diagnosis is:
   a. Mucous cyst
   b. Heberden's node   Ref. 30, pp. 729-730
   c. Rheumatic nodule   Ref. 43, p. 386
   d. Periarticular ganglion
99. X-ray examination of the joint would be expected to show:
   a. Marked demineralization of the sub-chondral bone
   b. Early degenerative hypertrophic arthritis   Ref. 30, pp. 729-730
   c. Characteristic findings of rheumatoid arthritis
   d. No pathologic findings
100. Accepted treatment would normally include:
   a. X-ray therapy
   b. Surgical excision with a full-thickness skin graft   Ref. 30, p. 730
   c. Amputation at the proximal interphalangeal joint
   d. Aspiration and injection with a cortisone derivative

TRUE OR FALSE (answers on pp. 276-277)

101. In the finger at the level of the proximal and distal interphalangeal joint the nerve will be volar to the artery.   Ref. 43, p. 174
   (T) (F)
102. Dorsal dislocation of the thumb at the metacarpophalangeal joint is routinely easily reduced by traction only.   Ref. 43, p. 183
   (T) (F)
103. Volkmann's ischemic contracture is invariably due to improper casting or constricting dressings.   Ref. 30, p. 245
   (T) (F)
104. Dejerine-Sottas disease is usually best treated by resecting the involved segment of the nerve.   Ref. 43, p. 389
   (T) (F)
105. Skin incisions should be in the skin creases on the palmar surface of the hand because they hide the scar, and it is more physiologic.
   (T) (F)   Ref. 43, pp. 145-150
                   Ref. 111, pp. 310-373, 1974
                   Ref. 132, 1-2:213-215, 1970
106. When applying an abdominal pedicle flap to the forearm or hand, it is permissible to maintain the desired rotation of the forearm with a Kirschner wire, transfixing the radius and the ulna.   Ref. 30, p. 275
   (T) (F)   Ref. 43, p. 176

107. Absence of or congenital defects in the ulna occur more frequently than do similar defects of the radius. Ref. 30, p. 69
(T) (F)

108. The Fowler technique of tenodesis for metacarpophalangeal joint stabilization in the intrinsic minus hand is activated by wrist flexion.
(T) (F) Ref. 43, p. 301

109. Although the sublimis tendons to either the ring or small fingers may be severed at the wrist, active flexion of these digits may occur because of intercommunication of the sublimis tendon below the wrist.
(T) (F) Ref. 43, p. 168

110. Primary closure with or without skin grafts is relatively less important in the hand than elsewhere in the extremities. Ref. 31, p. 550
(T) (F) Ref. 43, p. 164
Ref. 111, pp. 344-347, 1974
Ref. 127, 47-A:944, 1965
Ref. 127, 50-A:945, 1968

111. Experimental studies would seem to indicate that nerve repair with carefully placed perineural suture is superior to epineural suture.
(T) (F) Ref. 127, 49-A:669, 1967

112. Hydrofluoric acid burns of the hand are best treated with early injection of 10% calcium gluconate. Ref. 127, 52-A:931, 1970
(T) (F)

113. After synovectomy for rheumatoid arthritis, recurrence of the proliferative synovitis is expected in a high percentage of cases.
(T) (F) Ref. 111, pp. 310-374, 1972
Ref. 127, 51-A:15, 1969

114. Early care of burns of the hand should include immobilization until healed skin coverage is attained. Ref. 127, 48-A:655, 1966
(T) (F) Ref. 132, 1-2:311-319, 1970

115. Experimental studies show that primary nerve repair in clean wounds would be expected to give results superior to delayed repair.
(T) (F) Ref. 127, 50-A:965, 1968

116. The Doppler ultrasound flow detector is a useful tool in assessing blood flow to an ischemic extremity. Ref. 141, 135:373-378, 1972
(T) (F)

117. The primary pathology of tennis elbow is believed to be on a basis of tears in the connective tissues of the common extensor origin.
(T) (F) Ref. 127, 55-A:1177-1182, 1973

118. Internal neurolysis has been shown to improve results in the treatment of advanced carpal tunnel syndrome. Ref. 127, 55-A:733, 1973
(T) (F)

119. Nail plasty has been a successful procedure in correcting the "split nail" deformity caused by trauma to the nail matrix.
(T) (F) Ref. 111, pp. 361-362, 1972

120. Mallet finger deformity without avulsion of bone may be treated successfully by simple but persistent splinting in the extended position; however, this may require up to 10 to 12 weeks.
(T) (F) Ref. 127, 44-A:1061, 1962

121. List four methods for treatment of the ulnar claw hand.

   Ref. 31, pp. 442-480
   Ref. 43, pp. 295-306
   Ref. 112, pp. 23-27
   Ref. 127, 55-A:1667-1675, 1973

122. List four contraindications for surgical release of muscles or tendons in the patient with spastic contracture of the wrist and hand.

   Ref. 112, p. 175

123. List five changes occurring in rheumatoid arthritis of the hand that may contribute to ulnar deviation of the digits.   Ref. 112, pp. 64-67

   Ref. 127, 49-A:31, 299, 1967

124. List four methods of repair for fingertip amputations designed to maintain length.   Ref. 52, pp. 151-154

   Ref. 106, 66:109, 1969
   Ref. 111, pp. 359-360, 1972
   Ref. 127, 40-A:317, 1967
   Ref. 127, 52-A:559, 923, 1970

125. List four operative methods for treatment for pseudarthrosis of the carpal navicular.   Ref. 113, 33:56, 1963

   Ref. 127, 28:749, 1946
   Ref. 127, 30-A:98, 1948
   Ref. 127, 50-B:102, 110, 1968
   Ref. 132, 1-2:299-307, 1970

126. List five essentials to be considered before transferring a tendon in the hand.   Ref. 30, pp. 441-442

   Ref. 31, p. 410

127. List six causes that may account for the limitation of joint motion.

   Ref. 43, pp. 227-231

128. List four techniques or methods whereby radioulnar synostosis may be prevented or corrected.   Ref. 30, p. 276

129. List five alternative methods by which a patient with Kienböck's disease could be acceptably treated.   Ref. 30, p. 296

   Ref. 132, 1-2:299-309, 1970

130. List six surgical procedures that may be of benefit in the reconstruction of the hand following Volkmann's ischemic contracture.

   Ref. 30, pp. 255-256
   Ref. 112, pp. 150-154

131. List the functional loss to the wrist and hand when an ulnar nerve is damaged above the elbow.   Ref. 43, pp. 308-309

132. List four areas of nerve compression that may mimic the carpal tunnel syndrome.   Ref. 30, p. 263

   Ref. 43, p. 368
   Ref. 127, 48-A:211, 1966
   Ref. 129, 55:1197, 1958

133. List four methods of possible treatment when there has been traumatic loss of a metacarpal head.
Ref. 30, pp. 287-289
Ref. 132, 4-2:349-372, 1973
Ref. 142, 48:1113, 1968
134. List four types of nerve endings occurring within the hand. Ref. 30, p. 19
135. List six solid benign soft tissue tumors that arise in the hand.
Ref. 30, p. 721
Ref. 41, p. 1740
Ref. 43, p. 375
136. List five abnormalities noted in the function of the hand with intrinsic muscle paralysis.
Ref. 127, 55-A:1667-1675, 1973
137. List four methods of treatment for degenerative arthritis of the carpo-metacarpal joint of the thumb.
Ref. 111, pp. 350-351, 1972
Ref. 113, 43:347-356, 1972
Ref. 137, 47:252-257, 1971
138. List six contributing factors toward the etiology of carpal tunnel syndrome.
Ref. 111, pp. 336-337, 1972
Ref. 111, pp. 337-338, 1974
Ref. 127, 55-A:78-82, 1973
139. List five types of regional anesthesia that, when selectively used, will allow for most upper extremity surgery.
Ref. 132, 1-2:205-212, 1970
140. A 19-year-old man, 1 year after head trauma, presents with spastic pronation flexion contracture of the right forearm, wrist, and fingers with the thumb in palm. His cognition is acceptable. He has sensation to sharp objects, heat, and cold. After median and ulnar nerve blocks he demonstrates active wrist extension to 10°, and fingers extend to neutral passively. Prolonged splinting helped, but not enough. List six procedures that should be considered in restoration of the extremity.
Ref. 113, 41:439-445, 1970
Ref. 127, 52-A:253-268, 901-920, 1970
Ref. 127, 55-A:580-585, 1973
Ref. 127, 56-A:466-472, 1974

Pathology

JAMES M. BULLOCK, B.S., M.D.

MULTIPLE CHOICE, SINGLE ANSWER (answers on pp. 278-279)

Select the *one* answer that will best complete or answer each of the following statements or questions.

1. The most likely malignant tumor to arise from preexisting Paget's disease is:
   a. Chondrosarcoma   **Ref. 2, p. 92**
   b. Osteosarcoma   **Ref. 127, 48-A:9, 1966**
   c. Giant cell tumor   **Ref. 127, 49-A:102, 1967**
   d. Fibrosarcoma   **Ref. 127, 51-B:24, 1969**

2. The least likely malignant tumor to arise following irradiation of bone would be:
   a. Chondrosarcoma
   b. Fibrosarcoma   **Ref. 2, p. 96**
   c. Osteosarcoma   **Ref. 68, p. 492**
   d. Osteosarcoma and fibrosarcoma

3. Fibrous metaphyseal defects occur most frequently in the:
   a. Proximal femur
   b. Distal tibia   **Ref. 2, p. 273**
   c. Proximal humerus   **Ref. 43, p. 1359**
   d. Distal femur

4. The presence of glycogen granules within the cytoplasm of tumor cells may be an important adjunct in differentiating between:
   a. Reticulum cell sarcoma and neuroblastoma
   b. Chondroblastoma and chondrosarcoma   **Ref. 1, p. 1059**
   c. Ewing's sarcoma and reticulum cell   **Ref. 127, 41-A:349, 1959**
      sarcoma
   d. Liposarcoma and myxosarcoma

5. Reticulum cell sarcoma of bone occurs most frequently in the:
   a. Upper extremities
   b. Lower extremities   **Ref. 3, p. 230**

c. Flat bones

d. Vertebrae

6. Reticulum cell sarcoma occurs most frequently in the:
   a. Epiphyses of long bones
   b. Diaphyses of long bones   Ref. 3, p. 230
   c. Metaphyses of long bones
   d. Flat bones

7. Fibrous metaphyseal defect (nonosteogenic fibroma) occurs in approximately _____ of normal children.
   a. 5%
   b. 10%   Ref. 2, p. 273
   c. 33⅓%   Ref. 43, p. 1359
   d. 50%

8. In eosinophilic granuloma the peripheral blood eosinophilic count is:
   a. Elevated
   b. Decreased   Ref. 5, p. 197
   c. Normal
   d. Variable or normal and of no diagnostic value

9. Hand-Schüller-Christian disease is best treated with:
   a. Local resection of the lesions
   b. Antibiotics   Ref. 5, p. 194
   c. Radiation of involved areas
   d. Antileukemic drugs

10. The most common area of bony involvement of multiple myeloma is the:
    a. Pelvis
    b. Vertebral column   Ref. 5, p. 613
    c. Ribs   Ref. 127, 48-B:707, 709, 1966
    d. Skull

11. Following total nerve injury, a microscopic picture of increased fibrous tissue replacement of muscle would be expected after:
    a. 4 to 6 weeks
    b. 3 to 6 months   Ref. 4, pp. 127-130
    c. 6 to 12 months
    d. 18 months

12. The most common malignant tumor involving bone is:
    a. Osteosarcoma
    b. Metastatic carcinoma   Ref. 2, p. 263
    c. Multiple myeloma
    d. Ewing's sarcoma

13. Hand-Schüller-Christian disease, although highly variable in its form, shows an overall mortality close to:
    a. 10%
    b. 50%   Ref. 5, p. 194
    c. 90%
    d. 100%

14. Typical Letterer-Siwe disease occurs most frequently:
    a. At puberty
    b. Under 3 years of age   Ref. 5, p. 198
    c. Over 1 year of age   Ref. 22, p. 1162
    d. Over 5 years of age
15. The benign primary tumor (hamartoma) of bone occurring most frequently is:
    a. Chondroblastoma
    b. Osteoid osteoma   Ref. 43, pp. 1338, 1343
    c. Osteochondroma
    d. Enchondroma
16. Eosinophilic granuloma occurs most frequently in all but the:
    a. Skull
    b. Small bones of the hands and feet   Ref. 5, p. 195
    c. Vertebrae
    d. Long bones of the lower extremity
17. Periosteal new bone formation may be seen in all but one of the following lesions:
    a. Osteosarcoma
    b. Osteomyelitis   Ref. 49, p. 227
    c. Eosinophilic granuloma
    d. Scurvy
    e. Melorheostosis
18. Reticulum cell sarcoma of bone:
    a. Metastasizes early to the lung and other
       bones in contrast to Ewing's sarcoma
    b. Has a five-year survival rate of approxi-   Ref. 5, p. 647
       mately 50%   Ref. 43, pp. 1392-1393
    c. Should not be treated by irradiation only
    d. Is best treated with curettage and packing
       of the lesion with bone chips
19. A 32-year-old woman has a three-year history of a slowly enlarging, hard, multinodular painless lesion over the flexor surface of the thumb. The largest nodule measures 1.5 cm. There is x-ray evidence of marginal bone erosion. The most logical diagnosis would be:
    a. Glomus tumor
    b. Epidermal inclusion cyst of bone   Ref. 5, p. 683
    c. Enchondroma   Ref. 43, p. 375
    d. Giant cell tumor of the tendon sheath
20. Enchondromatosis is known as _____ disease.
    a. Albright's
    b. Ellis–van Creveld   Ref. 5, pp. 115, 142, 163
    c. Ollier's   Ref. 43, p. 1344
    d. Albers-Schönberg
21. A microscopic picture of Verocay bodies with an Antoni type A or type B pattern would be diagnostic of:
    a. Neurofibroma
    b. Neurilemmoma   Ref. 1, p. 1126-1127

c. Interdigital neuroma

d. Amputation neuroma

Ref. 43, p. 1443
Ref. 127, 49-A:1605, 1967

22. Pigmented villonodular synovitis:
    a. Develops from synovial tissue and may invade bone
    b. Results from repeated hemarthrosis causing permanent synovial changes
    c. Usually occurs in young adults with mild articular pain and swelling
    d. When treated with complete synovectomy, gives a reasonable chance of success

Ref. 43, pp. 1377-1378,
1441

23. Microscopically the rheumatoid nodule:
    a. Is easily distinguished from the nodules seen in rheumatic fever by the aggregation of histiocytes
    b. Is easily distinguished from tuberculoma because of the absence of giant cells
    c. Appears as a central area of collagen surrounded by a zone of histocytes intermixed with lymphocytes and occasional giant cells
    d. Is usually characterized by Antoni type A and B patterns of palisading

Ref. 5, p. 745

24. Which of the following is a generalized disease associated with a rheumatoid-like arthritis?
    a. Ulcerative colitis
    b. Reiter's syndrome
    c. Sarcoidosis
    d. Psoriasis
    e. All of the above

Ref. 106, 57:5-55, 1968

25. Which of the following is *not* true of the healing of cartilaginous defects?
    a. Hyaline cartilage does not heal with normal hyaline cartilage but mainly with fibrous tissue and fibrocartilage.
    b. In small, surgically produced injuries in experimental animals, superficial injuries sometimes heal with imperfect hyaline cartilage formation. In injuries extending through the subchondral plate, healing consists of the growth of granulation tissue into the defect with a greater or lesser transformation into fibrocartilage or abnormal hyaline cartilage.
    c. If a defect or a fracture through hyaline cartilage is held tightly together, it will heal by granulation tissue invasion.

Ref. 106, 64:56, 1969

26. Liposarcoma is *not* characterized by:
    a. A capsule that is easily dissected without additional invasion of surrounding tissue
    b. Amputation as the treatment of choice
    c. Rare lesions being in the thigh and buttocks
    d. Preexisting lipomas

    Ref. 5, p. 659
    Ref. 43, p. 1437
    Ref. 127, 48-A:229, 1966

27. The most lethal of all primary bone tumors is probably:
    a. Osteosarcoma
    b. Reticulum cell sarcoma of bone
    c. Ewing's sarcoma
    d. Chondrosarcoma

    Ref. 2, p. 159
    Ref. 43, p. 1409
    Ref. 68, p. 360

28. Chondrosarcoma arising in long bones occurs most frequently in the:
    a. Tibia
    b. Humerus
    c. Femur
    d. Radius and ulna

    Ref. 2, p. 25

29. Ewing's tumor occurs most frequently:
    a. Over 30 years of age
    b. Under 50 years of age
    c. Under 15 years of age
    d. Under 30 years of age

    Ref. 1, p. 1058
    Ref. 5, p. 628

30. Synovial chondromatosis occurs most frequently:
    a. In small joints
    b. In multiple joints
    c. Between 20 and 40 years of age
    d. As metaplasia

    Ref. 5, p. 767
    Ref. 43, p. 1441
    Ref. 127, 49-B:530, 1967

31. The most common finding among the multiple manifestations attributed to neurofibromatosis would be:
    a. Localized hypertrophy
    b. Scoliosis
    c. Café au lait spots
    d. Fibroma molluscum (verrucous type skin hypertrophy)

    Ref. 43, p. 1443
    Ref. 127, 32-A:601, 1950

32. Enchondromas occur most frequently in the:
    a. Epiphyses of long bones
    b. Metaphyses of long bones
    c. Diaphyses of long bones
    d. Flat bones

    Ref. 5, p. 527
    Ref. 43, p. 1344

33. Synovial sarcoma characteristically:
    a. Arises within a joint or tendon sheath
    b. Is most frequently seen in young adults
    c. Occurs with equal frequency in upper and lower extremities
    d. Has a cure rate of over 50%

    Ref. 5, p. 657
    Ref. 43, p. 1442

34. Chondroblastoma is known to metastasize:
    a. In over 50% of cases
    b. Rarely (no reported cases)   Ref. 3, p. 47
    c. Occasionally   Ref. 2, p. 17
    d. Never
35. Chondroblastoma is microscopically characterized by:
    a. A generous supply of giant cells
    b. Sheets of young chondroblasts, with areas   Ref. 43, p. 1344
       of calcification and paucity of adult hy-   Ref. 68, p. 48
       aline cartilage
    c. Abundant mitotic figures
    d. Pleomorphic multinucleated chondrocytes
       and chondroblasts within and about
       hyaline cartilage
36. Pigmented villonodular synovitis occurs most commonly in association
    with the _____ joint.
    a. Shoulder
    b. Hip   Ref. 43, p. 1377
    c. Knee   Ref. 127, 50-B:291, 1968
    d. Ankle
37. Enchondroma occurs most frequently in the:
    a. Cylindrical bones of the hands and feet
    b. Carpal and tarsal bones of the hands and   Ref. 5, p. 527
       feet   Ref. 43, p. 1343
    c. Proximal end of the humerus and femur
    d. Middiaphysis of long bones
38. Chondroblastoma is most frequently noted in the:
    a. Epiphyses of long bones
    b. Metaphyses of long bones   Ref. 5, p. 574
    c. Diaphyses of long bones   Ref. 68, p. 44
    d. Flat bones
39. Synovial osteochondromatosis:
    a. Occurs most frequently in the knee joint
    b. Is known to result from trauma   Ref. 5, p. 767
    c. Does not recur after total synovectomy   Ref. 43, p. 1441
    d. Occurs only within joints   Ref. 127, 49-B:532-533, 1967
40. Preservation of the integrity of a peripheral nerve by careful dissection
    would be most feasible in removal of:
    a. A neurilemmoma
    b. A plexiform neurofibroma   Ref. 1, p. 1126
    c. An interdigital neuroma   Ref. 43, p. 1443
    d. A malignant schwannoma   Ref. 127, 49-A:1609, 1967
41. Chondromyxoid fibroma occurs most frequently in the:
    a. Epiphyses of long bones
    b. Metaphyses of long bones   Ref. 5, p. 580
    c. Diaphyses of long bones   Ref. 68, p. 203
    d. Flat bones

42. Ganglions:
    a. Rarely reoccur because they are easily excised, being single lesions
    b. Routinely have a normal synovial membrane lining and no satellite cystic changes in the capsule
    c. Communicate with the joint space in less than 50% of cases
    d. Occur most frequently about the wrist, arising from the scaphoid lunate ligament

    Ref. 5, p. 767
    Ref. 30, pp. 721-722
    Ref. 32, p. 869

43. Chondrosarcoma most frequently occurs in:
    a. The pelvis, ribs, or proximal femur
    b. About the knee
    c. The diaphyses of long bones
    d. Small bones of the hands and feet

    Ref. 2, p. 23

44. The onion skin pattern of subperiosteal new bone formation, although not diagnostic, would be most likely in which of the following tumors involving long bones?
    a. Eosinophilic granuloma
    b. Reticulum cell sarcoma
    c. Ewing's sarcoma
    d. Osteosarcoma

    Ref. 2, p. 157
    Ref. 68, p. 354

45. Fibrosarcoma of bone occurs most frequently about the:
    a. Knee and elbow
    b. Periosteum
    c. Ankle
    d. Time of retirement

    Ref. 1, p. 1065
    Ref. 5, p. 602
    Ref. 43, p. 1435

46. Osteosarcoma is characterized by:
    a. The knee and the shoulder being the most common sites
    b. The lesion always arising de novo
    c. Histologic features showing no cartilage
    d. Early lymph node spread

    Ref. 2, p. 89
    Ref. 43, p. 1379
    Ref. 127, 48-A:7-9, 1966
    Ref. 127, 49-A:101, 1967

47. The diagnosis of fibrosarcoma of bone on x-ray examination may be strengthened by the presence of:
    a. Marginal sclerosis
    b. Nonerosion of the cortex
    c. Codman's triangle
    d. Evidence of preexisting bone infarct

    Ref. 1, p. 1065
    Ref. 127, 42-A:802, 1960

48. Which of the following tumors would be the *least* likely to metastasize?
    a. Osteosarcoma
    b. Fibrosarcoma of bone
    c. Ewing's sarcoma
    d. Fibrosarcoma of soft tissue

    Ref. 1, p. 1065
    Ref. 5, p. 668

49. Which of the following is *not* a characteristic of a discoid meniscus?
    a. Most cases occur unilaterally.
    b. It is usually seen in young people.   Ref. 106, 64:107-113, 1966
    c. It presents with classic clinical findings
       easily separated from other internal de-
       rangements.
    d. Microscopic examination reveals mucoid
       degeneration almost invaribly.
    e. An acquired lesion due to a lax meniscal
       femoral ligament is at the posterior at-
       tachment.

50. The most common intramedullary tumor of the spinal cord in adults is:
    a. Chordoma
    b. Ependymoma   Ref. 1, p. 1253
    c. Meningioma
    d. Glioblastoma

51. A 25-year-old white man has a history of dull aching pain in his right
    knee. X-ray examination reveals an expansive lesion of the entire distal
    shaft. There is a multilocular appearance, with a marked thinning of the
    intact cortex. Biopsy shows a microscopic picture of fiber bone spicules
    interspersed in a loose whirled field of spindle cells. There are occasional
    giant cells present. The most likely diagnosis would be:
    a. Metaphyseal fibrous defect
    b. Osteoblastoma   Ref. 5, p. 163
    c. Fibrous dysplasia   Ref. 43, p. 1357
    d. Osteosarcoma

52. The earliest microscopic evidence of skeletal involvement in rheumatoid
    arthritis usually is:
    a. Surface destruction of the articular
       cartilage by pannus formation
    b. Periosteal new bone formation along the   Ref. 5, p. 742
       shaft   Ref. 45, 36:14, 1964
    c. Fibrovascular granulation tissue formation
       beneath the subchondral plate causing de-
       struction of bone and the deep layers of
       articular cartilage
    d. Focal collections of chronic inflammatory
       cells deep within bone, with pseudocyst
       formation

53. The microscopic findings of all motor units to a muscle in the same stage
    of atrophy and the presence of empty Schwann tubes in the muscular
    nerves indicate:
    a. Anterior horn cell degeneration
    b. Progressive atrophic paralysis   Ref. 4, p. 704
    c. Amyotrophic lateral sclerosis
    d. Interruption of the motor nerve

54. A 54-year-old white woman gives a history of right chest pain for three months. During the past 2 weeks she has noted a mass that pulsates. X-ray examination reveals a destructive lesion of the sixth rib underlying the soft tissue mass. The likely diagnosis is:
    a. Osteoid osteoma
    b. Metastatic carcinoma of the thyroid   Ref. 1, p. 1069
    c. Metastatic carcinoma of the uterus   Ref. 2, p. 263
    d. Aneurysmal bone cyst
55. A tuberculous process of bone most frequently involves the:
    a. Hip joint
    b. Long bones   Ref. 5, p. 257
    c. Spine
    d. Flat bones
56. "Adamantinomas" occur most frequently in the:
    a. Tibia
    b. Femur   Ref. 2, p. 252
    c. Pelvis
    d. Humerus
57. Chondrosarcoma of the pelvis would be most likely to metastasize to the:
    a. Lung via ingrowth of the tumor into
       venous channels
    b. Regional lymph nodes   Ref. 5, p. 589
    c. Retroperitoneal space by dissection along   Ref. 127, 48-B:742, 1966
       tissue planes
    d. Other bones by arterial or venous channels
58. Enlargement of scattered muscle fibers with long chains of centrally placed muscle nuclei is microscopically characteristic of:
    a. Facioscapulohumeral Landouzy-Déjerine
       muscular dystrophy
    b. Myotonic dystrophy   Ref. 4, pp. 281-282
    c. Pseudohypertrophic muscular dystrophy
       of Duchenne
    d. Progressive dystrophic ophthalmoplegia
59. Which of the following is classified as a lipid storage disease?
    a. Gaucher's disease
    b. Hand-Schüller-Christian disease   Ref. 43, pp. 369-371
    c. Eosinophilic granuloma
    d. Letterer-Siwe disease
60. Presence of the zone phenomenon may be helpful in diagnosing:
    a. Juxtacortical osteosarcoma
    b. Chondroblastoma   Ref. 2, p. 279
    c. Myositis ossificans
    d. Multiple myeloma
61. The most common tumor to metastasize to bone in middle-aged women is that of the:
    a. Thyroid
    b. Cervix   Ref. 45, 11:202, 1958

c. Ovary

d. Breast

62. The most common primary malignant bone tumor is:
    a. Multiple myeloma   Ref. 2, p. 152
    b. Osteogenic sarcoma   Ref. 5, p. 612
    c. Chondrosarcoma   Ref. 127,48-B:703, 1966
    d. Ewing's sarcoma   Ref. 127, 49-A:101, 1967

63. A 60-year-old man has a lytic lesion of the eighth thoracic vertebral body that is proved to be metastatic squamous cell carcinoma. The most likely site of origin would be the:
    a. Oral pharynx
    b. Prostate   Ref. 1, p. 1070
    c. Eight-year draining sinus of chronic
       osteomyelitis of the tibia
    d. Lung

64. Frozen section, in the hands of an experienced pathologist, would be most reliable for diagnosing:
    a. Reticulum cell sarcoma
    b. Fibrosarcoma   Ref. 43, p. 1335
    c. Chondrosarcoma   Ref. 127, 39-A:74, 1957
    d. Chondroblastoma

65. Myositis ossificans is most likely to occur in the _____ muscles.
    a. Brachialis anticus and quadriceps femoris
    b. Brachialis anticus and deltoid   Ref. 2, p. 279
    c. Gluteal
    d. Semimembranosus and biceps femoris

66. The patient with solitary myeloma of bone would be expected to:
    a. Have a complete spontaneous regression
       of the disease
    b. Have an altered electrophoretic serum   Ref. 22, p. 1327
       protein pattern   Ref. 43, pp. 1397-1398
    c. Have an elevated serum calcium level   Ref. 127, 48-B:704, 705, 1966
    d. Eventually develop widespread involve-
       ment

67. To make the diagnosis of myositis ossificans microscopically:
    a. Inflammation of muscle must be present
    b. Skeletal muscle must be involved   Ref. 2, p. 280
    c. Periosteum must be involved
    d. A clean-cut zonal phenomenon of matura-
       tion is most helpful

68. The criteria for diagnosis of radiation-induced osteogenic sarcoma would include which of the following?
    a. It must be confirmed by microscopic ex-
       amination.
    b. It must arise from bone and have received   Ref. 127, 48-A:5, 1966
       at least 3,000 rads, five or more years
       prior to development of sarcoma.

c. The patient must have had an asymptomatic
latent period following irradiation therapy.
d. The bone must have been radiologically
normal prior to irradiation.
e. All of the above.

69. Giant cell tumor of bone is believed to originate in the:
   a. Diaphysis and secondarily involve the
      metaphysis
   b. Metaphysis and secondarily involve the   Ref. 2, p. 201
      epiphysis
   c. Metaphysis and secondarily involve the
      diaphysis
   d. Epiphysis and secondarily involve the
      metaphysis

70. Disappearing bone disease is most closely associated with:
   a. Hyperparathyroidism
   b. Aneurysmal bone cysts   Ref. 2, p. 234
   c. Hemangioma of bone   Ref. 127, 37-A:985, 1956
   d. Sickle cell anemia

71. Which of the following characteristics of chondroblastoma is *not* true?
   a. It commonly occurs in the second decade
      of life.
   b. It originates in the epiphysis.   Ref. 3, p. 33
   c. It is more common in females.
   d. The lesion is usually small.
   e. Pathologic fractures are uncommon.

72. Concerning osteoid osteoma, which of the following is *not* true?
   a. Pain is more severe at night.
   b. Tiny nerve fibers have been demonstrated   Ref. 3, p. 120
      microscopically in this tumor.
   c. The metaphysis is the most common site
      in long bones.
   d. The nidus is formed by a maze of closely
      situated osteoid trabeculae.
   e. The best treatment is block excision.

73. In an x-ray film of a vertebral body showing diminished bone density
   with either parallel vertical streaks or a honeycomb appearance, you
   would most likely suspect:
   a. Giant cell tumor
   b. Multiple myeloma   Ref. 3, p. 325
   c. Hemangiomas
   d. Osteoblastoma
   e. Fungal infection

74. Hemangiopericytomas are microscopically diagnosed by:
   a. Endothelial cells inside the reticulum sheath
   b. Silver stains that show the pericytes out-   Ref. 101, p. 72
      side the reticulum sheath but surrounded
      by reticulum fibers

c. The presence of mitotic figures

d. Proliferative pericytes

75. In adult rhabdomyosarcoma the primary location is usually in the deep tissues of the extremities, whereas in the juvenile form the location is in the musculature of the:

a. Pelvis

b. Head and neck   Ref. 101, p. 134

c. Flank

d. Hands and feet

76. The underlying pathologic defect in osteopetrosis is:

a. Defective resorption of bone

b. Exuberant bone formation   Ref. 69, p. 190

c. In the precartilage bone model

d. The inability to balance calcium and phosphorus metabolism

77. Diaphyseal sclerosis (Englemann's disease) is characterized by all but which of the following?

a. It starts in the femur and tibia.

b. There is subperiosteal thickening of bone.   Ref. 5, p. 175

c. Failure of resorption of the inner border of the cortex occurs.

d. The metaphysis and epiphysis become involved.

e. Decreased hematopoiesis may result in anemia.

78. Pulmonary hypertrophic osteoarthropathy is characterized by all of the following except:

a. Clubbing

b. Osteophytosis   Ref. 5, p. 340

c. Synovitis

d. Endosteal bone proliferation

e. Increased arteriovenous shunts and poorly oxygenated blood stimulating connective tissue proliferation

79. In pseudohypertrophic muscular dystrophy (Duchenne's) all of the following are true except:

a. Males affected at a rate approximately five times greater than are females

b. Muscle weakness usually beginning centrally and spreading to the extremities   Ref. 5, p. 807

c. SGOT and SGPT seldom elevated in the early stages of the disease

d. CPK enzymes helpful in following the progression of the disease

e. Decreased urine creatinine found in the symptomatic stages

80. In arthrogryphosis all but which of the following are true?
    a. It is characterized by multiple symmetric
       contractures developing in utero.
    b. Contractures in most cases are due to the   **Ref. 5, p. 827**
       shortening of extensor muscles.
    c. Muscles are hypotonic.
    d. Deep tendon reflexes are often absent.
    e. Electrical reactions are weak.

MULTIPLE CHOICE, MULTIPLE ANSWERS (answers on pp. 279-280)

Select one or more answers that will best complete or answer each of the following statements or questions.

81. Chondrosarcoma is more frequently _____; it occurs infrequently

    _____ the age of 30 years.
    a. De novo
    b. Secondary   **Ref. 5, p. 587**
    c. Before   **Ref. 127, 48-B:729, 1966**
    d. After

82. Desmoid tumors are characterized by:
    a. Occurring more commonly in males
    b. Often involving abdominal musculature   **Ref. 101, p. 19**
    c. Insidious infiltration
    d. Usually easy excision with a low rate of
       recurrence
    e. Tissue of true differentiated fibroblasts

83. In osteosarcoma, when a surgical specimen reveals lymph node metastasis, which is not common, the outcome is:
    a. Always fatal
    b. Guarded   **Ref. 127, 48-A:10, 1966**
    c. Improved with further radical measures
    d. Not helped by further radical surgery

84. Pseudogout or chondrocalcinosis is characterized by which of the following?
    a. Calcification of the menisci in the knee
    b. Calcification of triangular fibrocartilage   **Ref. 127, 48-B:56-58, 1966**
       in the radiocarpal joint
    c. Calcification of the symphysis pubis
    d. Recorded involvement of the acromio-
       clavicular joint
    e. False positive test for urate crystals intra-
       cellularly in the joint fluid

85. Juxtacortical chondroma is seen most frequently in _____ and _____
    carry a known malignant potential.
    a. Children
    b. Adults   **Ref. 68, p. 196**
    c. Does
    d. Does not

86. Enchondromatosis:
    a. Is usually considered to be hereditary
    b. Is usually considered to be a develop-
       mental type of chondrodysplasia
    c. May cause severe deformities, necessi-
       tating amputation
    d. May develop in flat as well as cylindrical bones

Ref. 5, p. 657
Ref. 43, p. 1344

87. Chondromyxoid fibroma occurs _____, and it is seen _____.
    a. More frequently in males than in females
    b. With approximately equal sex distribution
    c. Most frequently between the ages of 10 to
       30 years
    d. Nearly evenly distributed throughout all
       age groups

Ref. 1, p. 1047
Ref. 68, p. 203

88. In childhood leukemia, x-ray film changes often include:
    a. Osteolytic lesions
    b. Generalized rarefaction
    c. Growth arrest lines
    d. Premature epiphyseal closure
    e. Periosteal reaction

Ref. 3, p. 381

89. Giant cell tumor of the tendon sheath:
    a. Occurs most frequently in the hand
    b. Is the same as a true synovioma
    c. Usually dictates amputation as the
       treatment of choice, once the diag-
       nosis is established
    d. Routinely contains hemosiderin gran-
       ules and xanthoid cells

Ref. 2, p. 283
Ref. 5, pp. 683, 684
Ref. 43, p. 1375
Ref. 127, 51-A:78, 80, 1969

90. Liposarcoma:
    a. Is a well-encapsulated tumor that is
       amenable to local excision, usually with-
       out recurrence
    b. Is known to be adequately treated by
       radiotherapy only
    c. May be of variable cell type
    d. Should be treated by radical local ex-
       cision or amputation

Ref. 1, p. 1135
Ref. 43, p. 1437
Ref. 127, 48-A:229, 1966

91. Metaphyseal fibrous defects usually occur _____ the age of 15
    years and _____ have a known malignant potential.
    a. Over
    b. Under
    c. Do
    d. Do not

Ref. 2, p. 274
Ref. 43, p. 1359

92. Physaliphorous cells would be expected in a:
    a. Chordoma
    b. Osteogenic sarcoma
    c. Nucleus pulposus in an infant
    d. Chondroblastoma

Ref. 43, p. 1393

93. Juxtacortical chondroma is best controlled by _____ and is known to recur _____.
   a. Local excision
   b. Radical excision or amputation   Ref. 68, p. 196
   c. Infrequently
   d. Frequently

94. Parosteal sarcoma (juxtacortical osteosarcoma), when compared with osteosarcoma:
   a. Has a lower mortality rate when acceptably treated
   b. Has a higher mortality rate even when   Ref. 2, p. 891
      acceptably treated   Ref. 5, p. 562
   c. Shows no significant difference in its be-   Ref. 127, 48-A:24, 1966
      havior pattern   Ref. 127, 49-A:415, 1967
   d. Has a behavior pattern quite different, and exact diagnosis may alter treatment recommendations

95. Central fibrosarcoma of bone, when acceptably treated, carries a prognosis of survival:
   a. Greater than that of a fibrosarcoma arising in soft tissue
   b. Less than that of a fibrosarcoma arising   Ref. 2, p. 198
      in soft tissue   Ref. 43, p. 1387
   c. The same as a fibrosarcoma arising in soft tissue
   d. Greater than that of osteosarcoma

96. Osteosarcoma is most likely to occur in which two age groups?
   a. 1 to 10 years
   b. 10 to 20 years   Ref. 2, p. 92
   c. 30 to 40 years   Ref. 127, 48-A:6, 1966
   d. Over 50 years   Ref. 127, 49-A:102, 1967

97. Eosinophilic granuloma is more frequent in _____ and occurs most frequently _____ the age of 25 years.
   a. Males
   b. Females   Ref. 5, p. 195
   c. Over
   d. Under

98. Lesions of eosinophilic granuloma _____ usually characterized by periosteal new bone formation and cortical expansion. When occurring in long bones, there _____ a definite predilection for the epiphyseal and metaphyseal areas.
   a. Are
   b. Are not   Ref. 5, p. 195
   c. Is
   d. Is not

99. Osteochondroma may take on the neoplastic character of:
    a. Chondrosarcoma
    b. Fibrosarcoma   Ref. 5, p. 527
    c. Osteosarcoma
    d. Chondroblastoma
100. Accepted treatment of eosinophilic granuloma would usually include:
    a. Curettage
    b. Radiation therapy   Ref. 5, p. 198
    c. Total en bloc local resection
    d. Amputation
101. Solitary enchondroma is found most frequently _____ the age of
    25 years and _____ known as Codman's tumor.
    a. Over
    b. Under   Ref. 5, p. 527
    c. Is   Ref. 43, p. 1343
    d. Is not
102. Kaposi's sarcoma:
    a. Is a malignant lesion
    b. Usually arises on extremities   Ref. 1, p. 114
    c. Begins as a bluish macule or nodule   Ref. 43, p. 1439
    d. Is seen infrequently in the United States
    e. Microscopically has both vascular and
       fibrovascular elements
103. Which of the following stains would probably be of most help in differ-
    entiating between reticulum cell sarcoma and Ewing's sarcoma?
    a. Periodic acid–Schiff
    b. Hortega's silver stain   Ref. 5, p. 646
    c. Sudan III   Ref. 127, 41-A:349, 1959
    d. Basic fuchsin
104. The tumors most likely to be confused microscopically with Ewing's sar-
    coma would be:
    a. Osteosarcoma
    b. Reticulum cell sarcoma   Ref. 1, p. 1059
    c. Neuroblastoma   Ref. 68, p. 363
    d. Liposarcoma
105. Reticulum cell sarcoma of the bone is more frequent in _____.
    The tumor has an age preponderance in _____.
    a. Females
    b. Males   Ref. 4, p. 640
    c. Those over 30 years of age
    d. Relatively even distribution
106. Desmoid tumors are:
    a. More common in women
    b. Persistent, locally invasive, and may de-   Ref. 5, p. 688
       stroy an entire muscle group if not ade-   Ref. 43, p. 1443
       quately excised
    c. Usually treated successfully with wide
       adequate local excision

129

d. Known to metastasize occasionally

e. Microscopically anaplastic and easily mistaken for fibrosarcoma

107. Multiple endochondromas are most frequently seen _____ the age of 25 years and _____ believed to carry a known malignant potential after years of existence.

a. Over

b. Under   Ref. 5, p. 527

c. Are   Ref. 43, p. 1340

d. Are not

108. Synovial sarcoma:

a. Seldom recurs locally

b. Seldom metastasizes   Ref. 5, p. 657

c. Is best treated with radical local excision   Ref. 43, pp. 1441-1442 or amputation

d. Should include resection of local lymph nodes

109. According to Enzinger and Winslow, the types of liposarcoma that tend to recur locally and metastasize late are:

a. Round cell

b. Well differentiated   Ref. 1, p. 1136

c. Pleomorphic

d. Myxoid

110. Metaphyseal fibrous defects are usually located _____ in the _____ of long bones.

a. Eccentrically

b. Centrally   Ref. 2, p. 273

c. Diaphyses   Ref. 43, p. 1359

d. Metaphyses

111. Which of the following statements about aneurysmal bone cysts are true?

a. They usually occur in the diaphysis of long bone.

b. Radiologically they are expansile lesions.   Ref. 3, p. 357

c. Microscopically giant cells are rarely seen.

d. The recurrence rate following either excision or curettage with grafting is approximately 20% to 25%.

e. Radiation therapy may be very acceptable treatment for those surgically inaccessible lesions.

112. A diagnosis of internal derangement of the knee demands consideration of the following benign synovial lesions:

a. Osteochondromatosis

b. Pigmented villonodular synovitis   Ref. 127, 48-A:1350, 1351, 1966

c. Localized nodular synovitis

d. Hemangioma

e. Localized nodule fasciitis

113. Which of the following is (are) true of Volkmann's ischemia?
    a. It is more common in adults than in children.
    b. The first, most essential step is to recog- **Ref. 127, 48-B:635, 636, 1966** nize the early signs of ischemic damage.
    c. Early incision of the deep fascia and decompression of hematoma may prevent further tissue death.
    d. Treatment of ischemic contractures, by whatever means, are necessary, including lengthening of tendons and excision of fibrotic and all the totally destroyed muscle.
    e. Amputations rarely are necessary.
114. Nodular fasciitis is characterized by:
    a. A rapidly growing mass in the subcutaneous tissue of the upper extremity or trunk
    b. A histologic picture with plentiful **Ref. 127, 50-A:1204-1212, 1968** mitoses, bizarre spindle cells, and an invasive growth pattern frequently mistaken for malignancy, prompting unnecessary radical treatment
    c. Documented recurrences presumably related to incomplete excision
    d. Distinct histologic pattern resembling a reactive process
115. Achondroplasia is hereditary and transmitted as a mendelian dominant. Which of the following are characteristics of this disease entity?
    a. There is symmetrical shortening of all long bones at birth.
    b. The length of the vertebral column is **Ref. 49, p. 65** relatively normal so that dwarfism is due to short extremities.
    c. Fifty percent of the babies born with this defect die due to difficult delivery in a chondroplastic mother, a small contracted foramen magnum, or a diminutive thorax.
    d. Brachiocephaly is due to a nonprogressive hydrocephalus.
    e. There is marked atrophy of skeletal musculature.
116. Osteopetrosis is characterized by:
    a. Increased density of bone due to failure of resorptive mechanisms of calcified cartilage that interferes with a normal replacement of bone

b. Anemia due to osteoid encroachment on   **Ref. 49, p. 196**
    the marrow cavity and optic atrophy
c. A poor prognosis
d. Childhood death due to massive hemor-
    rhage and infection
e. A normal life span in most situations

117. Osteomalacia may be seen in which of the following?
    a. Calcium or vitamin D–deficient rickets
    b. Pregnancy   **Ref. 49, pp. 426-427**
    c. Fanconi syndrome
    d. Acidosis
    e. Steatorrhea or malabsorption syndrome

118. Pseudogout is characterized by which of the following?
    a. It simulates gouty arthritis by history.
    b. There is a highly associated incidence of   **Ref. 49, pp. 771-785**
    diabetes mellitus, hypertension, and ar-
    teriosclerosis.
    c. Uric acid levels are elevated.
    d. Serum levels of calcium phosphorous and
    alkaline phosphatase are normal unless
    there is concurrent disease such as hyper-
    parathyroidism.
    e. The synovial fluid in the acute attack
    has intracellular calcium pyrophosphate
    crystals that are best identified under
    polarized light.

119. Necrosis of the lunate was first observed in 1911 by Kienböck and has
    been associated with which of the following?
    a. Infection
    b. Appearance between 20 and 30 years of age   **Ref. 73, p. 104**
    c. A group of diseases known as aseptic
    necrosis
    d. Ulna abnormally shorter than the radius
    e. Repeated recurrent traumas that are more
    common in workers who utilize pneumatic
    tools

120. The increased size in the vertebral body, as seen on x-ray examination,
    may be seen in which of the following?
    a. Hemangioma
    b. Polyostotic fibrous dysplasia   **Ref. 73, pp. 271, 274**
    c. Metastatic hypernephroma
    d. Paget's disease
    e. Hodgkin's disease
    f. Morquio's disease

121. Spontaneous intervertebral fusion may occur as a result of which of the
    following?
    a. Scheuermann's disease
    b. Tuberculosis   **Ref. 73, pp. 280, 332, 333**

c. Fracture

d. Rheumatoid spondylitis

122. Pathologic abnormalities may be seen on x-ray examination of the pelvis in which of the following?

a. Iliac horn

b. Iliitis condensans   Ref. 73, p. 366

c. Hypoplasia of pubis

d. Craniocleidodysostosis

e. Regional ileitis

123. Which of the following are true about the pathologic changes seen in Dupuytren's contracture?

a. Most patients have one or more palmar nodules.

b. In a few patients there is a short inter-   Ref. 66, pp. 22, 23, 26
phalangeal band producing flexion de-
formity of the proximal phalangeal joint.

c. The palmar nodule lies in the subcutaneous fibrofascial layer and is attached
to the palmar aponeurosis; the interphalangeal band frequently bridges the
joint and intertwines itself among the
neurovascular bundle.

d. There is no connection between the interphalangeal band and the palmar nodules
in most situations; the palmar nodule,
once it occurs, results in rapid progression of the disease.

124. Which of the following are characteristics of the histopathology seen in Dupuytren's contractures?

a. Pacinian corpuscles are somwhat enlarged.

b. Small red cell extravasations and deposit   Ref. 66, p. 35
of iron pigments are commonly seen in the
hyperplastic foci.

c. Polymorphonuclear giant cells and eosin-
ophils demonstrate inflammatory nature.

d. Histologically similar hyperplastic tissue
is found to comprise knuckle pads and
plantar nodules of patients with strong
Dupuytren's diaphysis.

e. Progression of a Dupuytren's contracture
is from increased vascularity of the fibrofatty tissue to paravascular cellular proliferation, replacing fat into a hyperplastic
fibrous tissue and finely mature collagen
bands.

125. Which of the following are true about the pathogenesis of fat embolism?
    a. The source of embolic fat remains contested and could be from the marrow or from the lymphatics.
    b. Fat embolism may be a syndrome of intravascular coagulation defects. **Ref. 106, 65:221, 1969**
    c. Peltier believes that the emboli in the lungs produce a mechanical obstruction, the fat droplets are acted upon by lipase releasing fatty acids, and the delayed fatty acid release is responsible for the clinical and pathologic picture.
    d. Everyone agrees that pulmonary fat embolism per se is an important clinical entity in every case.
    e. It is possible to biopsy a petechia from the lateral chest or from other organs and demonstrate fat droplets in the petechiae.

126. Chondromyxoid fibroma is characterized by which of the following?
    a. It occurs predominantly between the ages of 10 and 30 years.
    b. This tumor is definitely capable of transforming to a chondrosarcoma. **Ref. 3, p. 50**
    c. It is usually associated with pain but not swelling.
    d. It is known as Codman's tumor.
    e. Myxomatous zones usually predominate in the microscopic field.

127. Which of the following are true of osteochondromas?
    a. They can involve any bone that develops from cartilage.
    b. They are the second most common benign neoplasms of bone. **Ref. 3, p. 59**
    c. Somewhere between 5% and 10% undergo malignant change.
    d. Chondrosarcoma would likely be the result of malignant change.
    e. They are usually not removed unless symptomatic.

128. Enchondromas are characterized by which of the following?
    a. They comprise roughly 10% of benign bone tumors.
    b. They are generally considered to arise from heterotopic cartilaginous cell nests in the metaphysis. **Ref. 3, p. 73**

c. Radiation is usually considered the best
   form of treatment.
d. They are located most often in the phalanges and metacarpals.
e. Malignant transformation is generally rare.

129. Which of the following statements concerning Maffucci's syndrome are
     true?
   a. Characterized by dyschondroplasia
   b. Characterized by hemangiomas   **Ref. 3, p. 81**
   c. Congenital but not hereditary
   d. High risk of development of chondro-
      sarcoma a major complication

130. Which of the following statements about nonossifying fibromas are true?
   a. No evidence of malignant transformation
      has been noted.
   b. They migrate away from the epiphysis.   **Ref. 3, p. 254**
   c. Radiologic accuracy of diagnosis is ap-
      proximately 100%.
   d. The best information seems to indicate
      the lesion arises as a developmental aber-
      ration at the epiphyseal plate.
   e. Periosteal reaction is often a gross feature.

SITUATION AND PROGRESSIVE THOUGHT (answers on p. 280)

Select the answer or answers that best apply in accordance with the information given in each of the following statements.

131. A 52-year-old white man, in otherwise good general health, has a history
     of recent right hip pain. X-ray examination reveals a mottled 8 cm cauli-
     flower-shaped tumor attached to the midportion of the right superior
     pubic ramus. The most likely diagnosis would be:
   a. Giant cell osteochon-
      droma   **Ref. 1, p. 1051**
   b. Chondroblastoma   **Ref. 2, pp. 22, 60, 66**
   c. Osteosarcoma   **Ref. 127, 45-A:1450, 1963**
   d. Chondrosarcoma   **Ref. 127, 48-B:729, 1966**

132. The chest x-ray film, intravenous pyelogram, cystogram, and blood
     chemistries were normal. You should advise:
   a. Watching the lesion for two months and
      then doing a repeat x-ray examination
   b. Incisional biopsy   **Ref. 1, pp. 1054**
   c. Needle biopsy   **Ref. 127, 48-A:1001, 1966**
   d. Wide en bloc excision of hemipelvec-   **Ref. 127, 48-B:753, 1966**
      tomy if necessary to give an adequate
      margin to the tumor

133. Prior to your consultation on the case, a needle biopsy had been performed. A reliable pathologist's report was cartilage tissue. You would advise:
   a. Reexamination of the patient at yearly intervals
   b. Open biopsy in another area to obtain additional tissue   Ref. 1, p. 1054
   c. Radiation therapy
   d. Wide en bloc excision or hemipelvectomy if necessary to give an adequate margin to the tumor and the biopsy site

   Ref. 1, p. 1054
   Ref. 127, 48-A:998, 1966
   Ref. 127, 48-B:753, 1966

134. The same patient comes to you four years after having received the recommended treatment of choice. A routine chest x-ray examination now reveals a right upper lobe density of 3 cm. The patient's other physical, laboratory, and x-ray findings are not remarkable. You should advise:
   a. Hemipelvectomy and referral to a thoracic surgeon, recommending right upper lobectomy
   b. Repeat biopsy of the site of the initial lesion
   c. Referral to a thoracic surgeon for investigation and consideration of right upper lobectomy
   d. Studies to prove the diagnosis of bronchiogenic carcinoma

   Ref. 4, p. 597
   Ref. 127, 45-A:1030, 1456, 1963
   Ref. 127, 49-B:74, 1967

135. A 65-year-old black man complains of low back pain. X-ray examination reveals a pronounced sclerosis of the L-2 vertebral body. No other abnormalities are noted. Which of the following would be *least* likely to produce this picture?
   a. Metastatic carcinoma of the lung
   b. Paget's disease
   c. Metastatic carcinoma of the prostate
   d. Hodgkin's disease

   Ref. 68, pp. 604-609
   Ref. 95, p. 58

136. The physical examination, chest x-ray film, and cystoscopy were unremarkable. The serum electrolytes and alkaline phosphates were normal. The acid phosphatase was within the upper limits of normal. You should advise:
   a. Radiation therapy
   b. Open biopsy
   c. Symptomatic care, with a back brace and repeat x-ray examination in one month
   d. Needle biopsy

   Ref. 43, pp. 1336, 1409
   Ref. 68, p. 15

137. On x-ray examination the involved vertebral body uniformly measured 2 mm greater in vertical and horizontal dimensions than the one above or below. The most likely diagnosis would be:
   a. Metastatic carcinoma of the bladder
   b. Paget's disease

   Ref. 5, p. 430

c. Metastatic carcinoma of the prostate

d. Hodgkin's disease

138. The patient was referred to you after a biopsy had been carried out. On reviewing the slides stained with hematoxylin and eosin, a mosaic pattern of the bone with irregular blue cement lines is noted. Which of the following could give this microscopic picture?

a. Irradiated bone

b. Chronic osteomyelitis   Ref. 1, p. 1029

c. Fibrous dysplasia   Ref. 68, p. 128

d. Reactive bone around metastatic cancer

139. A 23-year-old white woman in otherwise good health gives a four-year history of a slowly enlarging mass medial to the superior pole of the right patella. She denies having pain until the past few weeks. Physical examination reveals a 4 cm deep, mobile soft tissue mass. There is pain with full flexion of the knee but no apparent effusion. X-ray findings reveal the mass to be of water density, with clustered radiopacities. The *least* likely diagnosis would be:

a. Soft tissue chondrosarcoma

b. Synovial sarcoma   Ref. 5, pp. 657, 672, 687

c. Desmoid tumor   Ref. 68, pp. 564, 580, 582

d. Hemangioma   Ref. 95, p. 186

140. An open biopsy under tourniquet was performed. Frozen section showed irregular clefts and glandlike spaces lined with cuboid and columnar pseudoepithelial cells contained within a fibrosarcomatous stroma. There were small areas of calcification. This would be most characteristic of:

a. Myxosarcoma

b. Metastatic adenocarcinoma of the breast   Ref. 5, pp. 657, 658

c. Synovial sarcoma   Ref. 68, pp. 584-586

d. Rhabdomyosarcoma

141. The tumor would be best treated by:

a. Shelling it out with local excision

b. Radiation   Ref. 5, p. 657

c. Chemotherapy   Ref. 68, pp. 586, 587

d. En bloc radical excision or amputation,
with regional lymph node dissection

142. When the treatment of choice is carried out, a mortality rate of _____ would be expected.

a. 0%

b. Less than 20%   Ref. 1, p. 1150

c. Less than 50%   Ref. 5, p. 657

d. Over 70%   Ref. 68, p. 587

143. A 34-year-old man has a four-year history of progressive curvature of the back, with pain in his back and knees. Physical examination reveals a dorsal lumbar kyphosis, with marked limitation of motion. On x-ray examination there is noted to be narrowing of the disc spaces throughout the spine, with evidence of ankylosis. A likely diagnosis would be:

a. Paget's disease

b. Rheumatoid spondylitis   Ref. 5, p. 747

c. Degenerative disc disease, with secondary   Ref. 22, pp. 1899-1901
   spurring
d. Scheuermann's disease

144. The x-ray films also showed dense opacification of the discs. There were multiple periarticular opacities about the knees. A biopsy from the knee area showed dark pigmented articular cartilage, with dark cartilaginous nodules in the surrounding tissue. The pathologist reviewed the case and made the diagnosis of:
a. Hemochromatosis
b. Ochronosis   Ref. 5, p. 712
c. Porphyria   Ref. 95, pp. 173-174
d. Anthrocosis

145. The patient reported that his urine turned gray-black when standing for prolonged periods and that there was darkening of the sclera. This was due to:
a. Iron pigments
b. Coproporphyrin   Ref. 5, p. 712
c. Carbon-12   Ref. 22, pp. 1673-1674
d. Homogentisic pigments

146. The disease entity results from an inborn error in metabolism of:
a. Phenylalanine
b. Iron   Ref. 5, p. 712
c. Tyrosine and phenylalanine   Ref. 22 pp. 1673-1674
d. Porphyrin

147. A 20-year-old white woman has a mass over the posterior aspect of her right shoulder. She reports it is nonpainful but has progressed slowly in size over the past three to four years. Physical examination reveals a firm 3 × 5 cm mobile mass within the soft tissues. The *least* likely diagnosis would be:
a. Osteosarcoma
b. Synovial sarcoma   Ref. 5, pp. 691-694
c. Liposarcoma   Ref. 114, 86:351, 1961
d. Fibrosarcoma

148. Further examination reveals an additional mass previously unnoticed in the soft tissues of the buttocks. X-ray films reveal tumor masses of dense granular confluent nodular opacities. The most likely diagnosis would be:
a. Tumoral calcinosis
b. Osteosarcoma   Ref. 5, pp. 691-694
c. Chondrosarcoma   Ref. 127, 49-A:727, 1967
d. Myositis ossificans

149. Microscopically the pathologist would expect to see:
a. Progressively maturing bone from the outside toward the inside (zonal phenomenon) of the lesion
b. Dark-staining amorphous calcium salts   Ref. 5, pp. 691-694
   surrounded by foreign body giant cell   Ref. 127, 49-A:726, 1967
   reaction

c. Fiber bone and osteoid forming in a sarcomatous stroma

d. Sodium urate crystals, with foreign body giant cell reaction

150. The treatment of choice would be:

a. Radiation to both lesions

b. Local radical excision, with regional lymph node dissection

c. Excision of the mass for symptomatic and cosmetic reasons, warning the patient that similar lesions tend to occur locally and elsewhere

Ref. 5, pp. 691-694
Ref. 127, 49-A:729, 1967

d. Repeat x-ray films at monthly intervals to follow progression of size

TRUE OR FALSE (answers on pp. 280-281)

151. The prognosis of osteogenic sarcoma is correlated with histologic type and the size of the tumor as well as the mode of therapy.
(T) (F)   **Ref. 127, 48-A:20, 24, 1966**

152. Volkmann's ischemia of the lower limb most frequently involves the flexor hallucis longus muscle and then the muscles of the anterior compartment that are superficial, but the soleus and gastrocnemius are less frequently affected.   **Ref. 127, 48-B:629, 1966**
(T) (F)

153. It has been established that nerve involvement in Volkmann's contracture is due to ischemia itself and not due to fibrotic muscle compressing the nerves.   **Ref. 127, 48-B:631, 1966**
(T) (F)

154. Codman's triangle, periosteal new bone formation, is pathopneumonic of osteosarcoma and is never seen in osteomyelitis, hemorrhage, or metastatic cancer.   **Ref. 49, pp. 42, 49**
(T) (F)

155. Hurler's syndrome and Morquio's disease may be confused. The changes in the spine help to differentiate the two. Vertebral bodies are flattened in Morquio's disease, but are normal or heightened in Hurler's syndrome. In Hurler's syndrome the vertebral beak is inferior, whereas in Morquio's disease the beak is central.   **Ref. 49, p. 288**
(T) (F)

156. Radiographic signs of infantile scurvy are best seen at the end of rapidly growing bones and are characterized by the white line where the zone of temporary calcification widens and becomes densely calcified. Immediately proximal to this is a radiolucent zone that is the result of depressed cellular activity and the inability to form an organic matrix.
(T) (F)   **Ref. 49, p. 418**

157. A supracondylar process of the humerus is usually distal, anterior, and medial and can be confused with an osteochondroma but is not an exostosis, since the protuberance occurs regularly in various mammals and

may serve as the origin for supernumerary portion of the pronator teres muscle. **Ref. 73, p. 141**

(T) (F)

158. The appearance and behavior of recurrent Dupuytren's tissue is consistent with its origin from local fibrofatty tissue. **Ref. 66, p. 34**

(T) (F)

159. The first clinical evidence of joint involvement in rheumatoid arthritis is secondary to synovitis and pannus formation and there is no alteration of the articular cartilage matrix. **Ref. 106, 64:96, 1969**

(T) (F)

160. Reiter's syndrome is often confused with gonococcal arthritis and is best differentiated by mucocutaneous manifestations, e.g., eye inflammation.

(T) (F) **Ref. 106, 57:19, 1968**

161. The presence of multinucleated giant cells would rule out the diagnosis of metaphyseal fibrous defect. **Ref. 2, p. 274**

(T) (F) **Ref. 43, pp. 1359-1367**

162. Eosinophilic granuloma of the spine involves the disc space primarily and the vertebral body secondarily. **Ref. 5, p. 603**

(T) (F)

163. Gaucher's disease is characterized by an excessive production of histiocytes filled with a complex lipid—kerasin. **Ref. 5, p. 206**

(T) (F)

164. An elevated eosinophil count of the peripheral blood in the presence of a single lytic lesion in the metaphysis of a long bone is practically diagnostic of eosinophilic granuloma. **Ref. 5, p. 197**

(T) (F)

165. An abundance of multinucleated giant cells would rule out the diagnosis of unicameral bone cyst. **Ref. 2, p. 274**

(T) (F) **Ref. 43, p. 1333**

166. Pigmented villonodular synovitis, a histologically benign lesion, may invade soft tissue and erode bone. **Ref. 2, p. 276**

(T) (F) **Ref. 43, pp. 1378-1379**

Ref. 127, 50-B:306, 312, 1968

167. Even when x-ray evidence of chondrosarcoma is strong, a needle or small wedge biopsy should be carried out prior to en bloc excision.

(T) (F) **Ref. 2, p. 25**

168. Chondromyxoid fibroma is rarely diagnosed until over 5 cm in size.

(T) (F) **Ref. 5, p. 580**

169. Giant cell tumor of a tendon sheath (fibroxanthoma) is neoplastic and bears some relationship to degenerative joint disease. **Ref. 2, p. 282**

(T) (F) **Ref. 127, 51-A:85, 1969**

170. Pigmented villonodular synovitis is closely associated with, and in many cases is probably a precursor to, synovial sarcoma. **Ref. 2, p. 276**

(T) (F) **Ref. 43, p. 1441**

171. Although the histologic origin of chondromyxoid fibroma is believed to be similar to chondroblastoma, it more frequently involves joints.

(T) (F) **Ref. 5, p. 578**

Ref. 68, p. 203

172. Rickets is easily identified microscopically by the thickened zone of provisional calcification. Ref. 5, p. 652
   (T) (F) Ref. 55, pp. 101, 147

173. Absence of a history of trauma would practically rule out the diagnosis of myositis ossificans in a 16-year-old boy with a warm painful mass over the distal thigh. Ref. 2, p. 279
   (T) (F)

174. A microscopic differentiation between parosteal sarcoma and myositis ossificans rarely poses a problem to the pathologist. Ref. 2, pp. 91, 280
   (T) (F) Ref. 43, p. 1384

175. Giant cell tumor of bone is frequently treated by curettage and bone grafting; although it may recur locally, it does not metastasize.
   (T) (F) Ref. 2, p. 204

176. Anatomic studies carried out by Batson would seem to indicate that the high rate of metastasis to vertebral bodies was indeed due to a vast arterial anastomatic complex. Ref. 68, p. 592
   (T) (F) Ref. 117, 111:112, 138, 1940

177. Vertebra is the second most common bone involved as a primary site of origin of giant cell tumor bone. Ref. 2, p. 201
   (T) (F)

178. The microscopic picture of the periarticular structures in Felty's syndrome, Still's disease, rheumatoid arthritis, and rheumatoid spondylitis is frequently indistinguishable. Ref. 5, p. 747
   (T) (F)

179. Desmoplastic fibroma is a benign fibrous lesion that arises most frequently eccentrically in cortical bone about the knee. Ref. 68, p. 299
   (T) (F) Ref. 127, 50-A:491, 1968

180. To prevent excessive contracture muscle biopsy material should be allowed to dry slightly in a straightened position and then kept moist for a short period before placing in a fixative. Ref. 2, p. 710
   (T) (F)

181. Osteomas almost exclusively involve the skull and facial bones.
   (T) (F) Ref. 3, p. 117

182. Osteoblastomas are uncommon, solitary, benign, vascular osteoid-producing tumors that most often involve vertebrae and long bones.
   (T) (F) Ref. 3, p. 132

183. The lower posterior portion of the metaphysis of the femur is the single most common site of parosteal sarcoma. Ref. 3, p. 167
   (T) (F)

184. Most myeloma patients have abnormal proteins. The A-myeloma globulin is the fraction most commonly found elevated. Ref. 3, p. 203
   (T) (F)

185. The skull is the most common site of the first detectable bone metastases in Ewing's sarcoma. Ref. 3, p. 228
   (T) (F)

186. Albright's disease includes monostotic fibrous dysplasia, precocious puberty, and increased areas of skin pigmentation. Ref. 3, p. 270
   (T) (F)

187. Monostotic fibrous dysplasia is most commonly found in the ribs.
(T) (F)   Ref. 3, p. 270

188. Bone cysts have a higher incidence in males and a much higher pre-dilection for occurrence in the proximal rather than distal end of long bones.   Ref. 3, p. 346
(T) (F)

189. Squamous cell carcinoma is the most common malignancy to arise from chronic osteomyelitic sinuses.   Ref. 3, p. 387
(T) (F)

190. Chordoma arises from the primitive notochord and has a predilection for the distal and proximal extremes of the axial skeleton.   Ref. 3, p. 411
(T) (F)

191. Nodular fasciitis may easily be misdiagnosed as a sarcoma because of numerous mitoses related to rapid growth.   Ref. 101, p. 24
(T) (F)

192. Ganglions have synovial linings.   Ref. 101, p. 34
(T) (F)

193. Osteogenesis imperfecta is characterized by the inadequacy of collagen and osteoblasts.   Ref. 69, p. 167
(T) (F)

LIST (answers on p. 281)

194. List in order the organ or origin of the four malignant tumors that most frequently metastasize to bone.   Ref. 2, p. 262
Ref. 68, p. 593

195. List six fibrous lesions of bone occurring in children or young adults.
Ref. 43, pp. 1333-1334

196. List five pathologic entities that involve the reticuloendothelial system and are frequently classified as the "histiocytoses."   Ref. 22, p. 1569

197. List four tumors that have been reported to arise in preexisting Paget's disease.   Ref. 68, p. 469
Ref. 127, 49-A:102, 1967

198. List the five most common classified soft tissue sarcomas in order.
Ref. 43, p. 1432

199. List four benign lesions from which chondrosarcoma is reported to arise.   Ref. 2, p. 25
Ref. 5, p. 587
Ref. 68, p. 497

200. List five involvements that have been attributed to manifestations of neurofibromatosis.   Ref. 5, p. 175
Ref. 43, pp. 1444-1445
Ref. 127, 32-A:601, 1950

201. List three diseases of bone in which fiber bone makes up a major share of the pathologic underlying bony structure.   Ref. 55, p. 31

202. List seven lesions that contain giant cells and may be confused with giant cell tumor of bone microscopically.   Ref. 127, pp. 1333, 1352

203. List four tumors that may be osteoblastic when metastatic to bone.
Ref. 2, p. 261
Ref. 68, p. 604

Physical medicine and rehabilitation

WILLIAM H. ANDERSON, Jr., M.D.

MULTIPLE CHOICE, SINGLE ANSWER (answers on p. 281)

Select the *one* answer that will best complete or answer each of the following statements or questions.

1. The Hubbard tank, in which the entire body except the head and shoulders is immersed, should probably not exceed temperatures of:
   a. 98° F
   b. 104° F   **Ref. 91, p. 60**
   c. 110° F
   d. 115° F
2. The above-knee (AK) amputee should be instructed to ascend steps by:
   a. Using a reciprocal gait pattern
   b. Advancing the prosthetic limb first, bring-   **Ref. 15, p. 272**
   ing the sound limb up to it
   c. Advancing the sound limb first, bringing
   the prosthetic limb up to it
   d. Always carrying a cane to give additional
   support
3. When kneeling, the AK amputee should:
   a. Place the sound foot well behind the prosthetic foot and allow the sound knee to contact ground
   b. Place the sound foot well ahead of the   **Ref. 15, p. 269**
   prosthetic foot and allow the prosthetic knee to contact ground
   c. First crouch on all fours and then reposition on the prosthetic knee
   d. Never allow the knee mechanism of the prosthesis to contact ground

143

4. Persistent hip flexion deformity secondary to spasticity and interfering with function or hygiene is probably best treated by:
   a. Phenol injection of the femoral nerve
   b. Intrapelvic iliopsoas myotenotomy   **Ref. 106, 63:150-152, 1969**
   c. Release of the iliopsoas from its distal insertion
   d. Release of the origin of rectus femorus
5. The physiologic effect of local heat probably will not:
   a. Include elevation of superficial tissue temperatures
   b. Increase capillary pressure and vasodilatation   **Ref. 91, p. 58**
   c. Increase the rate of local metabolism and phagocytosis in areas of inflammation
   d. Vary greatly with the source, that is, infrared, paraffin baths, hot packs, or whirlpool baths
6. A patient with a painful knee and muscle weakness of the right lower extremity:
   a. Ascends and descends stairs progressing with the left leg first
   b. Ascends and descends stairs using a normal reciprocal pattern   **Réf. 64, p. 186**
   c. Ascends stairs progressing with the right leg first
   d. Descends stairs progressing with the right leg first
7. To ambulate most efficiently a right hemiplegic patient:
   a. Will walk using a reciprocal gait pattern
   b. Carries a cane in the left hand and progresses it with the left leg   **Ref. 64, pp. 188-189**
   c. Carries a cane in the left hand and progresses it with the right leg
   d. a and c
8. Concerning chest physical therapy for orthopaedic patients with concurrent chronic obstructive pulmonary disease:
   a. The positions used in postural drainage are based on the segmental anatomy of the lung
   b. Exercises should encourage a low tidal volume and a high frequency   **Ref. 74, pp. 677, 681-684**
   c. Exercises should encourage a slow maximal inspiration and rapid forced expiration
   d. Percussion and vibration are outmoded and should be replaced by IPPB

9. Studies concerning sexual function among spinal cord injury patients indicate:
   a. Total cord lesions preclude erection and coitus
   b. Lower motor neuron lesions preclude erection   **Ref. 67, p. 40**
   c. Eighty percent of patients may be able to perform coitus
   d. Patients with upper motor neuron lesions may be able to attain an erection but unable to ejaculate or sire children.

10. Autonomic cardiovascular changes associated with quadriplegia often include:
    a. Tachycardia at rest
    b. Bradycardia at rest   **Ref. 48, pp. 268-274**
    c. Decrease in pulse rate and increase in blood pressure with eating, drinking, defecation, or rectal stimulation
    d. Increase in pulse rate and decrease in blood pressure associated with bladder distention

11. In the normal infant the earliest age by which the tonic neck reflex can definitely be expected to have disappeared is:
    a. At birth (in a full-term infant)
    b. 8 weeks   **Ref. 58, p. 33**
    c. 6 months
    d. 1 year

12. A patient suffering a complete lesion of the spinal cord at the C-5 vertebral body level would be expected to have return of function after the healing and regenerative period to and including the _____ level only.
    a. C-4
    b. C-5   **Ref. 67, pp. 23, 30, 1969**
    c. C-6
    d. C-7

13. Use of a wheelchair on smooth, level ground requires an energy expenditure that is:
    a. Approximately half that of normal walking
    b. Comparable to that of normal walking   **Ref. 48, p. 197**
    c. Twice that of normal walking
    d. Four times that of normal walking

14. The energy cost of paraplegic ambulation using crutches is:
    a. Comparable to normal walking at the same speed
    b. Two to four times greater than normal walking at the same speed   **Ref. 48, pp. 196-197**
    c. Less with braces providing free ankle dorsiflexion than with braces with a rigid ankle
    d. Similar to the energy cost of using a wheelchair on smooth, level ground

15. Gait training of the newly fitted AK amputee should begin with:
    a. Standard properly fitted crutches
    b. Bilateral Canadian crutches   Ref. 15, p. 261
    c. No external assistance
    d. Parallel bars
16. In rising from a chair, the AK amputee should:
    a. Place the prosthetic foot behind the good
       foot, with the prosthetic knee bent 90°
    b. Place the good foot behind the prosthetic   Ref. 15, p. 259
       foot, with the good knee bent greater than
       90° and then bend the body forward
    c. Keep both feet even
    d. First kneel and then arise from the kneeling
       position
17. Concerning wheelchair transfers for the hemiplegic patient:
    a. Most transfers are made by moving toward
       the stronger or more normal side
    b. Perceptual defects will rarely prevent an   Ref. 74, pp. 430-431
       unassisted standing transfer if strength is
       adequate
    c. Voluntary hip extension or extensor spas-
       ticity on the involved side is usually re-
       quired for an unassisted standing transfer
    d. a and c are correct
18. Exercises utilizing submaximal effort against submaximal resistance, with
    repetition to fatigue, would best be prescribed to:
    a. Build muscle mass
    b. Increase range of motion   Ref. 91, p. 82
    c. Develop coordination
    d. Increase endurance
19. A slightly overweight 50-year-old woman has a one-year history of right
    knee pain. Initially she struck her knee on concrete. Examination at that
    time revealed no perceptible injury of bone, ligaments, or cartilage. Ef-
    fusion developed and pain persisted. Examination at this time revealed
    moderate effusion, patellar crepitus, laxity of the periarticular structures,
    and definite thigh atrophy. Aspirated fluid was not remarkable. X-ray
    examination showed early mild hypertrophic arthritis. The therapy pre-
    scription most likely to be of value would be:
    a. Whirlpool three times a day, with massage
       and elastic wrap
    b. Diathermy to the knee every day, with   Ref. 127, 31-A:396, 1949
       passive range of motion exercises   Ref. 136, 43:263, 1963
    c. Cylinder cast for 3 weeks, with straight-leg
       raising exercises
    d. Moist heat twice a day, followed by quadri-
       ceps resistive exercises to fatigue

20. The rehabilitation program for the geriatric amputee should be started:
    a. When the decision to amputate is made
    b. 2 to 3 days prior to amputation,   **Ref. 45, 37:63-64, 1964**
       depending on the condition of the patient
    c. 2 to 3 days after amputation, de-
       pending on the condition of the patient
    d. When the wound is healed
21. The ambulatory stroke patient exhibiting a strong flexion pattern with marked equinovarus deformity, would best profit from:
    a. Heel cord lengthening only
    b. Heel cord lengthening and transfer of the   **Ref. 106, 63:142-148, 1969**
       tibialis posterior tendon anteriorly
    c. Pantalar arthrodesis
    d. Heel cord lengthening and release of the
       long toe flexors and tibialis posterior, with
       a split anterior tibial tendon transfer
22. Patients with paraplegia and quadriplegia should be treated with a bowel program of:
    a. Digital elimination of fecal impaction every
       few days as needed
    b. Daily enemas in conjunction with laxatives   **Ref. 67, p. 67**
    c. Training with diet, stool softeners, and sup-   **Ref. 142, 48:754, 1968**
       positories until a regulated pattern has
       been established
    d. Self-regulation, since autonomic function is
       not usually affected; no unusual problems
       would be anticipated
23. The area of lower extremity deformity most likely to respond favorably to corrective surgery in the stroke patient would be:
    a. Hip
    b. Knee   **Ref. 106, 63:143, 1969**
    c. Hip and knee
    d. Foot and ankle
24. In regard to spasticity:
    a. The primary pathology is at the motor
       end plate
    b. The stretch reflex is deprived of its normal   **Ref. 118, 55:332-337, 1974**
       supraspinal modulation
    c. Damage to the pyramidal tract alone will
       produce spasticity
    d. The "clasp-knife" phenomenon is charac-
       teristic of both spasticity and decerebrate
       rigidity
25. The most common known cause of death in spinal cord injury patients is:
    a. Pneumonia secondary to respiratory paral-
       ysis
    b. Septicemia from pressure sores   **Ref. 67, p. 33**
    c. Depression and suicide   **Ref. 123, 85:73-77, 1961**
    d. Urinary tract infections and complications

Select one or more answers that will best complete or answer each of the following statements or questions.

26. Common lower extremity residual from stroke would include:
    a. Loss of selective muscle control
    b. Manifestation of primitive flexion and extension patterns
    c. Flexion and extension patterns influenced by position
    d. Equinovarus spastic deformity of the foot with associated clawing of the toes

    Ref. 106, 63:5, 17, 24-29, 113-152, 1969

27. The quadriplegic patient with triceps function and weak hands (C-7 level) would be expected to:
    a. Transfer from wheelchair to car independently
    b. Drive an automobile with hand controls
    c. Transfer from wheelchair to toilet independently
    d. Ambulate functionally with braces and crutches

    Ref. 67, p. 97, Appendix C

28. Urinary complications following spinal cord injury are best averted by:
    a. A program of intermittent catheterization started at the time of the initial injury
    b. Continued use of the Foley indwelling catheter with frequent irrigations
    c Early urinary diversion through any one of several operative techniques
    d. Utilization of constant long-term antibiotic therapy

    Ref. 67, pp. 25, 30
    Ref. 88, p. 134
    Ref. 142, 48:746, 1968

29. A patient has significant impairment of his body image 3 weeks after the onset of stroke. This problem:
    a. May significantly effect his balance
    b. May be easily compensated by a short-leg brace
    c. Results from a lesion in the nondominant hemisphere of the brain
    d. Precludes any attempt at gait training or ambulation

    Ref. 106, 63:23-31, 1969

30. During the initial posttraumatic period, "spinal shock" patients—those with spinal cord injuries—should:
    a. Not be moved from a stable supine position
    b. Be started on a scheduled turning and positioning program

    Ref. 67, pp. 25, 43, 48, 54, 62
    Ref. 88, p. 113

c. Receive special assessment for signs
and symptoms of airway obstruction or
respiratory distress
d. Be started on a range of motion program
31. Massage:
a. May be an effective means of relaxing
muscle tension and relieving pain
b. Is known to improve circulation and help   Ref. 74, pp. 382-385
reduce edema   Ref. 91, pp. 72-75
c. Will reduce local deposits of fat effectively
d. Will prevent muscle atrophy and increase
muscle strength
32. A four-point crutch gait:
a. Is slower than a two-point gait
b. Allows three points to be in contact with   Ref. 91, pp. 147, 150
the supporting surface at all times
c. Requires moving both crutches at the same
time
d. Is relatively unsafe and should only be used
for advanced crutch walkers
33. Intraneural or intrathecal phenol injections may prove valuable in the
rehabilitation of patients with:
a. Flaccid lower motor neuron
paralysis
b. Upper motor neuron spasticity   Ref. 106, 63:18, 87, 122-131, 134, 1969
due to stroke or cerebral palsy   Ref. 142, 48:752, 1968
c. Spasticity resulting from spinal
cord injury
d. Persistent pain
34. A maximal active effort against maximal resistance, with few repetitions
daily, would:
a. Be an advisable program to increase
muscle strength
b. Not be an advisable program for increasing   Ref. 91, pp. 82-83
coordination or speed
c. Be an advisable program for increasing
endurance
d. Be specific to increase range of motion
35. Concerning shoe modification and prescription, which is true?
a. A Thomas heel is extended forward
on the medial side.
b. A varus-correcting T strap should be   Ref. 76, pp. 431, 439, 448, 451
attached to the medial side of the shoe.
c. A SACH (solid ankle cushion heel)
can be used for patients with restricted
ankle motion.
d. If a heel wedge is used to correct a varus
tendency, it should be placed on the
medial side.

36. In regard to cardiac work and cardiac rehabilitation:
    a. Activity in a hot environment can increase the cardiac work requirement
    b. Emotional factors can increase the cardiac work requirement
    c. Sexual intercourse is usually contraindicated for at least six months after a myocardial infarction
    d. Walking at 2 mph on level ground is 2 to 3 "MET" activity

    Ref. 74, pp. 696-699

37. The electrical stimulation of denervated muscle:
    a. Can be performed effectively with interrupted direct current (square wave)
    b. Can be performed effectively with sinusoidal current at 25 cps
    c. Should be performed at least three or four times daily
    d. Must be started early (within a few days) after denervation occurs, to retard muscle atrophy

    Ref. 74, pp. 377-378

38. Concerning the systems of therapy used in cerebral palsy:
    a. The Fay-Doman-Delacato approach emphasizes patterns of motion related to animal movements on the ascending evolutionary scale
    b. Brunnstrom emphasizes control of synergistic movement patterns
    c. Bobath emphasizes bracing and corrective surgery
    d. Rood attempts to initiate muscle contraction by applying sensory stimuli

    Ref. 58, 47-70

39. A 65-year-old AK midthigh amputee is fitted with his first prosthesis. During the check-out and first instruction period, it is noted that he has knee instability at the "heel strike" position. Muscle examination, used as a guide for physical therapy, would most likely show:
    a. Iliopsoas weakness
    b. Failure of the hamstrings to attach properly
    c. Gluteus maximus weakness
    d. Quadriceps femorus weakness

    Ref. 82, p. 77

40. Long-term studies relating to mortality among amputees reveals _____ rate than would be expected in the general population.
    a. A significantly high mortality
    b. A greater increase in the suicide
    c. A greater increase of accidental death
    d. Death from degenerative vascular disease affecting the central nervous system and cardiac status at a higher

    Ref. 120, 13:27-36, 1969

Select the answer or answers that best apply in accordance with the information given in each of the following statements.

41. After an automobile accident, an otherwise healthy young man arrived on a stretcher in the emergency room. He complained, "I can't move my hands or legs." X-ray examination revealed a fracture dislocation at the C-5 to C-6 vertebral level. No other significant injuries were noted. Physical examination demonstrated flaccid paralysis from the level of the lesion downward, just as the patient said. Frequently overlooked but very important and encouraging sign(s) would be:
    a. Return of the bulbocavernosus and anal wink reflex within the first 24 hours
    b. Presence of the bulbocavernosus and anal wink reflex at the time of the first thorough neurologic examination, 6 hours after injury   **Ref. 67, pp. 29-30**
    c. Presence of perianal sensation
    d. Presence of Achilles tendon reflexes at 72 hours, indicating that the period of "spinal shock" was over and that progressive neurologic recovery could be expected

42. A halo was applied, giving three dimensional control, and reduction was carried out satisfactorily with traction on a Stryker frame. At 24 hours there was no evidence of neurologic return. Vital signs were stable. The patient's overall well-being and rehabilitation program would best be enhanced by:
    a. Removal of the halo, application of Vinke or Crutchfield tongs, and continuation on the Stryker frame for 6 weeks to prevent pressure sores and ensure no development of further nerve root damage
    b. Attaching the halo to a carefully applied body jacket and allowing the patient up on a tilt table the next day, as tolerated, progressing to wheelchair ambulation to accomplish the goals of physical and occupational therapy   **Ref. 67, pp. 22, 52, 74**
    c. Carrying out an immediate posterior decompression laminectomy, followed by traction (as in a) and awaiting return
    d. Removing the halo, transferring the patient to a hospital bed in a four-poster brace, at bed rest with indwelling Foley catheter, and starting a rehabilitation program as soon as possible after fracture healing has occurred

43. After the patient's admission to the intensive care unit, he demonstrated excessive restlessness with increased pulse and respiration. The likely cause would be:
   a. Pulmonary embolus
   b. Manifestations of "spinal shock,"   **Ref. 67, pp. 21, 25, 32, Appendix D** which will respond to transfusions of whole blood
   c. Decreased vital capacity because the patient is now dependent on intercostal musculature for respiration with resultant atelectasis
   d. Decreased vital capacity because the patient is now dependent on diaphragm and neck musculature only for respiration with resultant atelectasis

44. Eight weeks after injury the patient suddenly became anxious, started profuse sweating of face, neck, and arms, and complained of a pounding headache. The pulse was noted at 130. The most likely diagnosis is:
   a. Septicemia from ascending pyelonephritis
   b. Pheochromocytoma   **Ref. 67, pp. 38, 39**
   c. Hypertension secondary to autonomic   **Ref. 142, 48:753, 1968** dysreflexia
   d. Aftermath of "spinal shock"

45. The entity would best be treated by which one or more of the following?
   a. Check for plugged catheter or acute urinary retention.
   b. Check for fecal impaction.   **Ref. 67, pp. 38, 39**
   c. Elevate the patient's head.   **Ref. 142, 48:753, 1968**
   d. Administer ganglionic blocking agent such as Etamon, followed by spinal anesthesia if ineffective.

46. At two months the patient demonstrates preservation of good wrist extension but flaccid paralysis of other forearm muscles. He would be expected to improve his level of function and benefit most from:
   a. Long opponens hand splints
   b. No splinting   **Ref. 67, pp. 91-94, 168, Appendix C**
   c. Wrist-driven, flexor-hinge hand splints
   d. Myoelectric controlled, externally powered hand splints

47. A 36-year-old housewife has acute low back pain. She gives a five-year history of mild, but persistent, low back pain, with three or four acute episodes that required bed rest. There is no history of sciatica. She is judged to be emotionally stable and in otherwise good general health. She has been to several physicians without lasting relief. The physical

examination reveals marked paraspinous muscle splinting and limitation of flexion and full extension. The neurologic examination is unremarkable. X-ray films are not helpful. The most acceptable initial program of treatment would be:

    a. Bed rest, with ice packs twice a day, followed by bilateral straight-leg raising exercises to strengthen abdominal muscles

    b. Bed rest, with moist heat four times a day,   **Ref. 127, 31-A:396, 1949** followed by muscle massage

    c. Bed rest, with moist heat four times a day, followed by sitting up and straight-leg raising exercises

    d. Bed rest, pelvic traction, pelvic tilting, and low back stretching exercises twice a day

48. After the acute phase, to obtain and maintain relief from low back pain, which of the following would be considered most advisable?

    a. Specific exercises to strengthen the quadratus lumborum and erector spinae muscles

    b. Specific exercises to strengthen and main-   **Ref. 35, p. 70** tain the abdominal musculature   **Ref. 127, 31-A:396, 1949**

    c. Learning to control and maintain an anterior pelvic tilt while sitting and standing

    d. Learning to control and maintain a posterior pelvic tilt, that is, decreasing the lumbar curve, while sitting and standing

49. When exercising from a supine position, decreased lumbar lordosis will tend to be caused by contraction of the:

    a. Rectus abdominis

    b. Hamstrings   **Ref. 35, p. 70**

    c. Iliopsoas   **Ref. 127, 31-A:396, 1949**

    d. Gluteus maximus

50. A 30-year-old housewife is hospitalized with red, swollen, painful joints. She gives an eighteen-month history of migratory joint symptoms. Presently there is widespread involvement that affects all the major joints of all four extremities, including the hands and wrists. A diagnosis of rheumatoid arthritis is made. The patient cannot or will not move the joints herself because of pain. The treatment during the acute phase would be:

    a. Complete bed rest, with the patient in the position of comfort, using pillows under the knees, arms, and elbows when possible

    b. Diathermy and Hubbard tank treatments   **Ref. 75, pp. 705-707** twice a day, with passive exercises only to all involved joints

    c. Bed rest, with all involved joints splinted or padded in the position of function, and active assistive exercises twice a day

d. Alternating hot and cold packs to decrease
swelling four times a day, followed by passive and stretching exercises

51. Under an adequate medical regimen the acute symptoms subsided. The
patient continues to have some soft tissue swelling, and joint motion is
limited by mild pain in the last 15° to 20° of flexion and extension in
nearly all joints. The most beneficial program would now be:

a. Moist heat to the involved joints, followed
by passive exercise and stretching

b. Moist heat followed by active assistive ex-   **Ref. 75, pp. 707-708**
ercises

c. Splinting until all swelling and pain have
subsided

d. Any form of deep heat, followed by
progressive resistive exercises to prevent
atrophy of the supporting musculature

52. If the patient's problem were one of early rheumatoid spondylitis, the
most important exercises would be:

a. Abdominal strengthening and pelvic tilt
exercises

b. An aggressive program to maintain general   **Ref. 74, p. 561**
mobility of the dorsal and lumbar spine

c. Deep breathing exercises

d. Exercises to maintain range of motion of
neck and hips

53. A 12-year-old boy is referred to physical therapy for muscle training following the transfer of the tibialis anterior to the calcaneus. Early training
of the transplanted muscle should stress:

a. Strong isometric contractions

b. Strong isotonic contractions   **Ref. 38, pp. 11, 42**

c. Full active range of motion   **Ref. 127, 41-A:189-209, 1959**

d. Repeated voluntary muscle contractions   **Ref. 136, 25:160-164, 1945**
producing the desired movement

54. After the boy has learned to contract the transferred muscle at will:

a. Functional phasic use will automatically
follow

b. The movement should be integrated by   **Ref. 38, pp. 42, 111**
passive movement of the other joints   **Ref. 127, 41-A:189-209, 1959**
of the limb   **Ref. 136, 25:160-164, 1945**

c. Movement should be integrated with
phasic activity before weight bearing or
functional use is started

d. No additional amount of training will
change the phasic activity of the transferred muscle

55. A 45-year-old housewife without known underlying disease developed
a left flaccid hemiplegia. During examination a week later, early spastic-

ity is noted in both the left upper and lower extremities. Her general condition is stable. A Foley catheter is in place. The patient suffers from dysphasia, but cognition is good. Which of the following are believed true? The patient:

a. Will be dependent on Foley catheter drainage for an extended indefinite period

b. Should have been started on a bowel and bladder training program already

c. Should start on a bowel and bladder training program sometime in the next few weeks

d. May not have needed an indwelling Foley catheter initially

Ref. 106, 63:14-20, 39-52, 1969

56. Initial rehabilitative and preventive care should:

a. Be started in the form of positioning, splinting, frequent turning, and range of motion automatically at the time of admission to the intensive care unit by the nursing staff

b. Include frequent turning to prevent pressure sores, but splinting, special positioning, and range of motion should not be started until after the acute phase, about 3 weeks

c. Include an early, in-depth evaluation by the nursing staff, physical therapist, occupational therapist, psychologist, social service worker, and physician as a combined care team

d. Not allow sitting, standing, or attempted ambulation until cerebral edema has resolved, usually about 3 weeks

Ref. 106, 63:14-18, 39-52, 1969

57. She is again seen 6 weeks after onset of hemiplegia. On evaluation of the lower extremity in an upright position, a good flexion pattern is demonstrated. The extension pattern is poor with trace hip extensors and zero hip abductors. The proper brace that will give the necessary support for ambulation is:

a. Long-leg brace with drop-lock knees and solid ankle

b. Long-leg brace with drop-lock knees and dorsi-assist (Klenzak) ankle

c. Short-leg brace with dorsi-assist ankle with 90° upstop

d. No permanent bracing indicated as patient will not be a functional walker until hip extension and abduction strength is improved

Ref. 106, 63:32, 1969

58. When seen three months from the time of onset, she has gained considerable strength in a mass extension pattern, particularly about the hip. The foot drags and the knee gives way on attempted ambulation. With knee stability she is able to support weight on that extremity, however. The brace of choice would be:
   a. Long-leg brace with drop-lock knees and a solid ankle
   b. Long-leg brace with drop-lock knees and dorsi-assist (Klenzak) ankle   **Ref. 106, 63:38, 1969**
   c. Short-leg brace with dorsi-assist (Klenzak) ankle
   d. Short-leg brace with adjustable locked ankle

59. Over the ensuing several weeks, spacticity of the involved extremities increased. She complained bitterly of shoulder pain at rest. Examination showed the range of motion of the shoulder to be restricted. The pain was aggravated by attempts at abduction with external rotation. Tightness of the structures to the shoulder was palpable. No specific areas of tenderness were noted. The most likely cause of the complaints would be:
   a. Bicepital tendinitis
   b. Degenerative calcific tendinitis of the rotator cuff   **Ref. 106, 63:82-87, 1969**
   c. Painful frozen shoulder secondary to spasticity of the internal rotation of the shoulder
   d. Referred pain

60. The patient had been on an appropriate active therapy program for the shoulder without improvement and, in fact, seemed to be regressing. The recommendation of choice would be:
   a. Repeat psychologic evaluation
   b. Pectoral and subscapularis tendon releases   **Ref. 106, 63:82-87, 1969**
      followed by appropriate therapy
   c. Manipulation of the shoulder joint with the patient under anesthesia and injection with a cortisone derivative followed by an appropriate therapy program
   d. Stop range of motion to the shoulder; no further treatment indicated at this time

TRUE OR FALSE (answers on p. 282)

61. The halo may act as a useful device in maintaining position and alignment in cervical lesions, thus allowing early mobility of the patient with or without quadriplegia.   **Ref. 67, pp. 22, 52, 74**
   (T) (F)

62. Pregnancy is not likely in the female with spinal cord injury, and when it does occur, it is a grave hazard to the mother and child.   **Ref. 67, p. 40**
   (T) (F)

63. The proper position of the indwelling catheter to prevent the complication of penoscrotal abscess or fistula is to tape the catheter down to the thigh.   Ref. 67, pp. 38, 45
(T) (F)

64. Occurrence of pressure sores in paraplegic and quadriplegic patients is inevitable and to be expected.   Ref. 67, pp. 25, 55
(T) (F)   Ref. 142, 48:740, 1968

65. If a traumatic injury to the spinal cord results in immediate complete motor and sensory loss below the level of the lesion and persists for 24 hours, laminectomy is rarely if ever indicated.   Ref. 67, pp. 24, 30
(T) (F)   Ref. 88, p. 27

66. Isometric exercise often causes substantial elevation of systolic and diastolic blood pressure.   Ref. 48, p. 171
(T) (F)

67. Spasticity in the paraplegic patient may be effectively relieved temporarily through passive stretching exercises.   Ref. 75, p. 750
(T) (F)

68. Ambulation in the hemiplegic patient following stroke should be attempted only after voluntary control of the involved limb occurs.
(T) (F)   Ref. 64, p. 176

69. The use of the "tilt table" is outmoded in present-day physical therapy centers and should not be used.   Ref. 75, p. 750
(T) (F)

70. When putting on shirts and jackets, the upper extremity amputee will find it easier if he is instructed to put the sleeve on the sound limb first.
(T) (F)   Ref. 15, p. 16

LIST (answers on p. 282)

71. List five types of exercises prescribed and utilized in physical therapy.
           Ref. 91, p. 83

72. List four types of crutch gait.   Ref. 64, pp. 113-115

73. List four basic rehabilitation goals for the hemiplegic patient.
           Ref. 64, p. 21

74. List six complications arising from immobilization of the total patient.
           Ref. 64, p. 175

75. List five deformities of infancy and childhood that may be helped through physical therapy, positioning, and splinting.   Ref. 75, pp. 672-701

SECTION 8

Physiology and biochemistry

FLOYD G. GOODMAN, B.S., M.D.

MULTIPLE CHOICE, SINGLE ANSWER (answers on pp. 282-283)

Select the *one* answer that will best complete or answer each of the following statements or questions.

1. The organic matrix of bone is composed primarily of:
   a. Collagen
   b. Mucopolysaccharide   Ref. 55, p. 11
   c. Chondroitin sulfate
   d. Hyaluronic acid
2. Mineralized human bone matrix contains approximately _____ water.
   a. 2% to 5%
   b. 10% to 12%   Ref. 55, p. 14
   c. 18% to 20%
   d. 35% to 40%
3. The inorganic phase (bone mineral) comprises about _____ of dry decreased bone.
   a. 25%
   b. 48%   Ref. 55, p. 14
   c. 73%
   d. 92%
4. Vitamin K is important in the:
   a. Production of thrombin
   b. Production of prothrombin   Ref. 22, p. 1610
   c. Production of thromboplastin
   d. Production of fibrinogen
5. The major mucopolysaccharide in the organic matrix of bone is:
   a. Chondroitin sulfate
   b. Hyaluronate   Ref. 55, p. 3
   c. Hyaluronic acid
   d. Hydroxyproline

6. In 1883 Sir Thomas Barlow described the clinical entity _____, which bears his name:
   a. Vitamin D–resistant rickets
   b. Infantile scurvy   **Ref. 5, p. 372**
   c. Hyperostosis fetalis
   d. Pseudohyperparathyroidism

7. The abnormal accumulation of sphingomyelin within the reticuloendothelial cells bears the name of:
   a. Gaucher's disease
   b. Niemann-Pick disease   **Ref. 22, pp. 1572-1573**
   c. Letterer-Siwe syndrome
   d. Hand-Schüller-Christian disease

8. Electrophoretic analysis of a patient's serum in multiple myeloma would most likely show abnormalities in the:
   a. Albumin
   b. Alpha fraction   **Ref. 2, p. 152**
   c. Beta fraction   **Ref. 22, p. 1581**
   d. Gamma fraction

9. Citrate intoxication from numerous whole blood transfusions may lead to cardiac arrest. It manifests its effect primarily by:
   a. Direct blocking action on the cardiac chemoreceptors
   b. Antagonizing the effect of epinephrine   **Ref. 22, pp. 1516-1517**
   c. Complementing the effect of increased sodium released through hemolysis
   d. Lowering the level of serum calcium

10. The water content of mineralized bone is:
    a. Greater than in unmineralized osteoid
    b. Less than in unmineralized osteoid   **Ref. 55, p. 14**
    c. The same as unmineralized osteoid
    d. Independent and unrelated to the mineral content

11. Osteoblasts:
    a. Increase in number by direct mitotic division of existing osteoblasts
    b. Form the organic matrix of bone   **Ref. 55, pp. 18, 52**
    c. Form hydroxyapatite crystals at the zone of provisional mineralization
    d. Are the primary precursor cells of osteoclasts

12. The offending urate crystals seen in gouty tophus are:
    a. Calcium urate
    b. Uric acid   **Ref. 5, p. 732**
    c. Sodium urate
    d. Potassium urate

13. Hand-Schüller-Christian disease probably involves the abnormal metabolism of _____.
   a. Amino acid
   b. Lipid   **Ref. 5, p. 224**
   c. Carbohydrate
   d. Collagen
14. To control bleeding in a patient with hemophilia, it is usually necessary to raise the plasma level of antihemophilic factor in the patient's blood to at least:
   a. 20% to 25% of normal
   b. 30% to 40% of normal   **Ref. 22, p. 1606**
   c. 50% of normal
   d. 60% of normal
15. Unmineralized bone matrix contains approximately _____ water.
   a. 20%
   b. 40%   **Ref. 55, p. 11**
   c. 70%
   d. 90%
16. The bleeding tendency in hemophilia is due to a defect in:
   a. Factor VIII
   b. Factor XIII   **Ref. 22, p. 1605**
   c. Factor VII
   d. Factor V
17. Tetracycline retained over 48 hours within the joint fluid may be an additional diagnostic criterion for:
   a. Septic arthritis
   b. Rheumatoid arthritis   **Ref. 125, 193:581, 1965**
   c. Gouty arthritis
   d. Osteoarthritis
18. Vitamin K is produced in the:
   a. Parenchymal cells of the liver
   b. Chief cells in the small bowel   **Ref. 22, p. 1610**
   c. Intestinal tract by bacteria
   d. Through enzymatic activity on protein
      synthesis within the bowel wall
19. Widened epiphyseal cartilage plates are characteristic of vitamin D deficiency in the growing child. This is due to:
   a. Inadequate alkaline phosphatase at the
      epiphyseal line
   b. Failure of osteoid and cartilage to min-   **Ref. 5, p. 387**
      eralize
   c. Inadequate osteoid formation by osteo-
      blasts
   d. Increased chondroblast activity and
      cartilage production

20. Fibrous bone:
    a. Undergoes continual remodeling, with frequent changes in shape and volume
    b. Usually exists as a permanent part of the adult skeleton
    c. Is produced by osteoblasts that respond quite differently from those producing lamellar bone
    d. Shows definite osteoid seams and haversian systems

    Ref. 55, p. 27

21. The maximum effect of colchicine is attained in acute gouty arthritis with:
    a. 0.5 mg every 6 hours
    b. 0.5 mg every 3 hours
    c. 0.5 mg every hour
    d. 0.5 mg every hour until gastrointestinal symptoms develop

    Ref. 104, p. 247

22. In the early hours following trauma, with hemorrhage and death of tissue, the pH tends to:
    a. Rise to levels as high as 8.2
    b. Remain relatively constant but may rise or fall between 7.1 to 7.8
    c. Fall to levels as low as 6.9 to 7.2 and then shift to above-normal levels by the seventh to tenth day
    d. First rise, with the dissolution of bone salts, but then fall, with the formation of callus during the seventh to tenth day

    Ref. 127, 28:290-291, 1946

23. Which of the following activities has the greatest metabolic demand?
    a. Walking upstairs
    b. Walking downstairs
    c. Swimming
    d. Football

    Ref. 22, p. 1455
    Ref. 125, 167:216, 1958

24. The alkaline phosphatase at a fracture site would be expected to:
    a. Rise sharply during the first few hours following fracture and remain elevated until the fracture has healed
    b. Remain relatively constant during the initial 5 to 7 days and then rise steadily during callous formation
    c. Fall sharply during the initial 5 to 7 days and then rise sharply during the active phase of mineralization
    d. Remain constant throughout fracture healing; however, elevation of the serum alkaline phosphatase after the first 5 to 7 days would occur

    Ref. 127, 28:288-293, 1948

25. Generalized bleeding in the event of neoplasm involving bone should arouse your suspicions to:
    a. Hypofibrinogenemia
    b. Hypoprothrombinemia   **Ref. 22, p. 1612**
    c. Hypocalcemia
    d. Thrombocytopenia
26. Biochemical studies of a fracture hematoma 24 hours after injury would be expected to show significantly:
    a. Elevated alkaline phosphatase and
       pH and low inorganic phosphorous
       levels
    b. Elevated inorganic phosphorous and   **Ref. 127, 28:288-293, 1946**
       alkaline phosphatase levels and low
       pH levels
    c. Low pH, elevated inorganic phosphorous,
       and normal alkaline phosphatase levels
    d. Elevated inorganic phosphorous, alkaline
       phosphatase, and pH levels
27. Although the exact daily minimum requirement for ascorbic acid is unknown, an accepted figure is in excess of:
    a. 5 mg/day
    b. 10 mg/day   **Ref. 22, p. 1421**
    c. 15 mg/day
    d. 30 mg/day
28. Serum uric acid levels are elevated in the patient with gout because:
    a. The kidneys are unable to normally excrete uric acid
    b. The metabolic pathways for uric acid   **Ref. 104, p. 30**
       breakdown are blocked
    c. There is increased uric acid formation
       through a metabolic fault
    d. The intestine is unable to secrete uric acid
       normally
29. Any male with an acute onset of inflammation within a peripheral joint and a serum uric acid above _____ should be strongly suspected of having gout
    a. 4 mg
    b. 5 mg   **Ref. 104, p. 57**
    c. 6 mg
    d. 7 mg
30. Calcium comprises approximately _____ of the inorganic phase of bone.
    a. 12%
    b. 25%   **Ref. 55, p. 14**
    c. 38%
    d. 70%

31. Coumarin compounds:
    a. Act as competitive antagonists of vitamin K and impair the synthesis of prothrombin
    b. Act as chelating agents that bind free serum calcium, without which the second stage of coagulation cannot take place
    c. Inhibit the production of fibrinogen within the liver
    d. Inhibit the conversion of fibrinogen to fibrin

    Ref. 22, p. 1610

32. The periodicity of collagen is:
    a. 320 angstrom units
    b. 640 angstrom units
    c. 860 angstrom units
    d. 1,020 angstrom units

    Ref. 55, p. 12

33. Biochemical studies of a fracture site 10 days following injury would be expected to show:
    a. Elevated alkaline phosphatase and pH and low inorganic phosphorous levels
    b. Elevated inorganic phosphorous, alkaline phosphatase, and pH levels
    c. Elevated inorganic phosphorous and alkaline phosphatase levels and low pH levels
    d. Low pH, elevated inorganic phosphorous, and normal alkaline phosphatase levels

    Ref. 127, 28:288-293, 1948

34. Chondroitin sulfate, a mucopolysaccharide, is most plentiful in:
    a. Collagen
    b. Osteoid
    c. Fiber bone
    d. Hyaline cartilage

    Ref. 5, p. 14
    Ref. 55, pp. 11-16

35. A successfully fused segment of spinal column in a growing child would be expected:
    a. To equal in longitudinal growth any similar segment of unfused spine
    b. To not participate significantly in longitudinal growth of the spine
    c. To continue longitudinal growth throughout by interstitial remodeling at about 50% of normal growth rate
    d. To increase in length only through growth at its ends

    Ref. 127, 42-A:1411, 1960

36. Morquio-Ulrich disease may be differentiated from Hurler's disease and Morquio-Brailsford disease by:
    a. Increased excretion of keratosulfate, a mucopolysaccharide in the urine
    b. Presence of mucopolysaccharides in the urine

    Ref. 923, 46-A:741-745, 923, 1964

c. Storage of mucopolysaccharides and heparin monosulfate

d. Corneal opacities

37. Electromyographic studies in muscles supplied by a sectioned peripheral nerve would be expected to show:
    a. No motor activity
    b. Fibrillation   **Ref. 7, 16:250, 1959**
    c. Fasciculation
    d. Phenomenon of synchronization

38. The fat soluble vitamins are:
    a. A, B, E, and K
    b. A, D, E, and K   **Ref. 22, p. 1422**
    c. A, C, E, and K
    d. A, B, C, and K

39. Normal synovial fluid from a human joint would be expected to contain what number of nucleated cells?
    a. Less than 200/ml
    b. 200 to 500/ml   **Ref. 90, p. 3**
    c. 500 to 1,000/ml   **Ref. 127, 46-A:879, 1964**
    d. Over 1,000/ml

40. Chronic hypervitaminosis A appears to have its greatest effect on:
    a. Excessive cartilage cell proliferation
    b. Excessive osteoclast proliferation, with   **Ref. 5, p. 510**
       bone absorption
    c. Excessive enchondral bone formation and
       spurring, with widening of the epiphyses
    d. Excessive periosteal new bone formation

41. Skeletal muscle develops its greatest tension at:
    a. Resting length
    b. About 50% of resting length   **Ref. 57, pp. 37-38**
    c. About 80% of resting length
    d. About 120% of resting length

42. The most reliable guide to adequate vitamin D administration in vitamin D–resistant rickets is:
    a. Serum calcium
    b. Urinary calcium   **Ref. 127, 46-A:957, 963, 1964**
    c. Serum phosphorus
    d. Urinary phosphorus

43. Polymorphonuclear leukocytes numbering greater than _____ of the white cell count in synovial fluid would be an ominous sign.
    a. 0%
    b. 5%   **Ref. 127, 46-A:879, 1964**
    c. 10%
    d. 20%

44. In the progressive muscular dystrophies the serum _____ would be expected to be elevated.
    a. Aldolase
    b. Creatine-kinase   **Ref. 29, pp. 77, 80**

c. Creatinine

d. a and b

45. Electromyographic motor unit recordings showing longer duration and higher amplitude than normal would suggest:

    a. A high cord lesion

    b. Amyotrophic lateral sclerosis   **Ref. 7, 16:250, 1959**

    c. Peripheral nerve damage

    d. Chronic poliomyelitis

46. Phosphocreatine serves its greatest role in:

    a. Muscle metabolism during violent exercise

    b. Muscle metabolism during prolonged sub-   **Ref. 57, p. 38**
       maximal exercise

    c. Muscle metabolism during the resting
       phase

    d. Paying back the oxygen debt

47. The tension that can be developed in skeletal muscle per cross-sectional area is relatively constant for all mammals. This is found to be:

    a. 0.5 kg/cm^2

    b. 1 to 2 kg/cm^2 **Ref. 57, p. 40**

    c. 3 to 4 kg/cm^2

    d. 5 to 6 kg/cm^2

48. The intravascular calcium within the body is:

    a. Carried primarily as a calcium proteinate
       complex in the plasma

    b. Primarily concentrated within the red   **Ref. 28, pp. 716-718**
       blood cells

    c. Carried primarily in the plasma, about
       one half as a calcium proteinate complex

    d. Primarily concentrated within the plasma
       fraction as a calcium citrate complex

49. The patient with vitamin D–deficient rickets would be expected to demonstrate:

    a. Elevated serum phosphorus and alkaline
       phosphatase

    b. Elevated serum calcium and alkaline   **Ref. 28, p. 586**
       phosphatase

    c. Decreased serum calcium and phosphorus
       and elevated alkaline phosphatase

    d. Normal or low alkaline phosphatase

50. In enchondral bone formation, primary spongiosa is referred to as:

    a. Cancellous bone

    b. Mineralized chondroid cores overlain   **Ref. 5, pp. 26, 65**
       with primitive fiber bone

    c. Granulation tissue and young osteoblasts

    d. Mature bone formed from conversion of
       fiber bone

51. What percent of body calcium is within the skeleton?
    a. 40%
    b. 60%   **Ref. 62, p. 340**
    c. 85%
    d. 90%
52. Increase in serum alkaline phosphatase would probably not be seen in:
    a. Hyperparathyroidism
    b. Rickets   **Ref. 5, p. 416**
    c. Osteoblastic osteosarcoma
    d. Hypophosphatasia
53. The calcium concentration in relatively protein-free fluids such as spinal
    fluid would be expected to be:
    a. The same as the serum calcium level
    b. Higher than the serum calcium level   **Ref. 28, p. 718**
    c. About one fourth the serum calcium level
    d. About one half the serum calcium level
54. Synovial fluid with lowered glucose, poor mucin precipitate, decreased
    viscosity, and a white cell count of 100 cells per milliliter would be most
    indicative of:
    a. Traumatic arthritis
    b. Degenerative arthritis   **Ref. 127, 46-A:884, 1964**
    c. Gouty arthritis
    d. Rheumatoid arthritis
55. Paget's disease is characterized by:
    a. Increased serum calcium and alkaline
       phosphatase
    b. Decreased serum potassium and increased   **Ref. 5, p. 467**
       alkaline phosphatase
    c. Increased alkaline phosphatase and normal
       potassium and calcium
    d. Increased serum calcium and decreased
       serum potassium
56. Secondary hyperparathyroidism is most popularly believed to be a result
    of increased parathyroid hormone output resulting from:
    a. Inability to manufacture ammonium ions
       in the kidney
    b. Renal tubular defect and low phosphate   **Ref. 5, pp. 399, 403**
       retention
    c. Glomerular damage and phosphate reten-
       tion
    d. Decreased target cell response
57. Vitamin C deficiency most markedly affects:
    a. Formation of collagen and osteoid
    b. Production of chondroblasts   **Ref. 5, p. 371**
    c. Mineralization of cartilage spicules
    d. Diaphysis of long bones

58. ^{85}Sr, ^{86}Sr, ^{89}Sr, and ^{226}Ra have proved useful in the study of bone metabolism and the bone tissue interphase because these elements tend to replace _____ in the hydroxyapatite structure complex.
   a. Calcium
   b. Potassium   **Ref. 127, 45-A:1072, 1963**
   c. Sodium
   d. Phosphorus

59. The viscosity of synovial fluid is primarily due to:
   a. Hyaluronic acid
   b. Chondroitin sulfate   **Ref. 127, 46-A:878, 1964**
   c. Amino acids
   d. Protein

60. Growth hormone is believed to affect:
   a. Chondroblastic activity only
   b. Osteoblastic activity only   **Ref. 5, p. 429**
   c. Both
   d. Neither

61. The amount of synovial fluid that would be expected in a normal knee joint is approximately:
   a. 1 ml
   b. 5 ml   **Ref. 90, p. 3**
   c. 10 ml
   d. 20 ml

62. Milkman's syndrome is believed to be the adult form of:
   a. Renal rickets
   b. Vitamin D–refractory rickets   **Ref. 5, p. 394**
   c. Pseudohypoparathyroidism
   d. Idiopathic hypophosphatemia

63. Hypervitaminosis D may mimic closely:
   a. Hyperthyroidism
   b. Hyperparathyroidism   **Ref. 5, p. 503**
   c. Vitamin D–resistant rickets
   d. Hypervitaminosis A

64. The inorganic phosphorous levels at the site of fracture would be expected to:
   a. Remain stable during the first 10 days until osteoid is formed
   b. Fall sharply during the first few hours   **Ref. 127, 28:289, 1946**
      following fracture, correlating closely with the fall in pH
   c. Rise sharply during the first few hours following fracture, reaching the high point of concentration about the time pH is lowest
   d. Fall during the first 10 days and then rise, reaching the high point at the height of fiber bone formation

65. In vitamin D–refractory rickets, Fanconi syndrome in children, or Milkman's syndrome in adults, the site of apparent dysfunction is the:
   a. Kidney
   b. Intestinal mucosa   Ref. 5, pp. 394, 410
   c. Bone tissue level
   d. Serum calcium ion transport

66. High serum calcium, high alkaline phosphatase, low or normal phosphorus, and nephrolithiosis would be strongly suggestive of:
   a. Hyperparathyroidism
   b. Pseudohypoparathyroidism   Ref. 5, p. 440
   c. Hypoparathyroidism
   d. Pseudohyperparathyroidism

67. Uniform dwarfism, with failure of sexual and skeletal maturation but normal intelligence, is most indicative of:
   a. Hypothyroidism
   b. Hypoparathyroidism   Ref. 5, p. 431
   c. Hypopituitarism   Ref. 62, p. 310
   d. Hypoadrenalism

68. In hyperparathyroidism, blood chemistries would be expected to show:
   a. Increased calcium and phosphorus
   b. Increased calcium and decreased phos-   Ref. 5, pp. 443, 506
      phorus   Ref. 62, p. 341
   c. Decreased calcium and phosphorus
   d. Decreased calcium and increased phos-
      phorus

69. Retarded somatic development, retarded appendicular skeletal growth, short stature, and increased water-binding capacity of fibrous tissues are indicative of:
   a. Hyperadrenalism
   b. Hypopituitarism   Ref. 5, p. 432
   c. Hypoparathyroidism
   d. Hypothyroidism

70. Alkaline phosphatase would be expected to be below normal or normal in:
   a. Postmenopausal osteoporosis
   b. Osteomalacia and rickets   Ref. 5, p. 420
   c. Hyperparathyroidism
   d. Paget's disease

71. The atomic number of an atom is equal to the:
   a. Number of neutrons in the nucleus
   b. Number of protons in the nucleus   Ref. 127, 45-A:1068, 1963
   c. Number of protons and neutrons in the
      nucleus
   d. Number of electrons and protons within
      the atom

72. Succinylcholine has its primary effect by:
    a. Inhibiting the release of acetylcholine
    b. Blocking the action of acetylcholine on   **Ref. 59, pp. 604, 610**
       the muscle cell
    c. Depolarizing the muscle cell
    d. Blocking dephosphorylation of adenosine
       triphosphate and is effectively antagonized
       by neostigmine
73. Hyaluronate:
    a. Is a normal constituent of plasma
    b. Occurs in synovial joints and is known to   **Ref. 127, 46-A:876, 1964**
       be manufactured by the synovial mem-
       brane cells
    c. Crosses the membrane barrier gradient
       from the plasma to the synovial fluid by
       a "metabolic pump" mechanism
    d. Is an essential amino acid
74. Accelerated skeletal maturation, high turnover osteoporosis, and negative
    calcium and nitrogen balance, with usually normal serum calcium and
    phosphorus levels, are characteristic of:
    a. Hyperadrenalism
    b. Hyperpituitarism   **Ref. 28, p. 462**
    c. Hyperparathyroidism   **Ref. 55, p. 91**
    d. Hyperthyroidism
75. McArdle syndrome:
    a. Is the second most common form of mus-
       cular dystrophy
    b. Is not an inherited disease   **Ref. 22, pp. 1662-1663**
    c. Is due to a deficiency of muscle phosphorylase
    d. Is characterized by increased peripheral
       venous blood lactate after exercise
76. Curare has its primary effect by:
    a. Inhibiting the release of acetylcholine
    b. Inhibiting the formation of acetylcholine   **Ref. 59, pp. 601-603**
    c. Depolarizing the muscle cell
    d. Blocking the action of acetylcholine on the
       muscle cell
77. The secretory activity of the parathyroid gland, although not proved, is
    most popularly believed to be controlled by:
    a. Serum calcium levels
    b. Serum alkaline phosphatase levels   **Ref. 5, p. 452**
    c. Serum phosphorous levels   **Ref. 28, p. 721**
    d. An anterior pituitary hormone
78. The chemotherapeutic drug of choice in multiple myeloma is:
    a. Ethyl carbamate
    b. Melphalan   **Ref. 22, p. 1583**
    c. Triethylenemelamine
    d. Chlorambucil

79. All of the following have been found to have an increased incidence in hyperparathyroidism. The second most common associated finding is:
    a. Renal stones
    b. Bone disease   **Ref. 6, p. 680**
    c. Peptic ulcer
    d. Pancreatitis
80. The sum of the water derived from solid foods and the water of oxidation from metabolic processes is usually considered to equal about _____ per day for the average adult man.
    a. 400 ml
    b. 700 ml   **Ref. 6, p. 80**
    c. 1,000 ml
    d. 1,400 ml
81. It has been shown that muscles have a span of contraction that is approximately _____ of their fiber length.
    a. 27%
    b. 34%   **Ref. 81, p. 1137**
    c. 46%
    d. 57%
    e. 69%
82. The Blix curve:
    a. Demonstrates the active length-tension relationship of a muscle
    b. Demonstrates the passive length-tension   **Ref. 15, p. 167** relationship of a muscle   **Ref. 81, p. 1136**
    c. Demonstrates the combined effect of ac-   **Ref. 127, 48-A:363, 1966** tive and passive tension as related to length
    d. Demonstrates the electrical shift in potential across the muscle cell membrane
83. No increase in urinary phosphorus during 3 hours following intravenous injection of 200 units of parathyroid extract would be expected in:
    a. A normal individual
    b. Hypoparathyroidism   **Ref. 5, p. 457**
    c. Hyperparathyroidism   **Ref. 22, p. 1853**
    d. Pseudohypoparathyroidism
84. Mast cells are believed to be important in wound healing through the production of:
    a. Tropocollagen
    b. Mucopolysaccharides   **Ref. 6, p. 10**
    c. Ascorbic acid
    d. Fibroblasts
85. Disharmonious skeletal enlargement with tufting of the toes and enlargement of the nose, mandible, and frontal bosses are indicative of:
    a. Hyperthyroidism
    b. Hyperpituitarism   **Ref. 5, p. 429**
    c. Hyperadrenalism
    d. Hypergonadism

86. The defect in wound healing in ascorbic acid deficiency may be corrected by administration of ascorbic acid within:
    a. 24 hours
    b. 48 hours   Ref. 6, p. 10
    c. 7 days
    d. 14 days
87. The entity named idiopathic hypercalcemia is believed to be one and the same as:
    a. Hypervitaminosis A
    b. Caffey's disease   Ref. 5, p. 507
    c. Hypervitaminosis D
    d. Scurvy
88. Which of the following hormones are apparently not affected by ACTH?
    a. Deoxycorticosterone
    b. Corticosterone   Ref. 62, p. 321
    c. Aldosterone
    d. Hydrocortisone
89. A tenfold increase in urinary phosphate output above normal following an Elsworth-Howard test would be indicative of:
    a. Hyperparathyroidism
    b. Hypoparathyroidism   Ref. 5, p. 457
    c. Pseudohypoparathyroidism   Ref. 22, p. 1853
    d. Hypothyroidism
90. The offending cell in pituitary adenoma believed responsible for the increased production of growth hormone is the:
    a. Chief cell
    b. Acidophilic cell   Ref. 62, p. 302
    c. Chromophilic cell
    d. Basophilic cell
91. The decurarizing agent of choice is:
    a. Prostigmine
    b. Ephedrine   Ref. 59, p. 613
    c. Atropine
    d. Neostigmine
92. Oxygen consumption studies have shown that the highest efficiency in normal people occurs when walking:
    a. Under 1.5 mph
    b. 1.5 to 2.5 mph   Ref. 82, p. 163
    c. 3 to 3.5 mph
    d. Over 3.5 mph
93. In hyperparathyroidism you would expect to see:
    a. Increased urinary calcium and phosphorus
    b. Increased urinary calcium and decreased   Ref. 62, p. 341
       phosphorus
    c. Decreased urinary calcium and phos-
       phorus
    d. Decreased urinary calcium and increased
       phosphorus

94. Ascorbic acid is believed to be most closely associated with:
   a. Fibroblast production
   b. Collagen synthesis   **Ref. 6, p. 10**
   c. Mast cell proliferation   **Ref. 62, pp. 359, 360**
   d. Mucopolysaccharide production
95. Vitamin A in the normal diet is believed to contribute mainly to:
   a. Epiphyseal cartilage cell growth and
      maturation
   b. Production of osteoblasts   **Ref. 5, p. 510**
   c. Membranous bone formation
   d. Normal resolution of chondroid matrix
96. Although collagen may appear within the healing wound within 36
   hours, significant amounts are not present until:
   a. 48 hours
   b. 6 days   **Ref. 6, p. 10**
   c. 10 days
   d. 14 days
97. The half-life of ACTH in man is approximately:
   a. 15 minutes
   b. 14 hours   **Ref. 62, p. 322**
   c. 12 hours
   d. 24 hours
98. Atropine has its primary effect by:
   a. Inhibiting the muscarinic action of ace-
      tylcholine
   b. Inhibiting the adrenergic effect of epi-   **Ref. 59, p. 524**
      nephrine
   c. Acting on postganglionic sympathetic
      fibers
   d. Inhibiting the nicotinic action of acetyl-
      choline
99. A man weighing 70 kg consists of approximately _____ water.
   a. 40%
   b. 65%   **Ref. 81, p. 289**
   c. 80%
   d. 90%
100. Phytate:
   a. Promotes zinc absorption
   b. Inhibits zinc absorption   **Ref. 106, 103:213, 1974**
   c. Is present in high concentrations in meat
   d. Is present in low concentrations in
      legumes, unleavened bread, and cereal
      grains
101. Oral administration of 1-α-hydroxy–vitamin D was found to ameliorate
   the conditions of renal osteodystrophy. Anticonvulsant drugs hinder
   these effects, probably by:
   a. Reducing the effects of 1,25-dihydroxy–
      vitamin D on intestinal absorption of
      calcium

b. Reducing the solubility of 1-α-hydroxy–   Ref. 125, 234-1:52, 1974
      vitamin D in fat
   c. Interfering with the effects of 1,25-
      dihydroxy–vitamin D on renal reabsorp-
      tion of calcium
   d. Interfering with the conversion of 1-α-
      hydroxy–vitamin D to 1,25-dihydroxy–
      vitamin D in the liver

102. Pectus carinatum (pigeon breast) is commonly a feature of:
   a. Gaucher's disease
   b. Hand-Schüller-Christian disease   Ref. 127, 46-A:734, 1964
   c. Morquio-Ulrich disease
   d. Niemann-Pick disease

103. Cathepsin D, E, and B₁:
   a. Are lysosomal enzymes
   b. Are incapable of degrading cartilage   Ref. 127, 55-B:88-91, 1973
   c. Have not been isolated in human cartilage
   d. Have optimum activity in alkaline con-
      ditions

104. Administration of allopurinol for gout:
   a. Decreases urinary uric acid
   b. Decreases serum uric acid   Ref. 87, p. 235
   c. Abolishes uric acid stones   Ref. 39, p. 103
   d. All of the above

MULTIPLE CHOICE, MULTIPLE ANSWERS (answers on pp. 283-284)

Select one or more answers that will best complete or answer each of the
following statements or questions.

105. Local anesthetics such as lidocaine and procaine are believed to have
   their major effect:
   a. By depolarizing the nerve trunk
   b. On the motor end plate and terminal   Ref. 59, pp. 371, 374
      nerve receptors
   c. On the smaller nerve fibers first
   d. By blocking the shift in potential across
      the cell membrane that normally occurs
      during conduction

106. Factors influencing calcium absorption from the gastrointestinal tract
   are:
   a. Parathyroid hormone
   b. Gastrointestinal motility   Ref. 22, pp. 1287, 1290
   c. Fatty acid absorption   Ref. 28, p. 606
   d. None of the above

107. Increased urinary excretion of phosphoryl ethanolamine may be seen in:
   a. Hypophosphatasia
   b. Scurvy   Ref. 5, p. 416
   c. Hypothyroidism   Ref. 62, p. 220
   d. Normal individuals

108. Benemid in the treatment of gout:
    a. Acts as a strong anti-inflammatory agent
    b. Produces an analgesic effect   Ref. 104, p. 73
    c. Inhibits the tubular reabsorption of urates
    d. Tends to decrease serum uric acid levels
109. Heparin produces its anticoagulant effect by interfering with the:
    a. Formation of intrinsic thromboplastin
    b. Conversion of fibrinogen to fibrin   Ref. 22, p. 1612
    c. Formation of prothrombin
    d. Absorption of vitamin K
110. Osteocytes:
    a. Reproduce by mitotic division
    b. Do not ordinarily divide   Ref. 55, pp. 22, 23
    c. Depend on diffusion of nutritional ele-
       ments through canaliculi
    d. Have an average life span of 25 years
111. Hypophosphatasia is an inborn error of metabolism characterized by:
    a. Phosphoryl ethanolamine in the urine
    b. Decreased serum inorganic phosphate   Ref. 5, p. 416
    c. Low or low normal alkaline phosphate   Ref. 22, p. 1869
    d. Skeletal abnormalities resembling rickets
       or osteomalacia
112. Which of the following are uricosuric agents?
    a. Benemid
    b. Colchicine   Ref. 104, p. 187
    c. Salicylate
    d. Corticosteroids
113. The bleeding tendency in hemophilia type B (Christmas disease) may
    be controlled with:
    a. Fresh whole blood
    b. Stored whole blood   Ref. 22, p. 1608
    c. Fresh plasma
    d. Freshly frozen plasma
114. The serum studies in hypervitaminosis A would be expected to show:
    a. Normal calcium and phosphorous levels
    b. Elevated carotene levels   Ref. 5, p. 510
    c. Elevated vitamin A levels
    d. Elevated serum calcium and phosphorous
       levels and decreased alkaline phosphatase
115. Attacks of gout are known to be precipitated by:
    a. Parenteral penicillin
    b. Mercurial diuretics   Ref. 104, p. 143
    c. Fatty foods
    d. Wine
116. Low to normal serum calcium with an elevated serum phosphate and
    alkaline phosphatase would suggest:
    a. Hypoparathyroidism
    b. Hyperparathyroidism   Ref. 5, pp. 399, 452, 457

c. Secondary hyperparathyroidism

d. Vitamin D–resistant rickets

117. In multiple myeloma, which of the following laboratory tests would be expected to be abnormal?

a. Serum protein

b. Serum calcium   Ref. 22, p. 1581

c. Serum phosphorus

d. Acid phosphatase

e. Urinalysis

118. The recommended treatment of hypoparathyroidism includes:

a. Low dietary calcium and phosphorus

b. High dietary calcium and low phosphorus   Ref. 6, p. 680

c. Vitamin A supplements

d. Vitamin D supplements

119. Ascorbic acid is believed to be closely involved in the:

a. Conversion of proline to hydroxyproline

b. Metabolism of phenylalanine and tyrosine   Ref. 22, pp. 1445-1446

c. Preservation of folinic acid

d. Production of platelets

120. Which of the following may frequently be found in excess in the urine of patients with vitamin D–resistant rickets or Fanconi syndrome?

a. Phosphates and amino acids

b. Bicarbonates and potassium   Ref. 5, p. 410

c. Potassium, glucose, and glycine

d. Any of the above

121. Indicate the relative toxicity of the following, starting with the most toxic.

a. Procaine

b. Cocaine   Ref. 59, pp. 379-384

c. Lidocaine (Xylocaine)

d. Tetracaine (Pontocaine)

122. The chloride shift:

a. Is believed to account for the 3% increase in hematocrit from arterial to venous blood

b. Is primarily concerned with balancing the   Ref. 44, pp. 34-35 equilibrium caused by the transport of sodium and potassium ions when hemoglobin is oxygenated

c. Is predictable and adheres to the Donnan equilibrium theory

d. Concerns the replacement of the negative charge within the red blood cell at the capillary level when bicarbonate ion diffuses into the plasma

123. The mass number of an element:
    a. Is equal to the sum of the protons and neutrons within the nucleus
    b. Is equal to the sum of the protons and electrons within the atom   Ref. 127, 45-A:1068, 1069, 1963
    c. Will be the same for all isotopes of a given element
    d. Will change for each isotope, in keeping with the loss or addition of neutrons

124. The end product(s) of aerobic glycolysis in muscle metabolism is (are):
    a. Tricarboxylic acid
    b. Pyruvic acid   Ref. 57, p. 38
    c. Carbon dioxide and water
    d. Lactic acid

125. The gamma efferent system:
    a. Increases the sensitivity of the muscle spindle
    b. Motor neurons are regulated to a large degree by higher centers   Ref. 57, p. 67
    c. Is probably the mechanism by which spasticity is increased in the patient with cerebral palsy when nervous or under stress
    d. Acts directly on the extrafusal fibers

126. Patients with mild and moderate idiopathic scoliosis have been reported to have alteration in pulmonary function. Which of the following would be expected to show significant alteration from normal?
    a. Vital capacity
    b. Timed vital capacity and tidal volume   Ref. 127, 46-A:61, 1964
    c. Inspiratory capacity
    d. Expiratory reserve capacity

127. Alizarin red has been known for many years to stain bone in vivo. Recent studies have indicated that alizarin red:
    a. Is taken up in areas of new bone formation
    b. Inhibits new bone formation   Ref. 127, 46-A:505-508, 1964
    c. Reacts strongly with hydroxyapatite
    d. May interfere with collagen synthesis

128. Local anesthetics such as cocaine and procaine:
    a. Have a tertiary amino group in common
    b. In proper concentration may block only the sensory fibers without appreciably affecting the motor nerves   Ref. 59, pp. 372-375
    c. Act as central nervous system depressants
    d. Are detoxified primarily in the kidney

129. Succinylcholine:
    a. Is classified as a short-acting muscle relax-
       ant
    b. Should be administered only by the intra-   Ref. 59, p. 615
       venous route
    c. Is an effective antagonist to curare
    d. Is readily detoxified in the plasma by en-
       zymatic hydrolysis
130. The physiologic effect of ischemic vascular disease on lamellar bone in
    the lower extremity has been shown to include:
    a. Osteocyte death and filling of
       lacunae with mineral
    b. Plugging of haversian canals   Ref. 127, 39-A:898-900, 1957
    c. Microscopically identifiable areas of   Ref. 127, 46-A:807-809, 1964
       increased focal necrosis
    d. Early x-ray changes
131. Human synovial fluid normally contains:
    a. Concentrations of protein approximately
       double that of plasma
    b. Concentrations of protein approximately   Ref. 127, 46-A:879, 1964
       one-third that of plasma
    c. Fibrinogen and thrombin but not pro-
       thrombin or fibrin
    d. No protein with molecular weights above
       160,000
132. Tritiated thymidine:
    a. Is a desoxyribonucleic acid precursor
    b. Has proved to be an excellent tool in   Ref. 127, 45-A:529, 1072, 1963
       studying areas of cell division
    c. Localizes within the mitochondria
       of the dividing cell
    d. Is incorporated into the chromosomal
       network of the cells prior to mitotic
       division
133. Administration of systemic papain in young laboratory animals has been
    shown to:
    a. Stimulate epiphyseal growth and pro-
       liferation of cartilage cells
    b. Cause premature closure of the epiphyseal   Ref. 101, 45-A:25, 1963
       plates
    c. Cause depletion of the intercellular matrix
    d. Increase mucopolysaccharide levels in
       blood and urine
134. The stretch reflex:
    a. Utilizes the annulospiral endings of the
       muscle spindle as the sense organ re-
       ceptors
    b. Is initiated in the extrafusal fibers   Ref. 57, p. 66

c. Is primarily a polysynaptic reflex arc
d. Is the only known monosynaptic reflex arc in the body

135. Calcitonin reportedly:
    a. Is a pituitary hormone
    b. Is a parathyroid hormone   Ref. 54, p. 449
    c. Exhibits a depressing effect on excessively high serum calcium
    d. Is the circulating factor in the blood that controls the output of parathyroid hormone

136. Creatine:
    a. Plays an important role in its conjugated form as an energy donor in muscle contracture
    b. Is formed primarily within the muscle cell   Ref. 29, p. 72
    c. Undergoes a reversible reaction with creatinine
    d. Is formed primarily within the liver

137. Adenosine triphosphate:
    a. Is made up of adenine, ribose, and three phosphoric acid residues
    b. Is the principal intracellular carrier of   Ref. 57, pp. 36, 38, 201-202
    energy throughout the body
    c. Primarily depends on the hydrolyzation of phosphocreatine for its synthesis from adenosine diphosphate
    d. Stores the equivalent amount of energy as acetyl coenzyme A per mole

138. The inverse stretch reflex:
    a. Utilizes the Golgi tendon organ as the receptor
    b. Implies that the harder a muscle is   Ref. 57, p. 68
    stretched the stronger the reflex contraction
    c. May be initiated either by active or passive stretch
    d. Implies that relaxation of the muscle occurs as a protective mechanism when excessive severe stretch is applied

139. The deposition of calcium carbonate from solution is prevented by:
    a. Collagen
    b. Pyrophosphate   Ref. 127, 55-B:66
    c. Hydroxyproline
    d. Diphosphonates

140. Electromyographic tracings would be expected to show fibrillary potentials in:
    a. Muscular dystrophy
    b. High cord lesions   Ref. 7, 16:247, 1959

c. Lower motor neuron lesions

d. Acute poliomyelitis

141. Acetylcholine is the primary mode of impulse transmission:
    a. At the motor end plate
    b. In postganglionic parasympathetic fibers   Ref. 59, p. 466
    c. In autonomic preganglionic fibers
    d. In postganglionic sympathetic fibers

142. The end product(s) of anaerobic glycolysis is (are):
    a. Tricarboxylic acid
    b. Pyruvic acid   Ref. 57, p. 38
    c. Lactic acid
    d. Carbon dioxide and water

143. The normal cell:
    a. Carries an electropositive charge at its
       outer periphery
    b. Has an electronegative cytoplasm   Ref. 57, p. 12
    c. Carries an electronegative charge within
       the cell because of the increased negative
       chloride concentration
    d. Has a higher concentration of potassium
       inside the cell than outside

144. Factors influencing calcium absorption from the gastrointestinal tract
    are:
    a. Level and ratio of calcium and phos-
       phorus in the diet
    b. pH   Ref. 22, pp. 1287, 1289
    c. Vitamin D
    d. All of the above
    e. None of the above

145. The respiratory compensation of metabolic alkalosis would be expected
    to:
    a. Cause further increase in carbon dioxide
       concentration
    b. Cause increased bicarbonate ion concen-   Ref. 44, pp. 77-79
       tration
    c. Cause decrease in pH
    d. a and b, resulting in c

146. Energy expenditure by older men, when walking up to 3 mph, would
    be expected to:
    a. Be greater than in younger individuals
    b. Be less than in younger individuals   Ref. 82, p. 151
    c. Be about the same as in younger in-
       dividuals
    d. Correspond to an oxygen consumption
       level of 715 ml/min

147. Which of the following have been noted to be commonly associated with acromegaly and gigantism?
    a. Diabetes insipidus
    b. Diabetes mellitus   Ref. 5, p. 431
    c. Hyperthyroidism
    d. Hyperparathyroidism
148. A polyphasic electromyographic pattern is indicative of:
    a. Regenerating innervation
    b. Partial denervation   Ref. 127, 31-A:822, 1949
    c. Normal muscle innervation   Ref. 127, 44-A:1052, 1962
    d. Denervated muscle
149. Indicate in descending order the relative importance of the following mechanisms of carbon dioxide transport within the blood.
    a. Carbamino compounds within the plasma
    b. Carbonic acid within the plasma   Ref. 44, pp. 31-32
    c. Hemoglobin carbamino compounds within the erythrocyte
    d. Bicarbonate ions formed in the erythrocyte
150. Total body fluids in a man weighing 70 kg would probably be divided into quantities most closely resembling which of the following?
    a. Connective tissue and cartilage water— 2.5%
    b. Intracellular water—55%   Ref. 81, pp. 1049-1053
    c. Plasma water—15%
    d. Bone water—7.5%
151. A patient suffers from prolonged vomiting following anesthesia and develops a metabolic alkalosis. If this were uncompensated, the blood chemistries would be expected to show:
    a. Elevated pH and decreased carbon dioxide and bicarbonate ion concentration
    b. Increased carbon dioxide and bicarbonate ion   Ref. 44, p. 77
    c. Elevated pH and bicarbonate ion and normal carbon dioxide
    d. Normal bicarbonate and pH and depressed carbon dioxide
152. Ascorbic acid in the human being is necessary in the normal:
    a. Production of ground substance
    b. Production of collagen   Ref. 5, p. 376
    c. Production of cartilage   Ref. 22, p. 1445
    d. Mineralization of osteoid and cartilage
153. Hydroxyapatite crystals:
    a. Are a chemical compound
    b. Are of a specific size   Ref. 55, p. 15
    c. Are the basic lattice structure of bone
    d. Contain primarily calcium phosphate and hydroxyl ions

154. Carbonic anhydrase:
    a. Is an important enzyme in the Krebs cycle
    b. Catalyzes the mineralization of bone matrix in conjunction with alkaline phosphatase
    c. Is an important catalyst in the red blood cell and is concerned with the "chloride shift mechanism"
    d. Plays a primary role in acid base balance within the renal tubular cells of the kidney

    Ref. 44, pp. 34-37, 80-85

155. Fibrous bone:
    a. Usually has a lower mineral density than does lamellar bone
    b. Lacks uniform three-dimensional structure
    c. Has an increased number of osteocytes over lamellar bone per cubic millimeter
    d. May be easily identified microscopically using polarized light

    Ref. 55, pp. 29, 31

156. Pseudogout is characterized by:
    a. Rapid response to colchicine
    b. Calcification of articular cartilage
    c. Increased serum uric acid
    d. Intraleukocytic calcium pyrophosphate crystals in the aspirated joint fluid

    Ref. 5, p. 735

157. Which of the following would be expected to be useful in correcting the coagulation defect in a patient with hemophilia?
    a. Concentrates of antihemophilic factor VIII
    b. Freshly frozen plasma
    c. Stored whole blood
    d. Fresh packed cells

    Ref. 22, p. 1606

158. The osteoblast is believed:
    a. To reproduce itself by mitotic division as the primary mode of proliferation
    b. To have a life span of approximately 25 years when incorporated into bone as an osteocyte
    c. To be 50% less effective when produced at 60 years of age than when produced at 20 years of age
    d. To respond entirely differently when forming fiber bone than when forming lamellar bone

    Ref. 55, pp. 24, 27, 105

159. Calcium and phosphorus are reabsorbed through the convoluted tubules of the kidney. Parathyroid hormone inhibits the reabsorption of _____ and is believed to promote the reabsorption of _____.
    a. Calcium
    b. Phosphorus   Ref. 62, p. 341
    c. Both
    d. Neither

160. Creatinine is:
    a. An end product of normal muscle me-
       tabolism
    b. Not reabsorbed by the kidney tubule   Ref. 29, p. 74
       and is therefore useful as an indicator of
       gomerular filtration
    c. Produced primarily in the kidney
    d. Will have an increased urinary concen-
       tration in the muscular dystrophies

161. Which of the following is (are) examples of high turnover osteoporosis?
    a. Senile osteoporosis
    b. Postmenopausal osteoporosis   Ref. 55, p. 91
    c. Hyperadrenal cortical osteoporosis
    d. Thyrotoxic osteoporosis

162. The chronaxia of a given excitable tissue:
    a. Is a current equal to one half the rheobase
    b. Is a current equal to twice the rheobase   Ref. 57, p. 23
    c. Is the length of time required for a current
       equal to twice the rheobase to produce
       a response
    d. Is equal to the rheobase divided by the
       utilization time

163. Growth hormone:
    a. In animal experiments stimulates growth
       only as long as there is a fat reserve
    b. Has protein anabolic effect believed to be   Ref. 62, p. 304
       mediated through the action of insulin
    c. Causes a retention of water and phos-
       phates
    d. Causes decreased renal function

164. Pseudohypoparathyroidism is characterized by:
    a. Decreased parathyroid hormone output
    b. Decreased "target tissue response"   Ref. 5, p. 457
    c. Normal "target tissue response"   Ref. 62, p. 347
    d. Normal parathyroid hormone output

165. In vivo and in vitro studies of cartilage destruction in infectious arth-
    ritis indicate:
    a. The responsible substance is derived
       from the bacterial toxins
    b. The proteolytic enzymes are released   Ref. 127, 45-A:803, 1963
       from leukocytes

c. A combination of bacterial enzymes and pus are necessary for cartilage destruction

d. The mechanism of destruction is unknown

166. Epinephrine and norepinephrine have their adrenergic effect in the transmission of nerve impulses:
    a. At the motor end plate
    b. In postganglionic parasympathetic fibers   Ref. 59, pp. 423, 428, 486, 496
    c. In autonomic preganglionic fibers
    d. In postganglionic sympathetic fibers

167. In hyperadrenal cortical osteoporosis:
    a. The rate of new bone formation is normal, but resorption is increased
    b. Bone resorption rate is decreased   Ref. 55, pp. 92-93
    c. The rate of new bone formation is decreased and resorption is normal
    d. The rate of new bone formation is decreased

168. Fracture studies of the extremities of animals in the early postfracture period indicate:
    a. There is vasoconstriction in the arterial vascular bed of the fractured limb
    b. There is general vasodilatation in the involved limb   Ref. 127, 46-A:1267-1268, 1964
    c. The vascular bed of the opposite limb is unaffected
    d. There is vasoconstriction of the vascular bed of the opposite limb, with decreased blood supply

169. Curare has its primary effect:
    a. On the muscarinic effect of acetylcholine
    b. On the nicotinic effect of acetylcholine   Ref. 59, p. 606
    c. At the motor end plate
    d. On ganglions

170. Urinary hydroxyproline is considered an index of bone turnover. Sources contributing to elevated urinary hydroxyproline include:
    a. The ingestion of gelatin
    b. The synthesis of bone collagen   Ref. 127, 55-B:76, 1973
    c. The breakdown of nonosseous collagen
    d. The hepatic conversion of vitamin D to biologically active 25-hydroxy–vitamin D

171. The accumulation of cerebrosides in bone in Gaucher's disease may re sult in:
    a. Elaboration of osteoid formation
    b. Bone marrow depression and anemia   Ref. 7, 22:274, 1973
    c. Reduction of bone collagen formation
    d. Interference of intraosseous vascular flow with subsequent bone cell necrosis

172. Serum alkaline phosphatase:
    a. Is present in higher concentrations during the active growth period
    b. Arises primarily from bone, liver, and   Ref. 132, 3-3:551, 552, 1972 intestine
    c. Drops rapidly during the development of a malignant tumor in patients with Paget's disease
    d. In elevated concentration, generally can be considered an indication of bone forming activity due to growth, fracture healing, or skeletal disorder

173. The prime features of Silver's syndrome include:
    a. Congenital somatic asymmetry
    b. Round facies   Ref. 127, 55-A:1502, 1973
    c. Low birth weight
    d. Short stature

174. Disodium dichloromethylene diphosphonate (Cl_2MDP):
    a. Prevents soft tissue calcification
    b. Is effective when administered orally   Ref. 127, 55-B:68, 69, 1973
    c. Inhibits bone resorption
    d. Does not inhibit cartilage and bone mineralization

175. Intravenous administration of calcium:
    a. Safely and rapidly corrects hypocalcemia of renal osteodystrophy
    b. Is warranted in emergencies such as   Ref. 127, 56-A:373, 374, 1974 acute hypocalcemic tetany or impending cardiac failure
    c. Can result in nephrocalcinosis
    d. Should never be considered, since it may result in vascular calcification and cardiac arrhythmias

176. The early response of bone to immobilization:
    a. Is a decrease in vascular flow and mineralization during the first 10 days
    b. Is an increase in vascular flow and   Ref. 127, 54-A:119, 1972 mineralization during the first 10 days
    c. Is the maintenance of normal vascular flow and mineralization during the first 10 days

    d. Is a decrease in vascular flow and miner-
      alization after the fifteenth day

177. Woven collagen:
    a. Must be absorbed for lamellar deposition
    b. Serves as a framework for lamellar depo-   **Ref. 106, 116:46, 1976**
      sition
    c. Is a sign of rapid collagen formation
    d. Is a sign of retarded collagen formation

178. In addition to hypogonadism and retarded growth, zinc deficiency may
    result in:
    a. Increased activation of serum alkaline
      phosphatase
    b. Ectopic bone formation   **Ref. 106, 103:225-228, 1974**
    c. Delayed bone healing
    d. Birth of congenitally malformed children

179. Allopurinol:
    a. Increases production of uric acid
    b. Decreases production of uric acid   **Ref. 102, p. 550**
    c. Decreases total purine synthesis
    d. Increases total purine synthesis

SITUATION AND PROGRESSIVE THOUGHT (answers on p. 284)

Select the answer or answers that best apply in accordance with the information given in the following statements.

180. A 33-year-old white woman complains of pain over her left distal thigh.
    She gives a history of progressive anorexia, constipation, and polyuria.
    She complains of flank pain and muscle weakness. The serum calcium
    is elevated. Which of the following is the least likely?
    a. Vitamin D intoxication
    b. Multiple myeloma   **Ref. 22, pp. 1291, 1360, 1760-1761,**
    c. Hyperthyroidism   **1848-1849, 1581**
    d. Porphyria

181. On physical examination a tender thickening over the distal femur is
    noted. X-ray films reveal generalized porosis, with a lytic lesion of the
    distal femur and marked expansion of the thin cortex. The epiphysis is
    involved. The alkaline phosphatase is elevated. The elevated alkaline
    phosphatase tends to rule out:
    a. Paget's disease
    b. Multiple myeloma   **Ref. 22, p. 1581**
    c. Hyperparathyroidism
    d. Severe osteomalacia

182. A biopsy of the lesion of the distal femur shows a microscopic picture
    of an abundance of giant cells in a benign fibrous tissue stroma with
    altered blood pigments. The diagnosis is:
    a. Osteitis fibrosa cystica generalisata
    b. Osteitis fibrosa cystica disseminata   **Ref. 5, pp. 447-452**
    c. Giant cell tumor of bone
    d. Aneurysmal bone cyst

183. The treatment of choice is:
    a. Amputation at a high thigh level
    b. Removal of the parathyroid adenoma(s)   **Ref. 6, pp. 680-690**
    c. Curettement and packing of the lesion   **Ref. 22, p. 1850**
       with bone chips
    d. Radiation therapy to the involved area
184. A 57-year-old widow who lived alone was found semicomatose at the
    bottom of the stairs in her home. She reported she had fallen, probably
    2 days prior. A card in her purse identified her as a diabetic. She was
    tachypneic, had parched lips, and a smell of vomitus. The right lower
    limb was externally rotated and shortened, and there was a huge bruise
    over the thigh. X-ray films revealed a severe comminuted intertrochan-
    teric fracture. There was no evidence of trauma about the head. To
    best determine the acid-base status of the patient, place the following
    studies in the order of clinical usefulness.
    a. Carbon dioxide concentration and pH of
       venous blood plasma
    b. Plasma pH only   **Ref. 44, p. 114**
    c. Carbon dioxide concentration and pH of
       arterial blood plasma
    d. Alkali reserve
    e. Carbon dioxide concentration of plasma
       only
185. The blood sugar was drawn stat and was found to be 340 mg/100 ml.
    The other plasma chemistry findings would be expected to show:
    a. Lowered pH and elevated bicarbonate
       and carbon dioxide levels
    b. Lowered pH, bicarbonate, and carbon   **Ref. 44, pp. 97-98**
       dioxide levels
    c. Lowered carbon dioxide levels and ele-
       vated bicarbonate and pH levels
    d. Elevated pH and carbon dioxide levels
       and lowered bicarbonate
186. These findings and this history are a typical example of:
    a. An uncompensated metabolic acidosis
    b. A compensating respiratory acidosis super-   **Ref. 44, pp. 69-70, 97-98**
       imposed on metabolic acidosis
    c. A compensating metabolic acidosis super-
       imposed on a respiratory acidosis
    d. A compensating respiratory alkalosis su·
       perimposed on a metabolic acidosis
187. In the renal compensation of acid-base balance:
    a. The amount of acid excreted by the
       kidney can be calculated by knowing the
       pH and the 24-hour urine volume
    b. Passing of bicarbonate ion into the urine   **Ref. 44, pp. 82-92**
       is depended on extensively in the control
       of metabolic acidosis

c. Phosphate is utilized as the primary buffer

d. The quantity of ammonium ions increases proportionately to the rise in the pH of alkaline urine

188. A 7-year-old adopted white girl comes to the clinic with the complaint of muscle weakness and "numbness" of the fingers and hands. When exposed to cold, the exposed parts became "stiff" and the child is unable to move them. When eating ice cream or cold drinks, her throat and mouth will not function until allowed to warm. The most likely diagnosis would be:

a. Duchenne-type muscular dystrophy

b. Limb-girdle muscular dystrophy   Ref. 13, p. 244

c. Polymyositis   Ref. 29, p. 306

d. Paramyotonia congenita

189. The electromyogram for this disease would be expected:

a. To have a characteristic "dive bomber" sound

b. To show spontaneous fibrillation   Ref. 7, 16:250, 1959

c. To show no muscle activity   Ref. 13, p. 245

d. To show increased amplitude fasciculations

190. The most useful serum enzyme(s) used in the diagnosis of muscular dystrophy is (are):

a. Creatine-kinase

b. Phosphohexoisomerase   Ref. 29, p. 60

c. Aldolase

d. Lactic dehydrogenase

191. In the muscular dystrophies _____ urinary excretion is (are) decreased, whereas _____ excretion is (are) increased.

a. Creatinine

b. Creatine   Ref. 29, p. 74

c. Both

d. Neither

192. The affected child is known to have an unaffected brother. Assuming both were to marry normal mates, which of the following could be said?

a. Chances of affected offspring would be equal for both.

b. Fifty percent of the sister's offspring would   Ref. 13, p. 244 be theoretically affected.

c. Affected offspring will have no sex predilection.

d. The brother will have no affected offspring.

193. A 3-year-old black boy has a history of a healing epiphyseal fracture of the distal femur and a questionable bone growth disturbance. X-ray films of the long bones show general loss of mineralization and marked thinning of the cortex. There is abundant callous formation on the side of the fracture. This picture would be most compatible with:
   a. Morquio's disease
   b. Recently treated scurvy   Ref. 5, p. 373
   c. Achondroplasia
   d. Engelmann's disease

194. A biopsy of the distal femoral epiphysis was made on the uninjured side. Examination of the cortical bone showed an absence of haversian systems without normal lamellations and osteons. The osteoid seams were not unusually wide. The most probable diagnosis is:
   a. Vitamin D–resistant rickets
   b. Treated scurvy   Ref. 5, p. 158
   c. Osteomalacia
   d. Osteogenesis imperfecta

195. The epiphyseal area would be expected to show:
   a. Normal epiphyseal cartilage, chon-droblasts, and columnar formation; mineralization of the terminal inter-columnar chondroid bars; decreased osteoid, with a markedly diminished number of osteoblasts and osteoclasts; and decreased granulation tissue and persistence of the chondroblasts pushing into the metaphysis
   b. Normal epiphyseal cartilage to the zones of proliferation and columnar formation; marked irregularity at the spongiosa, with unorganized crowding of persistent mature chondroblasts ex-tending into the metaphysis; presence of an abundance of osteoid surrounding the islands of cartilage cells; and absence of a continuous line of provisional min-eralization

Ref. 5, pp. 132, 158, 375, 390
   c. Normal epiphyseal cartilage with normal chondroblasts and columnar formation; normal zone of provisional mineralization; and normal enchondral bone formation
   d. A narrowed epiphyseal plate; de-creased number of chondroblasts in disarray without evidence of progres-sive columnar formation or normal maturation; and random but scanty osteoid production and mineralization

196. This physiologic growth defect is primarily due to:
     a. Absence of adequate vitamin C
     b. Retarded rate of chondroblast prolifera-   **Ref. 5, pp. 153-161**
        tion and orderly cartilage formation
     c. Retarded rate of osteoblast proliferation
        and orderly osteoid formation
     d. Delayed rate and inability of the system to
        mineralize osteoid

197. The serum electrolyte pattern would be expected to show:
     a. Normal calcium and phosphorus and
        marked elevation of the alkaline phos-
        phatase
     b. Normal calcium, phosphorus, and alkaline   **Ref. 22, p. 1875**
        phosphatase
     c. Elevated calcium and alkaline phospha-
        tase and decreased phosphorus
     d. Decreased calcium and phosphorus and
        normal or slightly elevated alkaline phos-
        phatase

198. A patient with abnormal serum calcium and phosphorous levels was
     explored surgically for suspected parathyroid dysfunction. A somewhat
     enlarged gland was removed that showed upon frozen section monoto-
     nous sheets of large cells with distinct limiting membranes, dark-staining
     eccentrically placed nuclei, and almost clear cytoplasm. This would be
     most compatible with:
     a. Idiopathic (primary) parathyroid hyper-
        plasia
     b. Parathyroid adenoma   **Ref. 5, p. 452**
     c. Secondary parathyroid hyperplasia
     d. Pseudohypoparathyroidism

199. On receiving the pathologist's report, the surgeon should:
     a. Transplant the remainder of the tissue
        back within the neck
     b. Feel satisfied that the offending tissue has   **Ref. 5, p. 454**
        been removed and close the wound
     c. Carry out a radical neck dissection
     d. Dissect and remove the remaining glands

TRUE OR FALSE (answers on pp. 284-285)

200. The cell membrane is polarized, with the negative charge maintained
     on the outside and the positive charge inside.   **Ref. 57, p. 12**
     (T) (F)

201. The use of irradiated homogenous nerve grafts to replace peripheral
     nerve defects in dogs has not proved fruitful because of excessive for-
     eign body response and scar tissue formation.
     (T) (F)   **Ref. 127, 46-A:391-394, 1964**

202. Creatine and creatinine studies on urine and serum will not specifically differentiate neurogenic muscle disease from the progressive dystrophies. **Ref. 29, p. 52**
(T) (F)

203. There is well-substantiated evidence that estrogen in human beings acts as a stimulus to new lamellar bone formation. **Ref. 55, p. 44**
(T) (F)

204. Although many enzymes have been described within normal synovial fluid, hyaluronidase is not one of them. **Ref. 127, 46-A:879, 1964**
(T) (F)

205. Experimental ligation of the nutrient artery of the long bones in dogs would be expected to significantly lower the intramedullary pressure indefinitely. **Ref. 127, 46-A:787, 1964**
(T) (F)

206. Pseudohypoparathyroidism is synonymous with vitamin D–resistant rickets. **Ref. 5, pp. 410, 457**
(T) (F)

207. Excess vitamin C within the diet is known to produce severe toxic effects. **Ref. 22, p. 1447**
(T) (F)

208. Normal uric acid levels tend to be slightly higher in men than women.
(T) (F) **Ref. 104, p. 58**

209. Vitamin K would be effective in correcting a coagulation defect of blood secondary to administration of heparin. **Ref. 22, p. 1612**
(T) (F)

210. Collagen is considered a viable metabolizing constituent of the extracellular body compartment. **Ref. 55, p. 12**
(T) (F)

211. Primary gout is an inherited disease manifested as a congenital disturbance in uric acid metabolism. **Ref. 5, p. 729**
(T) (F)

212. Leukotoxin is believed to be an important component in the second collagen phase of wound healing. **Ref. 6, p. 11**
(T) (F)

213. With continued adequate doses of colchicine, serum uric acid levels would be expected to return to normal. **Ref. 104, p. 71**
(T) (F)

214. Effusion and increased intercapsular pressure with the knee joint causes a marked loss of effective quadriceps muscle control. This mechanism probably utilizes the pathways of the "inverse stretch reflex."
(T) (F) **Ref. 57, p. 68**
Ref. 127, 47-A:321, 1965

215. The presence of alkaline phosphatase is necessary for active mineralization of bone matrix. **Ref. 62, p. 219**
(T) (F)

216. It has been demonstrated that osteoclasts carry out bone destruction by phagocytosis. **Ref. 28, p. 714**
(T) (F)

217. Human growth hormone has been effective in significantly stimulating the growth of hypopituitary dwarfs.   Ref. 62, p. 308
     (T) (F)

218. Experimental evidence indicates that creatinuria in the muscular dystrophies is the result of a decreased normal metabolizing muscle mass rather than the cause.   Ref. 29, p. 75
     (T) (F)

219. Salicylates are known to enhance the uricosuric action of Benemid and may be used as adjuvant treatment.   Ref. 83, p. 82
     (T) (F)

220. Neurogenic muscle disease cannot be differentiated from the progressive muscular dystrophies by serum enzyme studies.   Ref. 29, p. 77
     (T) (F)

221. The older terms "renal rickets" and "secondary hyperparathyroidism" are synonymous.   Ref. 5, p. 399
     (T) (F)

222. Serum enzymes will be normal in the relatives of patients with progressive muscular dystrophy unless they too have clinical evidence of the disease.   Ref. 29, p. 69
     (T) (F)

223. The normal aging process has been found to significantly and predictably alter the organic components of human articular cartilage, predisposing it to degenerative arthritic changes.   Ref. 127, 46-A:1181-1183, 1964
     (T) (F)

224. Synovial fluid studies would seem to indicate that alkaline phosphatase is rarely elevated in association with destructive arthritic processes, whereas the opposite is true with acid phosphatase.
     (T) (F)   Ref. 127, 46-A:1737, 1964

225. The presence in fracture callus of multiple enzymes important in carbohydrate metabolism indicates that bone repair is dependent on carbohydrate metabolism to obtain structural intermediates and energy.
     (T) (F)   Ref. 106, 107:262, 1975

226. The incidence of osteomalacia in postgastrectomy patients has been found to be greater than that of the general public.
     (T) (F)   Ref. 132, 3-3:642, 1972

227. An increase in dietary calcium decreases the dietary requirement of zinc.   Ref. 106, 103:214, 1974
     (T) (F)

228. Lysosomes are located in increased number in rheumatoid synovium.
     (T) (F)   Ref. 127, 55-B:88, 1973

229. In animals, exogenous calcitonin counteracts the deleterious effects of cortisone on the skeleton.   Ref. 106, 90:208, 1973
     (T) (F)

230. Inhibition of collagen synthesis by proline analogues may prove to be beneficial in reducing tendinous scar formation in the future.
     (T) (F)   Ref. 127, 54-A:1507, 1972

231. Maffuci's syndrome dysplasia has not been known to undergo sarcomatous transformation.   Ref. 127, 55-A:1465, 1973
     (T) (F)

232. Urinary cyclic AMP (cyclic adenosine-3,5-monophosphate) is valuable in distinguishing between hypoparathyroidism and pseudohypoparathyroidism.   Ref. 132, 3-3:632, 1972
(T) (F)

233. Migratory polyarthritis is not commonly associated with idiopathic hemochromatosis.   Ref. 127, 55-A:1077, 1973
(T) (F)

234. Due to its effect on hepatic iron concentration, allopurinol should not be administered to immediate relatives of patients with idiopathic hemochromatosis.   Ref. 87, p. 685
(T) (F)

LIST (answers on pp. 285-286)

235. List six ways in which osteoporosis may theoretically occur.
                                                    Ref. 55, pp. 43, 84

236. List three common mechanisms by which diuresis occurs and give an example of a therapeutic agent to enhance each type of action.
                                                    Ref. 59, pp. 840-850

237. List six general factors influencing wound healing.   Ref. 6, pp. 11-14

238. List six methods that have been used to physiologically stimulate bone growth through the epiphyses.   Ref. 62, p. 308
                                                    Ref. 127, 45-A:15, 1963

239. List eight tests that would constitute a thorough routine examination of synovial fluid in joint disease.   Ref. 125, 193:581, 1965
                                                    Ref. 127, 46-A:881-882, 1964

240. List five mechanisms of molecular transfer across cell membranes.
                                                    Ref. 54, p. 52

241. List five factors influencing absorption of calcium from the gut.
                                                    Ref. 5, p. 37

242. List three proposed areas in which vitamin D may affect serum calcium levels.   Ref. 5, p. 37

243. List four sites of action of parathyroid hormone in affecting serum electrolyte levels.   Ref. 62, p. 341

244. List six local factors influencing wound healing.   Ref. 6, pp. 14-18

245. List five pathologic laboratory findings that may result from multiple myeloma.   Ref. 22, pp. 1581-1582

246. List the four major amino acids occurring in collagen.   Ref. 55, p. 13

247. List three proposed theories concerning the etiology of acetabular cysts.
                                                    Ref. 5, p. 747
                                                    Ref. 127, 45-A:682-686, 1963

248. List three forms in which radiation energy may be emitted from an isotope in the order of their magnitude, starting with the strongest. Identify the component particles in each form.
                                                    Ref. 127, 45-A:1070, 1963

249. List four methods or techniques frequently employed in the biologic assay or measurement of in vivo or in vitro radioactive materials.
                                                    Ref. 127, 45-A:1073, 1963

SECTION 9

Prosthetics and orthotics

JOHN GLANCY, C.O., and FLOYD G. GOODMAN, B.S., M.D.

MULTIPLE CHOICE, SINGLE ANSWER (answers on pp. 286-287)

Select the *one* answer that will best complete or answer each of the following statements or questions.

1. When the hand is in the position of function:
   a. The thumb is fully opposed
   b. The position of the hand is the same as at rest   Ref. 30, p. 10
   c. The wrist is at neutral position
   d. The thumb is in anatomic position
2. To duplicate the function of pinch (palmar prehension), the terminal device must open approximately:
   a. ¾ inch
   b. 1½ inches   Ref. 47, p. 114
   c. 2½ inches
   d. 3 inches
3. The average force used for carrying out pinch (palmar prehension) is:
   a. 1 pound
   b. 3 pounds   Ref. 47, p. 107
   c. 15 pounds
   d. 20 pounds
4. The terminal device in the upper extremity prosthesis attempts to duplicate:
   a. Push, pull, and pinch
   b. Pinch, pull, and grasp   Ref. 47, pp. 107-109
   c. Pinch, hook, and grasp
   d. Push, grasp, and hook
5. The Swanson postoperative hand splint was developed especially for:
   a. The surgical reconstruction of hands that have been severely crushed
   b. Finger joint arthroplasties, utilizing silicone rubber implants, for the arthritic hand   Ref. 124, 10:1-7, 1971

193

c. Any surgical procedure to the hand that requires dynamic finger-extension assist following the surgery

d. Any surgical procedure to the hand that requires dynamic finger-flexion assist following the surgery

6. A patient with a below-knee (BK) and patellar tendon-bearing (PTB) prosthesis was found to "drop off" (a shortening of the weight-bearing period, with quick accentuated knee flexion) at the time of "toe off." Which of the following would be an unlikely cause?

   a. Toe lever arm too short
   b. Flexible toe worn out   **Ref. 99, pp. 130-131**
   c. Keel length too short
   d. Overpull of the quadriceps muscle group

7. The only prosthesis in which flexion of the knee at "heel strike" is desirable is:

   a. Standard AK prosthesis
   b. Standard BK prosthesis   **Ref. 45, 37:43, 1964**
   c. PTB prosthesis
   d. Canadian hip-disarticulation prosthesis

8. The wrist-disarticulation amputee has a decided advantage over the medium below-elbow (BE) amputee because:

   a. Wrist flexion and extension are easily conserved
   b. Wrist flexion, extension, and radial and   **Ref. 15, p. 42**
      ulnar deviation are conserved
   c. Complete pronation and supination may be maintained
   d. Even though only about 60% of pronation and supination are maintained, these movements are important

9. The Dorrance 5X A terminal device refers to a:

   a. 5-inch opening split hook controlled with a cross strap anteriorly
   b. 5-inch opening split hook made of xenon   **Ref. 23, p. 79**
      alloy   **Ref. 120, 7-2:28, 1963**
   c. 5-digit prosthetic hand with thumb adduction
   d. Model No. 5 aluminum split hook, with a neoprene rubber insert

10. The replacement prosthesis for a 40-year-old housewife with a wrist disarticulation should:

    a. Be fitted about 10 days after surgery to eliminate troublesome postoperative edema
    b. Include a saddle-type harness to give her   **Ref. 15, p. 42**
       necessary maximum support

c. Include a strap-type elbow hinge to allow supination and pronation

d. Have a two-to-one step-up hinge to gain maximum flexion

11. The APRL replacement prosthesis name is derived from:
    a. Above-palm replacement loss
    b. Army Prosthetics Research Laboratories
    c. Atlantic and Pacific Rehabilitation Laboratories
    d. Angulation, pronation, rotation, and lamination

    Ref. 47, p. 110
    Ref. 79, p. 94

12. The APRL replacement prosthesis is:
    a. A voluntary opening and closing device
    b. The best known voluntary closing device
    c. A voluntary opening and automatic closing device
    d. The most popular terminal device

    Ref. 47, p. 111
    Ref. 79, p. 94

13. The split-hook terminal devices are:
    a. Unsatisfactory for heavy work
    b. Inefficient, requiring 10 pounds of pull for 1 pound of applied opening force
    c. The most efficient and will carry out all major functions
    d. Made only of stainless steel

    Ref. 15, p. 34
    Ref. 108, p. 34

14. Approximately 90% of hand function consists of:
    a. Hook
    b. Grasp
    c. Hook and grasp
    d. Palmar prehension (pinch)

    Ref. 47, p. 108
    Ref. 127, 45-A:933, 1963

15. The limb-deficient child requiring a prosthesis is best fitted:
    a. Before 1 year of age
    b. 18 to 24 months of age
    c. 3 to 4 years of age
    d. When he starts school

    Ref. 24, p. 63
    Ref. 108, p. 47

16. The congenital limb-deficient child is more likely to have involvement of:
    a. The left upper extremity over the right upper extremity by a 3 to 1 ratio
    b. The right upper extremity over the left upper extremity by a 3 to 1 ratio
    c. Both extremities about equally
    d. The lower extremities more frequently than upper extremities

    Ref. 24, p. 20

17. The AK suction socket is designed for major weight-bearing distribution to the:
    a. Soft tissues of the stump and thigh
    b. Ischial tuberosity
    c. Terminal end of the stump
    d. Terminal end of the stump and thigh

    Ref. 7, 7:232, 1950
    Ref. 108, p. 29

18. The AK amputee obtains greater power from the hamstrings and the abductors by fitting the amputation stump in:
    a. Slight extension and abduction
    b. Slight abduction and flexion   Ref. 15, pp. 310, 314
    c. Slight flexion and adduction   Ref. 79, pp. 84-85
    d. Slight flexion and external rotation

19. The abductor muscles of the hip are relatively unimportant in the contour and shaping of the thigh piece of the AK amputation prosthesis because:
    a. The abductors are above the level of the prosthesis socket
    b. They are unimportant in the gait of the   Ref. 15, p. 310
       AK amputee on the side of the prosthesis   Ref. 45, 37:39, 1964
    c. The quadrilateral socket automatically   Ref. 79, p. 85
       compensates for them
    d. None of the above

20. The anterior wall of the AK suction socket is depressed over the femoral vessels and nerves and:
    a. Provides protection for the femoral vessels and nerves
    b. Provides pressure, forcing the posterior   Ref. 15, pp. 299-300
       rim of the socket under the ischial   Ref. 45, 37:35, 1964
       tuberosity   Ref. 79, p. 84
    c. Provides stability by pressure against the tensor fasciae latae muscle
    d. Is of major importance to maintain the thigh in an adducted position

21. "Twisters" would be expected to be of greatest value in a brace for a patient with:
    a. Myelomeningocele
    b. Poliomyelitis   Ref. 10, p. 529
    c. Cerebral palsy   Ref. 127, 44-A:1466-1468, 1962
    d. Friedreich's ataxia

22. A BK amputee at midstance is found to have lateral bending of his body toward the side of amputation, with excessive deviation of his head toward the same side (greater than 1 inch). Which of the following is unlikely to be the cause?
    a. Prosthesis too long
    b. Hip abductor pathology or weakness   Ref. 79, p. 151
    c. Prosthetic foot set out too far laterally   Ref. 99, p. 130
    d. Prosthesis too short

23. The rigid, molded, polypropylene, BK orthosis is steadily becoming the orthosis of choice for bracing the flail foot-ankle complex in children with myelomeningocele. This is because:
    a. It has superior strength compared with metal braces
    b. It prevents unwanted motion in all   Ref. 127, 56-A:556-563, 1974
       three planes   Ref. 134, 26:14-16, 1972

c. It is able to support the shoe in stance
   phase.
d. It is easier to fabricate than is a metal
   brace

24. When prescribing a solid-ankle polypropylene BK orthosis for the patient whose knees and hips are symptom free, a smooth heel-toe gait can be facilitated by specifying in your prescription which of the following?
    a. The addition of a crepe sole to the shoe
    b. An orthopaedic shoe with a steel shank   Ref. 133, 13-4:37-38, 1959
    c. Lowering the heel on the involved side
       ¼ inch
    d. A cushion heel and rocker bar to the shoe

25. A 24-year-old man is fitted with a PTB prosthesis for a BK amputation. At midstance he is found to have an excessively wide base to his gait (greater than 2 inches). Which of the following is unlikely to be the cause?
    a. Hip abductor pathology or weakness
    b. Prosthesis too long   Ref. 79, p. 151
    c. Prosthetic foot outset too far laterally   Ref. 99, p. 130
    d. Prosthetic foot inset too far medially

26. The earliest recorded mechanical treatment of congenital clubfeet by molding and binding in a corrected position dates back to:
    a. Hippocrates (400 BC)
    b. Ambroise Paré (14th century)   Ref. 9, p. 485
    c. Scarpa (1781)
    d. Henry Neil (1825)

27. During "heel rise" a BK amputee with a PTB prosthesis is noted to go into knee extension. He complains of "unusual anterior knee pressure and difficulty going up inclines." Which of the following is unlikely to be the cause?
    a. Toe lever arm too long
    b. Shoe too tight on SACH type of foot, not   Ref. 79, p. 152
       allowing toe flexion   Ref. 99, pp. 130-131
    c. Toe lever arm too short
    d. Insufficient initial socket flexion

28. The polypropylene dorsiflexion-assist BK orthosis is not prescribed for the foot-ankle complex when the following is present:
    a. Paresis
    b. Paralysis   Ref. 134, 27-2:28, 1973
    c. Paresis with mild spasticity
    d. Paralysis with severe spasticity

29. The Denis Browne splint was originally devised for the correction of:
    a. Internal torsion of the tibia
    b. Congenital dislocation of the hip   Ref. 9, p. 485
    c. Equinus deformity in cerebral palsy
    d. Congenital clubfeet

30. Weak lumbricals in the presence of strong extensor digitorum communis would call for a basic opponens hand splint with the:
    a. Metacarpophalangeal extension assist
    b. Dynamic finger flexion assist **Ref. 14, p. 41**
    c. Lumbrical bar or metacarpophalangeal stop
    d. First dorsal interosseous assist

31. For the C-6 level quadriplegic with a wrist-driven hand orthosis, achieving optimum function and comfort can be difficult because:
    a. The extensor carpi radialis is rarely sufficiently innervated to provide adequate power for the orthosis to convert wrist extension to functional prehension
    b. Often the weight of the orthosis is more of a burden than a help to the patient, since he finds it too difficult to flex the wrist when wearing it
    c. Sometimes the flexor carpi radialis is also innervated and its activity tends to interfere with the function of the orthosis
    d. The stronger the extensor carpi radialis, the more forcefully the hand is pulled into radial deviation, thus causing malalignment between the hand and the orthosis

    Ref. 76, p. 213
    Ref. 100, p. 529, 1973

32. Edema of the stump on a person who wears a suction socket is a sign that the:
    a. Superior brim of the socket is not fitted snugly
    b. Socket is too tight on the distal part of the stump
    c. Superior brim of the socket is too high
    d. Venous return is restricted by a too tightly fitting socket

    Ref. 24, p. 184
    Ref. 99, pp. 114-148

33. The PTB orthosis is available with metal ankle joints or as a solid-ankle all-plastic unit. The orthosis of choice for a young adult male who has a delayed union fracture at midshaft of the tibia (due to a gunshot wound received six months ago) would be:
    a. The all-plastic solid-ankle PTB to ensure complete unweighting of the distal portion of the tibia below the fracture site
    b. The PTB with metal side bars and ankle joints limited to 5° of dorsiflexion and 5° of plantar flexion
    c. The PTB with free motion ankle joints, fitted to permit partial weight bearing on the foot

    Ref. 127, 49-A:874, 1967
    Ref. 127, 52-A:308, 1970
    Ref. 134, 28-4:5-11, 1974

    d. The all-plastic solid-ankle PTB to prevent
       motion in the ankle and subtalar joints
       and to ensure protection of the fracture
       site

34. The University of California Biomechanical Laboratory (UC-BL) shoe
    insert is used to treat foot conditions whose primary need is control of:
    a. Floor reaction forces
    b. Fixed valgus   **Ref. 122, 10-11:143-144, 1969**
    c. Lateral sheer forces   **Ref. 78, pp. 1-19, 1969**
    d. Force at "heel strike"

35. If suction suspension in the AK amputee is inadequate, the first auxil-
    liary suspension that should be tried is a:
    a. Rigid hip pelvic belt
    b. Shoulder harness   **Ref. 15, p. 343**
    c. Silesian bandage   **Ref. 108, p. 28**
    d. Flexible pelvic belt

36. The Milwaukee type of scoliosis brace achieves its effect primarily
    through:
    a. Constant thoracic pressure
    b. Traction   **Ref. 7, 16:210, 211, 1959**
    c. The wearer's postural reaction   **Ref. 127, 52-A:498-506, 1970**
    d. Immobilization after correction

37. The Glanbitz shoe modification is prescribed for:
    a. The cerebral palsy or myelomeningocele
       child with forefoot equinus or "drop"
    b. The cerebral palsy child with contracture   **Ref. 133, 12-1:21, 1958**
       of the Achilles tendon
    c. The myelomeningocele child with equino
       valgus foot
    d. The myelomeningocele child with a cal-
       caneous gait

38. The double-action ankle joint is the component of choice when brac-
    ing the traumatic paraplegic because it offers:
    a. Less motion in the anteroposterior plane
       when standing
    b. Clinical adjustability for setting optimum   **Ref. 134, 25-4:17, 1971**
       anteroposterior balance
    c. The durability of broader wearing surfaces
    d. A more positive anterior stop for swing-
       through gait

39. The basic philosophy of orthotic functional bracing and splinting is to:
    a. Correct preexisting deformities such as
       contractures
    b. Immobilize the diseased or healing parts   **Ref. 30, p. 180**
    c. Provide stability for the temporarily disabled part
    d. Provide better functional position and
       power to the long-term disabled patient or
       extremity

40. The basic opponens hand splint is a satisfactory functional splint:
    a. For loss of abduction and extension of the thumb
    b. For radial nerve palsy   Ref. 14, p. 41
    c. Following traumatic amputation of the thumb
    d. When there is absence of active thumb opposition but presence of abduction and extension

41. The straight-hook, noncanted, lyre-shaped terminal device is preferable in most cases to the canted terminal device because:
    a. It allows better grasp of round objects
    b. It performs the function of "hook" better   Ref. 47, pp. 109-110
    c. It allows the amputee to carry out farm and heavy work more efficiently
    d. The statement is false, since canted terminal devices are preferable except in approximately 8% of patients who usually do desk work

42. A patient with an AK amputation fitted with a quadrilateral, total-contact suction socket is found to drop off at "heel off" position. An unlikely cause would be:
    a. Toe lever arm too short on SACH foot
    b. Toe break too far posterior on conven-   Ref. 40, p. 9
       tional foot   Ref. 79, p. 160
    c. Socket placed too far forward at knee
    d. Dorsal stop bumper too strong or toe break too far anterior on conventional foot

43. The conventional foot and ankle:
    a. Depend on compressible rubber bumpers for dorsiflexion and plantar flexion
    b. Allow inversion and eversion   Ref. 15, p. 368
    c. Have no ankle motion but allow cushioning at "heel strike" and toe flexion at "toe off"
    d. Give good ankle contour for women in high heels

44. The contour of the abdominal panel of the molded girdle of the Milwaukee scoliosis brace increases abdominal pressure, and in so doing it:
    a. Utilizes the increased pressure to reduce lordosis
    b. Adds to the mediolateral stabilization of   Ref. 76, p. 292
       the spinal column
    c. Adds to the ability of the neck ring to unweight the spinal column
    d. Provides a flat surface for the attachment of the anterior bar

45. The foot that cannot dorsiflex beyond the neutral position, i.e., 90° to the tibia, is subject to abnormal stress beyond midstance because:
    a. It delays heel rise by as much as 90%
    b. The tibia cannot rotate forward its normal   **Ref. 133, 13-4:38, 1959**
       15° prior to heel rise   **Ref. 8, 20:138, 1971**
    c. The patient must substitute by internally rotating the foot
    d. The patient must substitute by circumducting the foot
46. The major cause of lower extremity amputation is:
    a. Atherosclerosis
    b. Atherosclerosis with diabetes   **Ref. 82, pp. 22-23**
    c. Trauma
    d. Tumor
    e. Infection
47. Oxygen consumption studies have shown that the normal well-fitted AK amputee walking at moderate speed requires:
    a. Approximately 20% less energy than does a normal person
    b. Requires 5% less energy than does a   **Ref. 82, p. 147**
       normal person
    c. Requires the same amount of energy as does a normal person
    d. Requires about 20% more energy than does a normal person
48. The well-fitted AK amputee would have difficulty walking forward upstream while trout fishing because:
    a. Hip musculature would be nonfunctional in manipulating the thigh socket
    b. The force of the current would not   **Ref. 15, p. 358**
       allow gravity and momentum to carry   **Ref. 120, 7-2:20-21, 1963**
       the lower limb segment of the prosthesis forward
    c. It is impossible for AK amputees to walk on the rough ground encountered in trout streams
    d. The distal segment of the AK prosthesis has a specific gravity of less than 1 and would float
49. Rotation of the foot is noted at the time of "heel strike" in an AK amputee fitted with a quadrilateral suction socket. The most likely cause would be:
    a. Heel too stiff on a SACH foot or plantar bumper too stiff on a conventional foot
    b. Toe lever arm too long   **Ref. 40, p. 4**
    c. Heel too soft on a SACH foot   **Ref. 79, p. 158**
    d. Toe break too far posterior

50. Knee stability in the geriatric AK amputee:
    a. Presents its greatest problem at "toe off"
    b. Is no longer a problem since the intro- Ref. 82, pp. 75-77, 88-89
       duction of the hydraulic knee, which is
       now prescribed almost routinely
    c. Is usually not a problem if good quad-
       riceps tone is maintained in the preop-
       erative and postoperative periods
    d. Is aided at "heel strike" by a soft plantar
       flexion bumper or a soft heel on the
       SACH foot

51. The abducted gait in the AK amputee with a quadrilateral suction socket
    would probably not result from:
    a. Crotch galling (painful raw areas) due to
       inadequately compensated hip flexion con-
       tractures or the ischium slipping off the
       seat
    b. Prosthesis too long   Ref. 7, 7:235, 1950
    c. Prosthesis too short   Ref. 40, p. 3
    d. Terminal stump pain   Ref. 79, p. 159

52. A smooth noiseless deceleration period of the swing phase is desirable
    for the AK amputee; however, if excessive terminal impact occurs, it
    is unlikely to be caused from:
    a. Increased shank velocity due to improper
       gait habit or excessive knee extension aid
    b. Increased shank velocity due to a light-   Ref. 40, p. 7
       friction setting   Ref. 79, p. 162
    c. The older amputee receiving reassurance   Ref. 120, 7-2:20, 1963
       that the knee is fully extended from the
       impact
    d. Friction set too heavy on conventional
       constant-friction knee unit

53. Lateral trunk bend toward the side of the prosthesis at midstance in the
    AK amputee would probably not result from:
    a. Inadequate adduction of the socket wall
    b. Prosthesis too short   Ref. 7, 7:235, 1950
    c. Foot outset too far   Ref. 40, p. 2
    d. Pain over the lateral proximal femoral
       area

54. A lateral gape at the outer brim of the PTB socket would probably not
    result from:
    a. Foot inset too far
    b. Stump shrinkage   Ref. 99, p. 86
    c. Excess lateromedial tilt of the socket
    d. Foot outset too far laterally

55. A 25-year-old man has a high AK amputation. The stump extends only 1½ inches below the level of the perineum. The stump has good contour and no deep crevices, scars, or contractures. There is some conjecture among the clinic team as to the type of appliance because of the short stump. The best prescription would be:
   a. A saucer-type prosthesis
   b. A Canadian hip socket molded to accom-   **Ref. 120, 4-2:61-63, 1957**
      modate the hip in full flexion
   c. To resect the distal 3 inches of bony
      stump and then fit with a Canadian hip
      prosthesis, using the usual molded socket
   d. Quadrilateral suction socket

56. The Canadian hip prosthesis has been relatively successful because:
   a. The hip joint is placed at the same level,
      both vertically and horizontally, as the
      acetabulum
   b. The hip joint is placed anteriorly, utilizing   **Ref. 79, p. 114**
      a 2½- to 3½-inch horizontal shaft, giving   **Ref. 120, 4-2:27, 32, 1957**
      superior strength and contributing to
      knee stability
   c. The hip joint is multicentric, dividing the
      stress equally among two or more centers
      of rotation
   d. The hip joint is a variation from the tilt-
      ing-table prosthesis, utilizing the track
      and roller joint and allowing a smooth,
      flowing gait.

57. The paraplegic with iliopsoas muscle control intact (L-3 level) would be expected to carry out:
   a. Physiologic ambulation only with long-leg
      braces and crutches
   b. Functional ambulation with long-leg   **Ref. 67, Appendix C**
      braces and crutches
   c. Brace-free ambulation
   d. Functional ambulation with short-leg
      braces and crutches

58. Recent studies in the treatment of leg fractures would tend to substantiate that _____ is the treatment of choice.
   a. Bed rest followed by cast immobilization,
      crutch walking, and nonweight bearing
   b. Early ambulation in a walking long-leg   **Ref. 106, 66:159-172, 1969**
      cast progressing to immediate full weight   **Ref. 127, 49-A:855, 1967**
      bearing
   c. Open reduction and plate fixation
   d. Intermedullary fixation

59. Which of the following statements is believed true concerning the limb-deficient child?
    a. Training should start at about 3 years of age.
    b. Training should start with detailed coun- **Ref. 120, 10:36-50, 1966**
       seling of the parents shortly after birth.
    c. Upper extremity fitting should be initiated when the child has attained sitting balance.
    d. Development of foot activities and dexterity should not be encouraged, as this will detract from acceptance of the prosthesis in the upper extremity amelic child.

60. The quadriplegic patient most likely to benefit from a myoelectric control externally powered orthotic device would have a level of function:
    a. C-3 or above
    b. Elbow flexion only, C-5 or above **Ref. 67, p. 169, Appendix C**
    c. With good wrist extensors (C-6)
    d. Good wrist extension, fair triceps, but with absence of sublimis or profundus function (C-7)

MULTIPLE CHOICE, MULTIPLE ANSWERS (answers on p. 287)

Select one or more answers that will best complete or answer each of the following statements or questions.

61. Recent developments in plastic materials have resulted in dramatic increase in their orthotic use because of the following advantages:
    a. Intimate fit
    b. Light weight **Ref. 134, 26-1:14-18, 1972**
    c. Ease of cleaning **Ref. 127, 56-A:556-563, 1974**
    d. Improved cosmesis **Ref. 134, 29-1:5, 1975**

62. The UC-BL dual axis ankle control system is reported to have its main advantage in:
    a. Durability and maintenance of alignment
    b. Accommodating subtalor as well as **Ref. 122, 10-11:97-234, 1969**
       ankle joint motion
    c. Providing secure, stable push-off in absence of plantar flexion power
    d. Allowing increased freedom about the ankle with subjective reports of increased level of functional activity with decreased energy consumption

63. When bracing the child with Legg-Perthes disease, the involved femur should be held in:
    a. Slight external rotation
    b. 10° of abduction **Ref. 120, 2-2:37-39, 1968**
    c. 30° to 45° of abduction **Ref. 134, 22-2:51, 56, 1968**
    d. Internal rotation

64. Which of the following are the main advantages of Polysar in its recent application to prosthesis?
    a. Immediate formation of the socket
       directly on the stump is possible.
    b. Minor adjustments are easily carried   **Ref. 122, 10-11:83-89, 1969**
       out.
    c. It maintains shape and position well.
    d. Metal and other attachments hold
       securely.

65. Appropriate bracing for the paraplegic with iliopsoas function (L-3 level) would include:
    a. Drop-lock or bail-lock knee hinges
    b. Locked ankles   **Ref. 67, p. 171**
    c. One piece, extended foot plate and stirrup
    d. Allowing the center of gravity to fall pos-
       terior to the hip and knee joints and an-
       terior to the ankle joint to maintain inde-
       pendent balance

66. The paraplegic patient with abdominal musculature giving pelvic control (T-12 level) would be expected to carry out:
    a. A wheelchair existence without ability to
       stand or ambulate with braces or crutches
    b. Physiologic ambulation with aid of long-   **Ref. 67, Appendix C**
       leg braces and crutches
    c. Functional ambulation with short-leg
       braces and crutches
    d. Functional ambulation with long-leg
       braces without need for crutches

67. A well-fitting plastic torso jacket that provides increased abdominal intracavity pressure, bilateral "shelves" between the iliac crests and the rib cage, and effective control of lumbar lordosis, offers the most protection to a child's paralyzed lumbar region when standing or when seated? Why?
    a. When standing because the combination
       of the above components of the jacket
       partially unweights the lumbar spine by
       bypassing some of the weight of the
       thorax directly onto the pelvis and down
       to the floor via the lower limbs
    b. Equally effective whether standing or sit-   **Ref. 76, pp. 283-284, 293**
       ting because the components described   **Ref. 70, pp. 134-138**
       are constant factors of control to the
       lumbar region, regardless of the
       positioning of the lower limbs
    c. Less effective when seated because the
       lower limbs are no longer receiving the
       trunk's weight, and the lumbar region
       is then subjected to chair reaction forces
       through the pelvis

d. More effective when seated because when standing, unweighting of the lumbar spine is accomplished by the upper limbs via the child's crutches, and the jacket's contribution is therefore superfluous

68. Spinal supports in the form of a lumbrosacral corset or chairback brace have been found to:
    a. Alter the duration of the swing phase of gait
    b. Decrease muscle myoelectric activity of the back muscles during gait   **Ref. 127, 52-A:51-60, 1970**
    c. Increase the myoelectric activity during normal gait
    d. Have little effect on myoelectric activity of back muscles during normal gait

69. The anterior wall of the total-contact suction socket for the AK amputee should be _____ the medial wall and _____ the lateral wall in width.
    a. Lower than
    b. Higher than   **Ref. 15, p. 299**
    c. Wider than   **Ref. 79, p. 84**
    d. Narrower than

70. The total-contact quadrilateral AK suction socket:
    a. May allow the patient to be completely harness free
    b. Usually eliminates the formation of an adductor roll   **Ref. 24, p. 184**
    c. Tends to minimize the development of stump edema
    d. Requires daily cleansing of the valve

71. The constant-friction (conventional) knee:
    a. Is outmoded and seldom prescribed any more
    b. Has an adjustable tension screw that may be set with a special tool by the amputee   **Ref. 15, p. 360** **Ref. 120, 7-2:21, 1963**
    c. Is stable when standing because the axis of rotation is behind the TKA (trochanter, knee, ankle) line
    d. The most frequently prescribed knee prosthesis

72. The hydraulic knee and foot unit:
    a. Damps excess heel rise (flexion at knee) and decelerates the leg at "heel strike"
    b. Allows immediate knee flexion at "heel strike," with plantar flexion of the foot   **Ref. 16, p. 320**
    c. Dorsiflexes the foot in swing phase and allows plantar flexion when sitting
    d. Has adjustable control for heel height

73. Cineplasty, the use of a skin-lined tunnel through the belly of a muscle to provide motor power for prosthetic devices:
    a. Was popularized and improved by a German surgeon named Sauerbruch prior to and during World War I
    b. Is a recent idea since the Korean War that was popularized by Vanghetti and made possible by modern surgical techniques
    c. Works best on the lower extremity because of the tremendous power of the hamstrings
    d. Is usually reserved for BE amputees only, using the biceps muscle

    Ref. 30, p. 623
    Ref. 43, p. 879
    Ref. 108, p. 50
    Ref. 127, 40-A:1389-1400, 1958

74. It is generally agreed that cineplasty:
    a. Should be carried out at the 6- to 8-year age level when otherwise indicated
    b. Should not be carried out until ages 11 to 13 years
    c. Is of greatest benefit because of development of a sense of "fine pinch" and great power for heavy work with the APRL terminal device
    d. Is of particular advantage, as it requires no shoulder harness and can be used in nearly any position·

    Ref. 15, p. 115
    Ref. 23, pp. 161-163
    Ref. 24, p. 46
    Ref. 127, 39-A:59, 1957

75. Insufficient toe-out in the alignment of a well-fitting, AK brace will:
    a. Not cause any malpositioning as long as the brace is aligned to match the patient's external tibial torsion
    b. Cause the patient's foot to be held in varus when standing and sitting
    c. Force the foot into varus when the patient sits, which externally rotates the knee so that it can align itself with the mechanical knee joints
    d. Force the foot into valgus, which causes the knee to rotate internally between mid-stance and toe-off

    Ref. 8, 20:135-136, 1971

76. The functional long-leg brace is contraindicated in cases of:
    a. Severe trunk muscle weakness
    b. Flail hip
    c. Panarthrodesis
    d. Any severe bilateral involvement

    Ref. 45, 37:98-109, 1964

77. Basic studies on human locomotion report that transverse rotation of the tibia is directly related to the valgus/varus rotations of the foot during stance phase—one cannot occur without the other. Can the lack of ac-

commodation for external tibial torsion in a brace have any effect on these synchronous motions of the foot-ankle complex?

a. No, because the fit of the calf band, shoe, and uprights is not intimate enough to block transverse rotations of the tibia in stance phase

b. Yes, since the uprights are attached to the shoe, they serve to block the normal transverse rotation in a medial direction that occurs between heel strike and flat foot

Ref. 8, 20:134-135, 1971
Ref. 72, pp. 455-462
Ref. 122, 10-11:135, 1969

c. No, because the full magnitude of medial rotation of the tibia occurs during swing phase and therefore the brace cannot have any effect on this motion

d. Yes, since failure to accommodate forces the foot into a valgus position and prevents the abrupt reversal in direction of the foot and tibia that normally begins at midstance

78. The use of rigid splints following trauma or surgery of the hand is usually indicated in cases of:
a. Dupuytren's contracture
b. Fracture
c. Tendon repair
d. Skin grafting

Ref. 30, pp. 628-630

79. The chairback brace best limits:
a. Flexion
b. Extension
c. Lateral motion
d. Torsion

Ref. 9, p. 211

80. Initial flexion built into the AK amputee prosthetic socket:
a. Is bad for the gait pattern, hinders control of the prosthesis, and should be avoided whenever possible
b. Adds to voluntary knee control
c. Is primarily limited in amount by cosmesis
d. May be acceptable up to 30° to 35° in short amputee stumps

Ref. 15, pp. 313-315

81. An AK amputee fitted with a quadrilateral total-contact suction socket is noted to have excess lumbar lordosis at "heel off." A likely cause would be:
a. Hip flexion contracture without sufficient allowance in the socket
b. Painful ischial seat
c. Posterior displacement of shoulders for increased balance
d. Heel lever arm too long

Ref. 40, p. 9
Ref. 79, p. 160

82. The William's back brace is designed to:
    a. Prevent and correct lordosis
    b. Prevent flexion of the lower lumbar spine   Ref. 9, p. 213
    c. Give dorsolumbar support
    d. Prevent lateral movement in the lumbo-
       sacral area
83. The orthopaedic corset should:
    a. Have its greatest constriction at the waist
    b. Support and lift the abdomen   Ref. 9, p. 241
    c. Be well molded around the pelvis and buttocks
    d. Exert the greatest pressure posteriorly at
       the top and bottom
84. A cable-controlled hook:
    a. Cannot be used with a figure-of-eight har-
       ness
    b. Is contraindicated when there is lack of   Ref. 14, p. 349
       sensation in the involved extremity
    c. Is contraindicated in the presence of an
       uncontrolled flail shoulder and elbow
    d. May be useful to the patient with a para-
       lyzed hand
85. The thumb-post attachment to the basic opponens hand splint:
    a. Should not be used in the presence of
       spasticity or flaccidity
    b. Is indicated only where there is some pre-   Ref. 14, pp. 197-199
       existing muscle control
    c. Tends to immobilize the metacarpopha-
       langeal and interphalangeal joints, hold-
       ing the thumb in opposition with the pad
       exposed to the opposing surface of the
       index and middle fingers
    d. Provides fingernail prehension
86. A long opponens hand splint:
    a. Does not extend beyond the wrist
    b. Is helpful in controlling radial and ulnar   Ref. 14, p. 42
       deviation of the wrist
    c. Is helpful in controlling undesired flexion
       or extension at the wrist
    d. Is contraindicated when there is spasticity
       or flaccidity of the wrist flexors
87. Lateral prehension is carried out with the thumb _____ and pro-
    vides _____ than does ordinary pinch.
    a. Pressing against the radial side of the in-
       dex finger
    b. Opposing the tips of the index and ring   Ref. 30, p. 12
       fingers
    c. More strength
    d. Less strength

88. Large grasp is _____ and requires an opening of approximately _____.
   a. Used more frequently than fingertip pre-
      hension
   b. Used less frequently than palmar pre-   **Ref. 47, p. 114**
      hension
   c. 1½ inches
   d. 3 inches
89. A wrist flexor unit that allows up to 50° flexion of the terminal device:
   a. Is usually indicated in the unilateral wrist-
      disarticulation amputee
   b. Allows the bilateral amputee to button   **Ref. 120, 7-2:27, 31, 1963**
      his shirt, shave, etc.
   c. Is always needed by the unilateral BE
      amputee
   d. Is indicated in the shoulder-disarticulation
      amputee to compensate for loss of mobil-
      ity at the shoulder and elbow
90. The flexor hinge hand splint:
   a. May transfer power from wrist to fingers
   b. May transfer power from finger to finger   **Ref. 14, pp. 57-63**
   c. Stabilizes wrist, thumb, and interphalangeal
      joints, allowing motion only at the metacar-
      pophalangeal joints
   d. Rules out unwanted finger motion
91. The Munster-type elbow socket:
   a. Dates back to the Civil War and is now
      outmoded
   b. Is a preflexed form-fitted socket designed   **Ref. 23, p. 46**
      for the short BE amputee   **Ref. 120, 8-2:4-14, 1964**
   c. Uses a step-up elbow hinge
   d. Lacks stability but retains forearm prona-
      tion, supination, and flexion
92. Whip in the prosthetic foot of the AK amputee may:
   a. Result from socket rotation of more than 1
      inch on a loose fit of the stump
   b. Result from improper alignment of the   **Ref. 7, 7:235, 1950**
      knee joint axis   **Ref. 40, p. 8**
   c. Frequently result from a prosthesis that   **Ref. 79, p. 161**
      is too long
   d. Be a manifestation of faulty walking habits
93. Circumduction in the swing phase of the AK amputee:
   a. Is not uncommon with wooden sockets and
      may result from excess thickness of the
      medial brim
   b. May result from inadequate seating of the   **Ref. 7, 7:235, 1950**
      stump within the socket   **Ref. 40, p. 2**
   c. Could result from too much friction in the **Ref. 79, p. 161**

knee joint, causing the amputee to increase the swing of the prosthesis to gain extension

d. Is most frequently caused by an adduction contracture

94. In the geriatric amputee population:

a. AK amputations outnumber BK amputations by more than a 2 to 1 ratio

b. Bilateral amputees occur in about 35%

c. Men outnumber women by nearly a 4 to 1 ratio

d. Fifty percent of amputees may be expected to use their prostheses for more than six months if a proper fitting and rehabilitation program is carried out

Ref. 82, p. 27

95. A soft rubber-cushion heel insert, as seen in the SACH foot, would be of value:

a. To reduce shock at "heel strike" in patients with ankle fusion

b. To increase knee stability in lower extremity bracing when a weak quadriceps is present

c. To reduce calf-band pressure for a brace wearer walking on uneven ground

d. To alleviate metatarsal pressure in the rheumatoid foot

Ref. 47, pp. 84, 91

SITUATION AND PROGRESSIVE THOUGHT (answers on p. 287)

Select the answer or answers that best apply in accordance with the information given in the following statements.

96. A 40-year-old executive of stable weight and good general health suffered a traumatic amputation 10 inches below the knee when hit by a sliding piece of sheet steel while touring a plant. He is referred to you. At initial surgery the stump wound is found to be sharp and clean. Initial procedures to provide the optimum functional stump would include:

a. Circular amputation followed by skin traction

b. Revision at a higher level, resecting the fibula approximately ¾ inch proximal to the tibia

c. Revision at a higher level (as described by Ertle) and myoplastic attachments

d. Revision at a higher level with equal lengths of tibia and fibula and myoplastic attachments

Ref. 33, pp. 16-24
Ref. 122, 10-9:4-13, 1968

97. If primary closure of the wound was carried out, the dressing of choice would be:
    a. Nonrestrictive pressure dressing overlain with Ace wrap
    b. Skin traction for first 5 to 7 days   Ref. 115, 116:429-432, 1968
    c. Immediate postoperative fitting   Ref. 116, 40:222-226, 251-260, 1967
       prosthesis   Ref. 136, 50:10-18, 1970
    d. Plaster splints over nonrestrictive   Ref. 142, 48:215-226, 1968
       pressure dressing, holding knee in flexion to give comfort

98. Four days after the accident the patient complains bitterly of a sharp cramping pain in the absent large toe. You would advise the patient:
    a. To rest and not worry for the pain will be gone when the wound is healed
    b. That you or the family will make   Ref. 15, pp. 208-215
       arrangements for a psychiatric   Ref. 119, Supple. 54, pp. 9-23, 1962
       consultation   Ref. 120, 2-1:4, 1955
    c. That the pain is not unusual and that it usually recurs with decreasing frequency and severity but infrequently occurs after a year
    d. Reassure the patient as to the nature of the pain and then inject the area of the posterior tibial nerve with Xylocaine and alcohol and treat symptomatically

99. The most desirable prosthesis would be a:
    a. Standard BK prosthesis with side joints, thigh lacer, and conventional ankle joint
    b. Standard BK prosthesis with side joints,   Ref. 15, p. 375
       thigh lacer, and SACH foot   Ref. 120, 7-2:18-20, 1963
    c. PTB prosthesis with a knee cuff and SACH foot
    d. PTB prosthesis with a hydracadence knee unit

100. A 16-year-old boy suffered a traumatic amputation of the right upper extremity 2 inches above the elbow in a farm accident. The boy wishes to return to helping his family with the farm work. As a part of the clinical team, you would advise which of the following components, that is, terminal devices?
    a. A voluntary closing, automatic locking prosthetic hand
    b. An APRL voluntary closing unit   Ref. 47, p. 115
    c. A canted split hook of stainless steel with a neoprene insert such as a Dorrance 5X
    d. A straight lyre-shaped split hook of aluminum with a neoprene insert

101. Wrist unit:
    a. Step-up wrist rotation unit
    b. A flexion unit   **Ref. 15, p. 32**
    c. A wrist-disarticulation friction-rotation unit   **Ref. 47, p. 115**
    d. A locking wrist rotation unit
102. Forearm and elbow:
    a. Double shell forearm with a flexible elbow
    b. Double shell forearm with a variable ratio outside   **Ref. 15, p. 76**
       the elbow
    c. Single shell forearm with a locking lever elbow
       hinge
    d. Single shell forearm with an internal elbow
103. Harness:
    a. AE figure-of-eight harness
    b. BE chest strap harness with a leather shoulder   **Ref. 15, p. 142**
       saddle
    c. AE chest strap harness with a leather shoulder
       saddle
    d. Shoulder cap with a triple harness
104. A 5-year-old white boy of normal mentality with cerebral palsy is referred to the brace clinic. Statistically the child's involvement is most likely to be:
    a. Ataxic paraplegia
    b. Athetotic upper extremity diplegia   **Ref. 127, 44-A:1447-48, 1962**
    c. Spastic lower extremity monoplegia
    d. Mixed-type hemiplegia
    e. Spastic hemiplegia
105. The patient is found to have a spastic triplegia involving the left upper and both lower extremities. When he walks, the right ankle is in 30° equinus and 10° varus. The mother states that late in the afternoon the boy is able to get the heel down completely flat when standing. On physical examination, clonus is noted. With gentle, steady pressure, however, the foot comes up to plus 5° dorsiflexion without varus. For this individual problem, which orthotic appliance would be most advisable?
    a. No bracing needed, as the child gets his
       foot down at the end of the day and will
       improve with age
    b. Low quarter shoe with a reverse Thomas   **Ref. 7, 10:303, 1953**
       heel and ⅛-inch lateral heel wedge   **Ref. 127, 44-A:1463, 1962**
    c. Double upright short-leg daytime brace,
       with Klenzak ankles set at medium ten-
       sion on a high quarter shoe
    d. Single upright short-leg brace, with a
       Phelps ankle set at plus 5° dorsiflexion
       on a high quarter shoe to be worn at
       night

106. The patient appears to have a good balance, but he walks with mild scissoring and 20° internal rotation of both lower extremities. There is bilateral adductor spasm; however, 25° abduction is easily obtained passively. The findings of the left foot are a mirror image of the right. As a part of the clinic team, you would advise:
    a. No treatment or bracing needed at this time
    b. Bilateral double upright long-leg braces, with an external rotating strap and droplock knees, and shoe and ankle as in previous answer   Ref. 127, 44-A:1467-68, 1962
    c. Bilateral cable twisters with a pelvis band, attached to the ankle and shoe as in previous answer
    d. Adductor tenotomy followed by 6 weeks in abducted long-leg casts

107. On examination of the upper extremity, the elbow and shoulder function is found to be satisfactory. The wrist at rest assumes the position of full pronation, 40° flexion and 30° ulnar deviation. The thumb is held in the loosely gripped palm. The patient can actively bring the wrist to a neutral position and rotation; however, the fingers do not fully extend and the thumb remains partially adducted. Stereognosis is good and the boy can pick up a pencil with some difficulty. Passively, the fingers do not fully extend when the wrist is extended. The orthotic device most likely to be of help is a:
    a. Wrist-driven flexor hinge hand splint, with thumb stabilizer for daytime wear
    b. Reverse knuckle-bender splint, with above-the-wrist extension for nighttime wear   Ref. 7, 9:244-46, 1952
Ref. 127, 44-A:1473, 1962
    c. "Hand sandwich" night splint
    d. Cock-up (spoon type) wrist splint for day and nighttime wear

108. A 74-year-old white man suffers from arteriosclerosis of the lower extremities, which is worse on the left. During the past 6 weeks there have been gangrenous changes of the large, third, and fourth toes, with ulceration and infection. The skin over the heads of the metatarsals seems warm to the touch and of good nutrition. However, there is no dorsalis pedis, posterior tibial, or popliteal pulse. The treatment of choice would be which of the following?
    a. Perform an immediate open amputation of the three involved toes, followed by hot soapy soaks three times a day, and intermittent elevation. After controlling the infection, treat definitively with a Symes amputation.

b. Control the infection by dry sterile dress-   Ref. 43, pp. 839-840, 847
ings, tepid soapy foot baths, and draining   Ref. 45, 16:199-202, 1960
of abscesses when necessary, followed
definitively by a transmetatarsal amputation.

c. BK amputation is the definitive treatment,
since absence of pulses about the foot rules
out the success of a lower amputation.

d. An AK amputation is the definitive treatment, since the absence of popliteal and
ankle pulses with one episode of gangrene
rules out the success of a lower amputation.

109. A midthigh AK amputation was performed. There were no complications and no contraindications for prosthetic fitting. The most satisfactory prescription would be a:

a. Total-contact quadrilateral suction socket,
hydracadence knee unit, and double
axis ankle

b. Total-contact quadrilateral socket with   Ref. 15, pp. 360-363
silesian bandage or pelvic belt, variable-   Ref. 82, pp. 52, 63, 67, 120
friction knee unit, and conventional single
axis foot

c. Quadrilateral open-end socket, pelvic belt,
. and constant-friction knee unit with lock
and a SACH foot

d. Plug-fit socket with constant-friction
knee unit and a SACH foot

110. The AK total-contact socket provides:

a. Improvement of proprioception

b. Reduction of mechanical impairment of   Ref. 122, 10-17:203, 1972
circulation   Ref. 108, p. 30

c. Reduction of motion between stump and
socket

d. Relief of pressure on ischial area

111. The patient had worn his prosthesis successfully for nearly a year when
a small skin nodule was noted at the rim of the socket over the adductor tendons. This increased in size until it was 1 cm in diameter.
It became tender, sensitive, and finally ulcerated. By this time several
other nodules had appeared. The most likely diagnosis would be:

a. Sebaceous cysts

b. Early squamous cell carcinoma   Ref. 120, 7-1:23, 1963

c. Epidermal inclusion cysts

d. Verrucous hyperplasia

112. A young male adult, whose foot was severely crushed eighteen months
ago, returns to you because his foot is becoming too painful to walk
on. The initial damage had required a triple arthrodesis, and due to
the loss of the distal third of his os calcis, a flap and skin graft was
performed. When pressure is applied to the ball of his foot, he com-

plains of severe pain across his instep. X-ray films show the triple arthrodesis to be intact. An all-plastic PTB solid-ankle orthosis with a cushion heel and rocker bar would be the best orthotic choice primarily because:

a. The patient is more likely to wear it continuously due to its light weight and cosmetic appearance

b. The cushion heel and rocker bar provide him with a heel-toe gait that would be quite natural in appearance

c. The PTB portion partially unweights the forefoot and the heel, whereas the rigidity of the ankle, insert portions, and rocker bar resist floor reaction forces from mid-stance to toe-off

d. The cushion heel absorbs the floor reaction forces between heel strike and toe-off, thus eliminating the stress causing the pain

Ref. 133, 13-4:37-38, 1959
Ref. 134, 28-4:6-11, 1974

113. When the axes of the ankle joints of a conventional brace are aligned perpendicular to the parasagittal line of a limb, the mechanical axis is not congruent to the axis of the anatomic joint. This is because the normal range of external tibial torsion that is present places the anatomic ankle axis at an oblique angle to the parasagittal line and to a straight line of forward progression of the body. During certain phases of the normal walking cycle, rotations occur in the sagittal plane about the axis of the ankle joint. These rotations of the anatomic and mechanical joints must occur simultaneously to achieve a normal heel-toe gait. However, the incongruity between the anatomic and mechanical joints dictates that simultaneous rotation of the two is a physical impossibility. Yet with such malalignment, a heel-toe gait appears to be the rule rather than the exception. What then must be occurring that makes the impossible seem possible?

a. Since the malalignment between the anatomic and mechanical axes blocks rotary motion about the anatomic axis, the heel-toe gait being observed is apparent rather than real

b. Whereas it is true that the incongruity between the joint axes prevents anatomic rotation in the sagittal plane, normal transverse rotation of the tibia serves as an adequate substitute.

Ref. 122, 10-11:138-139, 1969
Ref. 72, p. 461
Ref. 8, 20:134-135, 1971

c. The normal valgus rotation of the foot, which occurs within the subtalar joint between foot-flat and midstance, is forced to continue on through push-off, instead of its normal reversal into a varus direction between midstance and push-off.

d. The normal elasticity of the ligaments and musculature about the ankle joint allows sufficient accommodation for the incongruity without hindrance to rotation in the sagittal plane.

114. What effect may be expected from a brace that fails to accommodate for the amount of external tibial torsion that is present in a child with cerebral palsy who has mild-to-moderate spasticity in the foot-ankle complex?

   a. Likely to produce an additional factor of excitation to those factors that are operative in causing the spasticity

   b. No effect, since in the first instance upper motor neuron damage is the cause of the spasticity Ref. 122, 10-11:138-139, 1969

   c. Little or no effect because the proprioceptors in these regions would not be receiving stimuli denoting adverse conditions

   d. No effect, as externally applied stimuli cannot affect clonus

115. What effect may be expected from the long-term wearing of a brace that is aligned without accommodation for external tibial torsion, when the wearer is a growing child?

   a. Bony wedging in the form of a fixed valgus deformity of the foot

   b. A gradual correction of any excessive external tibial torsion that the child may present Ref. 8, 20:134-135, 1971
   Ref. 122, 10-11:138-139, 1969

   c. Little if any effect, due to the normal adaptivity of the foot-ankle complex

   d. Generally, adverse effects not likely, since there is a lack of intimacy in the fit of shoes

TRUE OR FALSE (answers on p. 287)

116. A metatarsal bar should be fitted so that the anterior margin is directly below the contact point of the metatarsal heads and should not elevate the sole of the shoe from the floor. Ref. 47, p. 80
   (T) (F)

117. Because of the restriction of elbow flexion, the Munster-type socket is contraindicated in the patient who cannot position his contralateral arm near his mouth. Ref. 79, p. 144
   (T) (F)

118. In most cases movement of the lumbosacral area can be effectively controlled by properly selected braces. Ref. 127, 39-A:111, 1957
   (T) (F)

119. The Williams and Bell posture back braces are primarily designed to correct excess lordosis.   **Ref. 9, p. 212**
    (T) (F)

120. Experience with the PTB prosthesis and the AK total-suction quadrilateral thigh socket has demonstrated that pressure over neurovascular bundles cannot be tolerated.   **Ref. 45, 37:35, 1964**
    (T) (F)   **Ref. 79, p. 84**

121. The newer valves in suction sockets are of such design that they only need to be cleaned every few months.   **Ref. 24, p. 222**
    (T) (F)

122. The amputee should wash his stump daily. In most cases morning is best.   **Ref. 120, 7-2:35, 1963**
    (T) (F)

123. The prosthetic socket may be wiped but should never be washed with soap and water, as this may damage the inside lining.   **Ref. 15, p. 245**
    (T) (F)

124. Stump socks should be washed with soap and warm water daily as soon as they are removed.   **Ref. 120, 7-2:35, 1963**
    (T) (F)

125. The Milwaukee scoliosis brace has its primary corrective effect through constant corrective pressure on the rib cage and chin.
    (T) (F)   **Ref. 7, 16:210, 211, 1959**
                                                                            Ref. 127, 52-A:498-506, 1971

126. The Taylor back brace would be acceptable for splinting multiple low thoracic vertebral compression fractures.   **Ref. 9, pp. 214-219**
    (T) (F)

127. Most back problems can be adequately treated with properly fitted support garments.   **Ref. 9, p. 242**
    (T) (F)   **Ref. 127, 39-A:137, 1957**

128. Castings for the hemipelvectomy and hip-disarticulation sockets should be made under weight-bearing conditions.   **Ref. 120, 4-2:41, 1957**
    (T) (F)   **Ref. 120, 8-1:5-9, 1964**

129. A BK amputee would not be a candidate for a PTB prosthesis if the stump were shorter than 4 inches unless knee joints were added.
    (T) (F)   **Ref. 120, 7-2:18-20, 1963**

130. The power for controlling the terminal device in the BE amputee through a figure-of-eight shoulder harness is properly derived by abduction of the contralateral shoulder.   **Ref. 15, p. 132**
    (T) (F)

131. The shoe-clasp dorsiflexion-assist BK brace may not be prescribed for foot-drop conditions that are expected to be of relatively short duration.
    (T) (F)   **Ref. 134, 27-2:24, 1973**

132. Judicious placement of a rocker bar under the sole of a shoe can affect the timing in which knee flexion will occur beyond midstance.
    (T) (F)   **Ref. 133, 13-4:37-40, 1959**

133. The lack of substantial quadriceps power is a contraindication to the use of a rocker bar.   **Ref. 133, 13-4:37-40, 1959**
    (T) (F)

134. The parapodium is not prescribed for the young child with myelo-meningocele whose level of lesion is above L-3.　　Ref. 85, p. 20
(T) (F)　　　　　　　　　　　　　　　　　　Ref. 120, 15-2:36-47, 1970

135. Crutches may be prescribed prophylactically for the L-3 to L-4 level myelomeningocele patient for long-term protection from lumbar root compression.　　　　　　　　　　　　　　Ref. 118, 36:255, 1955
(T) (F)

136. External tibial torsion and toe-out are one and the same in reference to checking the proper alignment of a leg brace to the anatomic ankle joint.　　　　　　　　　　　　　　　　Ref. 8, 20:134-135, 1971
(T) (F)

137. In bracing the paralyzed trunks of children who are nonambulatory, a major problem is that chair-reaction forces are not controlled by standard spinal bracing techniques.　　Ref. 131, 9-3:13-14, 1975
(T) (F)

138. The Boston system for the nonoperative control of scoliosis utilizes a prefabricated polypropylene girdle.　　　　　Ref. 34, 29:7, 1975
(T) (F)

139. The Lenox-Hill brace is designed to control abnormal rotation of the knee joint.　　　　　　　　　　　Ref. 127, 55-A:899-922, 1973
(T) (F)

140. The knee is considered a polycentric joint because the center of rotation traverses from a distal anterior position to a proximal posterior position with flexion.　　　　　　　　　　　Ref. 122, 10-18:92, 1972
(T) (F)

LIST (answers on pp. 287-288)

141. List the three basic components necessary in the harness of a body powered AE prosthesis.　　　　　　　　　Ref. 10, pp. 112-116

142. List five basic hand splints used frequently in the treatment of trau-matic lesions or structural deformities.　　　Ref. 30, pp. 150-180

143. List three systems for controlling externally powered upper extremity prostheses.　　　　　　　　　　　Ref. 127, 55-A:1493, 1973
Ref. 122, 10-19:104-123, 1973

144. Immediate postsurgical prosthetic fittings, although seldom contra-indicated, are not consistently performed. List four advantages of im-mediate postsurgical prosthetic fittings.　　　　　Ref. 23, p. 34

145. List six pads that are commonly used with the Milwaukee brace.
Ref. 76, p. 315

146. List seven types of suspension devices for the lower extremity am-putee.　　　　　　　　　　　　　　　Ref. 15, pp. 342-353
Ref. 99, pp. 72, 113
Ref. 120, 7-2:21, 1963
Ref. 122, 10-13:127, 1970

147. List three types of prostheses that have been designed for the patient with hip disarticulation.　　　　　　Ref. 120, 4-2:22-25, 1957

148. List five types of ankle joints that might be prescribed in lower extremity bracing.

Ref. 7, 14:338-339, 1957

Ref. 7, 10:284-288, 1953

Ref. 9, p. 521

Ref. 127, 44-A:1460, 1962

149. List six contraindications to limb fitting in the geriatric lower extremity amputee.

Ref. 82, p. 26

150. List four types of knee joint units.

Ref. 15, p. 359

SECTION 10

Surgical principles

JOHN D. KENNEY, M.D.

MULTIPLE CHOICE, SINGLE ANSWER (answers on p. 288)

Select the *one* answer that will best complete or answer each of the following statements or questions.

1. Despite elimination of patients with positive skin or eye tests, as high as _____ of persons given equine tetanus antitoxin may be expected to have delayed systemic reactions.
   a. Less than 1%
   b. 5%   Ref. 125, 188:626, 1964
   c. 10%
   d. 15%
   e. 20%
2. Because of the vitamin deficiency that it produces, isoniazid should be given in combination with which vitamin?
   a. C
   b. A   Ref. 43, p. 16
   c. D
   d. B_1
   e. B_6
3. Access to the ankle joint in treating osteochondromatosis is probably best obtained through which surgical approach?
   a. Posteromedial (Colonna-Ralston)
   b. Posterolateral (Gatellier-Chastang)   Ref. 43, p. 62
   c. Dorsolateral (Ollier)
   d. Posterior (Kocher)
   e. Medial (Koenig-Schaefer)
4. When performing a tendon transfer, one should attach the tendon to its new location in such a way that it is under about _____ of the elasticity of the muscle.
   a. 50%
   b. 60%   Ref. 43, p. 1519

221

c. 80%   **Ref. 127, 40-A:633, 1958**
d. 100%

5. In nerve injuries other than those caused by a sharp cutting edge the most advisable time for repair is _____ after injury.
   a. 24 hours
   b. 1 week   **Ref. 43, p. 1754**
   c. 2 to 3 weeks   **Ref. 127, 53-B:349, 1971**
   d. 6 to 12 weeks

6. Mild delirium, vacillating disorientation, hyperactive deep tendon reflexes, and flattening or inversion of the T waves on the electrocardiogram are indicative of:
   a. Hyperkalemia
   b. Hypokalemia   **Ref. 6, pp. 83, 312**
   c. Hypercalcemia   **Ref. 92, p. 106**
   d. Hypocalcemia
   e. Water intoxication

7. The average renal loss of potassium ion per day in a normal patient is approximately:
   a. 20 mEq
   b. 30 mEq   **Ref. 6, p. 100**
   c. 40 mEq   **Ref. 92, p. 103**
   d. 50 mEq
   e. 60 mEq

8. Which of the following is not recommended for repair of a 1.5 cm longitudinal tear in the wall of an artery?
   a. Excision of the segment and grafting
   b. Excision of the segment and primary   **Ref. 43, p. 54**
      anastomosis   **Ref. 127, 53-A:56, 1971**
   c. Excision of the wound edges and closure
      of the defect in a transverse manner
   d. Excision of the wound edges and closure of
      the defect along the long axis of the vessel

9. Pain in the throat radiating up behind the ear and an earache in a patient with a nasogastric tube in place should alert you to the possibility of:
   a. Esophageal stenosis
   b. Foreign body gastritis   **Ref. 6, p. 282**
   c. Laryngeal inflammation
   d. Incipient esophageal perforation

10. When injected into superficial tissues, the incidence of slough is highest when using which of the following?
    a. Pontocaine
    b. Nupercaine   **Ref. 80, p. 12**
    c. Xylocaine
    d. Metycaine
    e. Novocain

11. Which of the following is the most toxic when used as a local anesthetic agent?
    a. Xylocaine
    b. Novocain   **Ref. 80, p. 12**
    c. Pontocaine   **Ref. 92, p. 194**
    d. Intracaine

12. The incidence of fat embolism is _____ with intramedullary fixation of fractures than with other types of treatment.
    a. Higher
    b. Lower   **Ref. 43, p. 486**
    c. The same   **Ref. 127, 56-A:1327, 1974**
    d. Higher only if carried out during the first 48 hours following injury

13. The current recommended dose of human tetanus immune globulin is _____ units, depending on the severity and duration of the wound.
    a. 100 to 200   **Ref. 92, p. 396**
    b. 250 to 500
    c. 1,500
    d. 3,000

14. Which of the following should be given to a patient who has been taking a rauwolfia derivative and develops hypotension, bradycardia, and a low pulse pressure during general anesthesia?
    a. Thiopental sodium
    b. Norepinephrine   **Ref. 42, p. 88**
    c. Metaraminol   **Ref. 92, p. 2105**
    d. Atropine
    e. Epinephrine

15. Unit for unit, which form of tetanus antitoxin gives protective levels of circulating antibodies for the longest period of time?
    a. Equine
    b. Bovine   **Ref. 125, 188:626, 1964**
    c. Human
    d. No significant difference

16. The acute postoperative onset of arthritis involving a single joint, especially if the area is swollen, red, or warm, should lead you to suspect:
    a. Hematogenous osteomyelitis
    b. Rheumatoid arthritis   **Ref. 43, p. 14**
    c. Gout
    d. Thrombophlebitis
    e. Bursitus due to calcium mobilization from bone

17. The treatment of choice in the answer to 16 is:
    a. Systemic antibiotics, usually given intravenously
    b. Steroids, despite their effect on wound   **Ref. 43, p. 14**
       healing   **Ref. 127, 54-A:357, 1972**

c. Small doses of aspirin

d. Injection of the painful area with
   analgesics

e. Colchicine, either intravenously or orally

18. The most valid method of making a diagnosis of fat embolism is:

    a. EEG changes

    b. Fat droplets in the sputum   Ref. 43, p. 6

    c. Fat droplets in the urine   Ref. 127, 56-A:1327, 1974

    d. Arterial Po_2 of less than 70 mm Hg

    e. Clinical evaluation

MULTIPLE CHOICE, MULTIPLE ANSWERS (answers on p. 288)

Select one or more answers that will best complete or answer each of the
following statements or questions.

19. When screws are used for internal fixation of a fracture, they should be
    inserted at right angles to the long axis of the bone when possible be-
    cause:

    a. This position allows more efficient
       apposition of the fracture fragments when
       weight is applied   Ref. 43, p. 483

    b. Placement at a right angle to the fracture   Ref. 127, 34-A:219, 1952
       line allows reabsorption of bone along
       the screw track, with subsequent loosening
       of screws

    c. Fracture of the screw is common when the
       angle of shear is approximately 90°

    d. Less motion occurs at the fracture site,
       with less chance of pseudarthrosis

    e. The angle of entrance into the medullary
       canal is an important consideration in
       endochondral bone formation

20. Arthrodesis of the hip should combine which of the following to give the
    best functional result in an adult?

    a. Full extension

    b. 20° of flexion   Ref. 43, p. 1143

    c. Slight adduction

    d. 15° of abduction

    e. Neutral rotation

21. The treatment of fat embolism should include which of the following?

    a. Oxygen therapy

    b. Immediate surgical fixation of any long   Ref. 43, p. 6
       bone fracture   Ref. 127, 56-A:1327, 1974

    c. Anticoagulant doses of heparin

    d. Subanticoagulant doses of heparin

    e. Steroids

22. Which of the following are the best anesthetic agents to use in a patient with bronchial asthma?
    a. Methoxyflurane
    b. Cyclopropane   **Ref. 42, p. 87**
    c. Nitrous oxide   **Ref. 92, p. 199**
    d. Thiopental sodium
    e. Halothane
23. Campbell's method of treating nonunion of a fracture, as now practiced, includes which of the following?
    a. Excision of all the intervening
       pseudarthrosis scar
    b. Opening both ends of the medullary canal   **Ref. 43, p. 751**
    c. Packing of endosteal bone from the cortical   **Ref. 127, 47-A:180, 1965**
       graft in the medullary canal
    d. Packing of cancellous bone about the
       fracture
    e. Preparation of a bleeding cortical bone bed
       for the cortical graft that is fixed with
       screws
24. Which of the following antibiotics are bacteriocidal?
    a. Penicillin   **Ref. 92, p. 330**
    b. Methicillin   **Ref. 127, 47-A:290, 1965**
    c. Tetracycline
    d. Cephalosporin
    e. Erythromycin
25. Of the following, which signs are useful in diagnosing a transfusion reaction while a patient is undergoing general anesthesia?
    a. Urticaria
    b. Abnormal capillary bleeding   **Ref. 6, p. 175**
    c. Tachycardia, hypotension, and increased bleeding   **Ref. 92, p. 136**
    d. Fever
    e. Dark color of the blood despite adequate
       oxygenation of the patient
26. The proper dosage for antigas gangrene serum is _____ units given
    by the _____ route.
    a. 10,000
    b. 25,000   **Ref. 43, p. 494**
    c. 50,000
    d. Intramuscular
    e. Intravenous
27. When fusing a shoulder, the most commonly recommended position is
    _____ of true abduction, _____ of flexion, and _____ of
    internal rotation.
    a. 10°
    b. 25°   **Ref. 127, 56-A:913, 1974**
    c. 40° to 50°
    d. 15° to 20°
    e. 25° to 30°

28. In a patient receiving multiple transfusions of whole blood, _____ of calcium gluconate should be given after the _____ unit of blood.
    a. 500 mg
    b. 1,000 mg   **Ref. 6, p. 177**
    c. Second or third   **Ref. 92, p. 138**
    d. Fourth or fifth
    e. Fifth or sixth

SITUATION AND PROGRESSIVE THOUGHT (answers on pp. 288-289)

Select the answer or answers that best apply in accordance with the information given in the following statements.

29. A 17-year-old black boy weighing 70 kg has a deep palmar laceration, but is in good health otherwise and has no allergies. He states he fell in an alley and cut his hand on an unknown object. He reports having eaten just prior to the accident. Intravenous regional anesthesia of the extremity utilizing lidocaine (Xylocaine) is selected as the anesthetic of choice. This type of anesthesia:
    a. Has its major effect through anoxia, which is maintained by a tourniquet
    b. Cannot be maintained effectively   **Ref. 127, 46-A:809-816, 1964**
       and safely for more than about one
       third the normal tourniquet time
    c. Requires a higher concentration than is usual for local anesthetics
    d. Is usually best carried out utilizing a two-tourniquet system
30. The usual recommended concentration is:
    a. 0.5%
    b. 1%   **Ref. 127, 46-A:811-816, 1964**
    c. 2%   **Ref. 92, p. 193**
    d. 5%
31. The routine quantity of a 2% solution is utilized. The initial anesthetic is satisfactory. Unfortunately, after 5 minutes of operating time, the tourniquet suddenly deflates. Assuming the total dosage was released into the circulation, this would constitute approximately _____ of the toxic dosage.
    a. 50%
    b. 75%   **Ref. 59, pp. 377, 384**
    c. 100%   **Ref. 127, 46-A:811-816, 1964**
    d. 200%
32. The early toxic effects most likely would be:
    a. Central nervous system stimulation, with restlessness and tremor proceeding to convulsions
    b. Cardiac arrest   **Ref. 59, p. 377**
                                                                   Ref. 92, p. 195

c. Continued hyperventilation, with
developing respiratory alkalosis and
carpopedal spasm
d. Cardiac irregularity, perhaps leading to
fibrillation
33. The recommended treatment should include maintenance of an airway and:
a. Central nervous system stimulants
b. Barbiturates   **Ref. 59, p. 377**
c. Artificial respiration   **Ref. 92, p. 195**
d. Respiratory stimulants

TRUE OR FALSE (answers on p. 289)

34. Wounds infected with streptococci generally do not tend to form abscesses.   **Ref. 6, p. 64**
(T) (F)   **Ref. 92, p. 335**

35. In the treatment of clostridial infections, hyperbaric oxygen has been shown to have a beneficial effect.   **Ref. 127, 52-A:830, 1970**
(T) (F)

36. The success of a transfer of the tendon of a stance phase muscle to a swing phase function is predictable, since muscle reeducation is possible.   **Ref. 127, 41-A:189, 1959**
(T) (F)

37. In spinal anesthesia the autonomic fibers are affected first, since these nerves have the largest area per unit volume of axon and therefore are the most sensitive of all the nerves.   **Ref. 61, p. 7**
(T) (F)

38. Regarding the position of a shoulder arthrodesis, the correct amount of humeral rotation is of greater importance than is the degree of abduction.
(T) (F)   **Ref. 43, p. 1185**
                                                   Ref. 127, 56-A:913, 1974

39. Chloramphenicol has been shown to be capable of suppressing tetanus antibody formation after booster immunization with tetanus toxoid.
(T) (F)   **Ref. 130, 273:367-369, 1965**

40. Surgical treatment of tuberculosis ideally should be postponed until the lymphocyte-monocyte ratio is greater than five, since this indicates a state of adequate host resistance.   **Ref. 43, p. 1088**
(T) (F)

41. Tetanus toxoid should not be given at the same time as human tetanus antitoxin, since the latter will inhibit host antibody formation.
(T) (F)   **Ref. 92, p. 326**

42. In a grossly contaminated wound, antigas gangrene serum is of great prophylactic value.   **Ref. 92, p. 338**
(T) (F)

43. When used as a bone graft, cancellous bone unites more rapidly than does the same quantity of cortical bone.   **Ref. 43, p. 51**
(T) (F)   **Ref. 127, 47-A:179, 1965**

44. List two reasons why, when repairing a nerve secondarily, you should approach the proximal and distal portions rather than attacking the divided ends directly. **Ref. 43, p. 1756**

45. List five practical methods that might be utilized in closing the gap between two ends of a divided nerve without grafting. **Ref. 43, p. 1758**

46. List six complications or errors in technique or judgment that may give a poor result in foot and ankle stabilizations. **Ref. 127, 20-A:609, 1938**
Ref. 127, 32-A:1, 1950
Ref. 127, 47-A:340, 1965

47. List four methods that may be utilized to stabilize joints.
Ref. 43, pp. 1235, 1520

48. List five general types of surgical procedures that have been advocated for the treatment of tuberculosis. **Ref. 105, p. 107**

49. List five indications for the postoperative use of antibiotics. **Ref. 43, p. 14**

50. List four methods of treating scars. **Ref. 43, p. 213**

51. List two circumstances in which the use of steroids for the treatment of shock are indicated. **Ref. 42, p. 88**
Ref. 43, p. 5

52. List five indications for bone grafting. **Ref. 43, p. 46**

53. List four ways in which tourniquet paralysis may result. **Ref. 43, p. 21**

SECTION 11

Trauma

NEWTON B. WHITE, M.D.

MULTIPLE CHOICE, SINGLE ANSWER (answers on pp. 289-290)

Select the *one* answer that will best complete or answer each of the following statements or questions.

1. Posterior fracture dislocation of the hip is an emergency, and multiple attempts at closed reduction are:
   a. Rewarding
   b. Less damaging than surgical intervention   **Ref. 127, 56-A:1103, 1974**
   c. Contraindicated
   d. Open to discussion in some centers
   e. Humanitarian

2. In a prospective study reported in 1974 it was established that cephalothin _____ when used prophylactically for wounds associated with open fractures.   **Ref. 127, 56-A:532, 1974**
   a. Produced a significantly lower infection rate
   b. Was equally effective with combined dosages of penicillin and streptomycin
   c. Was ineffective in preventing infections (when the culture taken at triage was positive)
   d. Produced a high incidence of side effects
   e. Had no appreciable effect

3. Generally, the posterior malleolar fragment in a trimalleolar fracture must be replaced if it involves _____ the articular surface of the joint.
   a. One eighth
   b. One fourth   **Ref. 37, p. 263**
   c. One fifth
   d. One third

4. Nerve injury at the time of dislocation of the shoulder most frequently involves which of the following nerves?
   a. Radial
   b. Ulnar   **Ref. 36, p. 354**
   c. Median   **Ref. 127, 38-A:957, 1956**
   d. Axillary

5. Closed treatment of displaced fractures of both bones of the forearm in adults may be expected to yield poor functional results in _____ of cases.
   a. 10%
   b. 30%   **Ref. 127, 31-A:755, 1949**
   c. 50%
   d. 70%
   e. 90%

6. The mechanism of injury in Pott's fracture is:
   a. Eversion and external rotation
   b. Inversion and internal rotation   **Ref. 37, p. 250**
   c. Forced dorsiflexion and internal rotation
   d. Forced plantar flexion and internal rotation

7. A patient with a fracture of the lunate and scaphoid with moderate comminution is best treated by:
   a. Excision of the scaphoid and reduction of the lunate
   b. Excision of the lunate and reduction of   **Ref. 127, 47-A:915, 1965**
      the scaphoid
   c. Excision of the proximal carpal row
   d. Arthrodesis of the wrist
   e. Reduction of the dislocation and internal fixation of the lunate and scaphoid

8. Displaced transcervical and cervicotrochanteric fractures of the femur in children should be treated by:
   a. Closed reduction and cast fixation
   b. Gentle closed reduction and traction   **Ref. 132, 3-1:1675, 1972**
   c. Gentle closed reduction and pin fixation followed by spica cast protection
   d. Any of the above where feasible
   e. None of the above

9. Fracture of the greater tuberosity of the humerus occurs in about _____ of shoulder dislocations.
   a. 10%
   b. 20%   **Ref. 107, p. 482**
   c. 30%
   d. 40%
   e. 50%

10. Which of the factors listed below will not give early warning or aid in the diagnosis of fat embolism?
    a. Monitoring of blood gases
    b. Petechiae   **Ref. 127, 56-A:1327, 1974**

c. Change in the level of conciousness

d. Respiratory distress

e. Hyperpyrexia, tachypnea, and tachy-
cardia

11. The treatment of an undisplaced fracture of the base of the fifth metatarsal should be:

a. Elastic wrap and a shoe with a stiff sole

b. Partial weight bearing with crutches
until tenderness disappears   **Ref. 42, p. 1122**

c. Short-leg cast for 4 weeks

d. Physical therapy to promote callous
formation and to maintain ankle function

12. Pott's fracture is a:

a. Trimalleolar fracture of the ankle

b. Transcondylar fracture of the humerus   **Ref. 43, p. 509**

c. Linear shaft fracture of the tibia

d. Bimalleolar fracture of the ankle

e. Lateral tibial plateau fracture

13. The use of a cane on the side opposite that on which a valgus osteotomy of the femur has been performed is advised, since this will decrease the weight borne by the femoral head about _____ pounds for each pound of pressure exerted on the cane.

a. 2

b. 4   **Ref. 43, p. 788**

c. 6

d. 8

e. 10

14. Which of the following nerves has been reported as being most commonly injured in fractures of both bones of the forearm?

a. Ulnar

b. Median   **Ref. 127, 39-A:91, 1957**

c. Radial

d. Mixed injury

15. The most frequent site of dislocation in the cervical spine is between:

a. C-3 and C-4

b. C-4 and C-5   **Ref. 43, p. 620**

c. C-5 and C-6

d. C-6 and C-7

e. C-7 and C-8

16. In a child with a malunited fracture of the femoral shaft in which there is 1¾-inch shortening, reconstruction should not be attempted until the fracture is at least _____ months old.

a. 3

b. 5   **Ref. 43, p. 719**

c. 7

d. 9

17. The minimum amount of traction recommended for reduction of dislocations of C-6 and C-7 is _____ pounds.
    a. 6
    b. 8   Ref. 43, p. 618
    c. 10
    d. 15
    e. 18
18. A trimalleolar fracture is known as _____ fracture.
    a. Barton's
    b. Pott's   Ref. 43, p. 513
    c. Cotton's
    d. Jefferson's
19. In a stellate fracture of the patella with four major fragments the _____ portion is the most important and should be preserved if possible.
    a. Proximal
    b. Distal   Ref. 43, p. 539
    c. Medial
    d. Lateral
20. In luxatio erecta the _____ nerve is most commonly injured.
    a. Radial
    b. Median   Ref. 42, p. 401
    c. Ulnar   Ref. 77, p. 261
    d. Musculocutaneous   Ref. 107, p. 477
    e. Axillary
21. The highest spinal cord lesion usually compatible with life is at the _____ level.
    a. C-2
    b. C-3   Ref. 9, p. 515
    c. C-4
    d. C-6
22. In luxatio erecta the arm is held in full:
    a. Flexion
    b. Extension   Ref. 28, p. 401
    c. Abduction   Ref. 77, p. 261
    d. Adduction   Ref. 107, p. 477
23. The inability to carry out Kocher's third maneuver in reducing a dislocated shoulder usually indicates:
    a. Failure of reduction
    b. Misdiagnosed posterior dislocation   Ref. 42, p. 394
    c. Associated fracture
    d. Tear of the rotator cuff
24. The incidence of aseptic necrosis of the femoral head after fracture of the neck of the femur is generally reported as being:
    a. 5% to 10%
    b. 10% to 20%   Ref. 42, p. 825
    c. 25% to 40%   Ref. 125, 153:536, 1953
    d. 55% to 60%
    e. 75% to 80%

25. Differentiation of spinal shock from traumatic shock is often possible in that in the former there is:
   a. A slow, strong pulse
   b. Absence of thirst   **Ref. 65, p. 295**
   c. Warm, dry skin
   d. Alertness
   e. All of the above

26. In the tibial collateral ligament syndrome the medial meniscus is often thickened or has an old tear and frequently is displaced:
   a. Anteriorly
   b. Posteriorly   **Ref. 127, 36-A:88, 1954**
   c. Medially
   d. Laterally

27. Following arterial repair of the antecubital fossa, swelling of the extremity should be minimized and an effort made to keep the limb temperature in the range of _____ for the first few days after operation.
   a. 50° to 60° F
   b. 60° to 70° F   **Ref. 140, 31:62, 1952**
   c. 70° to 80° F
   d. 80° to 90° F

28. On the basis of experimental studies, meniscal tears may be expected to heal if:
   a. They are of the bucket-handle variety
   b. The tear involves only the central-anterior   **Ref. 127, 18:333, 1936**
      segment
   c. The posterior horn is damaged centrally
   d. The tear communicates with the synovium
      laterally

29. The second most common elbow fracture in children is:
   a. Supracondylar fracture
   b. Condylar fracture   **Ref. 119, 49:213, 1944**
   c. T type condylar fracture
   d. Monteggia fracture
   e. Fracture of the radial neck

30. Division of the brachial artery proximal to its radial and ulnar bifurcation may be expected to result in loss of a portion of the extremity in _____ of cases.
   a. Less than 1%
   b. 5%   **Ref. 117, 123:534, 1946**
   c. 15%
   d. 25%
   e. Greater than 25%

31. The most frequent neural injury associated with a supracondylar fracture of the humerus is contusion or laceration of the _____ nerve(s).
   a. Radial
   b. Median   **Ref. 42, p. 495**
   c. Ulnar   **Ref. 107, p. 131**
   d. Median and ulnar
   e. Median and radial

32. Which of the following humeral fractures is most commonly seen in adults?
   a. T or Y fractures of the distal humerus
   b. Transcondylar fractures   **Ref. 43, p. 647**
   c. Fracture of the capitulum
   d. Comminuted fracture of either or both condyles

33. If return of hand or forearm muscle function has not occurred after _____ months from the time a closed fracture of the humeral shaft was sustained, the nerve involved should be explored.
   a. 1
   b. 1½   **Ref. 42, p. 436**
   c. 3
   d. 6
   e. 12

34. Supracondylar T fractures of the humerus are best exposed:
   a. Anterolaterally (Henry)
   b. Laterally (J type of Kocher)   **Ref. 127, 22:278, 1940**
   c. Medially
   d. Posterolaterally (Campbell)

35. The most frequent complication of fractures of the humeral shaft is injury to the:
   a. Brachial artery
   b. Brachial vein   **Ref. 42, p. 436**
   c. Radial nerve
   d. Median nerve

36. The upper limit of time after which reversal of circulatory changes in Volkmann's ischemic contracture is unlikely is _____ hours.
   a. 6
   b. 12   **Ref. 42, p. 495**
   c. 18
   d. 24

37. Permanent loss of muscle function may be expected after peripheral nerve damage if reinnervation does not occur within _____ months from the time of injury.
   a. 3
   b. 9   **Ref. 65, p. 77**
   c. 12
   d. 15
   e. 18

38. A positive McMurray test is differentiated from normal clicks and snaps in that it is usually noted when the knee is beyond _____ of flexion.
   a. 50°
   b. 60°   **Ref. 42, p. 911**
   c. 70°   **Ref. 121, 29:407, 1942**
   d. 80°
   e. 90°

39. The use of the Lottes nail for treatment of fractures of the tibia should generally be reserved for fractures of the _____ one third of the bone.
    a. Proximal
    b. Middle   **Ref. 125, 155:1039, 1954**
    c. Distal
    d. Proximal and middle
    e. Middle and distal

40. Low-velocity gunshot wounds involving the knee joint should be treated by:
    a. Excision of the wounds of entrance and
       exit, dressing, and antibiotics
    b. Excision of the wounds of entrance and   **Ref. 127, 56-A:1047, 1974**
       exit, exploration of the knee joint, and
       removal of osteocartilaginous and metallic
       debris through judiciously chosen incisions
    c. a, plus tetanus prophylaxis
    d. b, plus tetanus prophylaxis, antibiotics, and dressings

41. A contaminated wound is usually considered to be infected after _____ hours.
    a. 3
    b. 6   **Ref. 43, p. 490**
    c. 12
    d. 18
    e. 24

42. The Hill-Sachs lesion in recurrent shoulder dislocations is in reality:
    a. A degenerative change in the articular cartilage
    b. An old fracture   **Ref. 43, p. 455**
    c. A defect in the capsule
    d. A congenital malformation

43. In a dislocation of the subtalar joint the forefoot is usually displaced:
    a. Anteriorly
    b. Posteriorly   **Ref. 43, p. 413**
    c. Medially   **Ref. 127, 36-A:299, 1954**
    d. Laterally

44. An old unrecognized dislocation of the distal radioulnar joint is usually best treated by:
    a. Liebolt reconstruction of the joint ligaments
    b. Bunnell stabilization of the joint   **Ref. 43, p. 431**
    c. Darrach procedure
    d. Arthrodesis of the radius and proximal carpal row

45. A traumatic hip fracture-dislocation where there is a posterior acetabular fragment so large as to preclude stability after reduction of the dislocation is classified as:
    a. Grade I
    b. Grade II   **Ref. 43, p. 416**
    c. Grade III
    d. Grade IV

46. The preventive measures concerning gas gangrene would not include:
    a. Recognition of wound factors such as type
       and degree of tissue damage and degree
       of contamination
    b. Adequate and thorough débridement   **Ref. 127, 56-A:1445, 1974**
    c. Use of antibiotics to allow minimal
       débridement, coverage of the bone, and
       primary closure
    d. Delayed closure of wounds in which
       contamination or tissue damage is great
47. The pathogenesis of Volkmann's ischemic contracture is:
    a. Complete or partial arterial occlusion
    b. Complete or partial venous occlusion   **Ref. 4, p. 416**
    c. Damage to one or more peripheral   **Ref. 121, 28:239-260, 1940**
       nerves, with alteration of the reflex arc   **Ref. 127, 6:331, 1924**
    d. Not fully understood
48. A tear of the medial collateral ligament in conjunction with a depressed
    fracture of the lateral tibial plateau may be suspected if, with abduction
    stress, the medial joint space opens more than _____ by comparison
    with the normal side.
    a. 0.5 mm
    b. 1 mm   **Ref. 127, 42-A:13, 1960**
    c. 1.5 mm
    d. 2 mm
    e. 2.5 mm
49. The most common injury incident to Volkmann's ischemic contracture of
    the forearm is:
    a. Fracture at the wrist
    b. Fracture of both bones of the forearm   **Ref. 4, p. 416**
    c. Fracture of the proximal end of the humerus
    d. Fracture of the distal end of the humerus
50. In a traumatic knee dislocation the structure most commonly injured
    is the:
    a. Anterior cruciate ligament
    b. Posterior cruciate ligament   **Ref. 127, 45-A:900, 1963**
    c. Medial collateral ligament
    d. Lateral collateral ligament
    e. Joint capsule
51. Fractures of the femur in children usually occur at what level?
    a. Proximal third
    b. Middle third   **Ref. 26, p. 129**
    c. Distal third
    d. Femoral neck
52. The earliest skeletal radiologic sign of infection of the hip joint after
    internal fixation of the hip fracture is:
    a. Increased size of the acetabulum
    b. Sequestration of a portion of the femoral head   **Ref. 43, p. 602**
    c. Bone absorption around the fixation device
    d. Narrowing of the joint space

53. Recurrence of a shoulder dislocation is most common in the age group of:
    a. Less than 20 years
    b. 20 to 30 years   **Ref. 127, 38-A:957, 1956**
    c. 40 to 50 years
    d. Over 50 years
54. Preoperative reduction of a subtrochanteric fracture is usually not successful because:
    a. The proximal fragment is rolled externally, as the capsule tends to "unwind"
    b. The pull of muscles attached to the proxi-   **Ref. 43, p. 577**
       mal fragment causes it to flex, externally rotate, and abduct
    c. Involvement of the calcar femoralis by the fracture will not allow engagement of the fragments
    d. Medial displacement of the distal fragment due to muscle pull cannot be overcome with the patient awake
55. Bryant's overhead traction for femoral fractures in infants:
    a. Is safe at all times
    b. Can be used for children weighing 25   **Ref. 132, 3-1:1691, 1972**
       pounds or more
    c. Is reserved for children over 2 years of age
    d. None of the above
56. In general, if instability of the knee is greater than _____, as compared with the normal knee, conservative therapy will not suffice.
    a. 5°
    b. 10°   **Ref. 43, p. 923**
    c. 15°
    d. 20°
57. Considering fractures in general, the body compensates least well for which of the following deformities?
    a. Angulation
    b. Overriding   **Ref. 26, p. 3**
    c. Rotation
    d. Comminution
58. Reversal of the normal carrying angle after a supracondylar fracture of the humerus is primarily a _____ deformity.
    a. Varus
    b. Valgus   **Ref. 26, p. 30**
    c. External rotation
    d. Anterior angulation
    e. Posterior angulation
59. The second most common position of the humeral head in a shoulder dislocation is:
    a. Anterior
    b. Posterior   **Ref. 42, p. 389**
    c. Inferior
    d. Superior

60. The treatment of a fresh fracture of the radial head with gross displacement in a child should be:
    a. Closed reduction and plaster immobilization
    b. Nothing except a sling for comfort   **Ref. 26, p. 57**
    c. Open reduction and internal fixation with
       a threaded wire, followed by plaster casting
    d. Open reduction without internal fixation,
       followed by plaster immobilization
    e. Excision of the radial head

61. The most frequent joint to be dislocated is the:
    a. Shoulder
    b. Elbow   **Ref. 43, p. 389**
    c. Proximal radioulnar
    d. Ankle

62. With increasing age the radial head gradually becomes larger in circumference than the neck of the radius; therefore "nursemaid's elbow" rarely occurs after _____ years of age.
    a. 2
    b. 4   **Ref. 42, p. 534**
    c. 5   **Ref. 141, 98:573, 1954**
    d. 8

63. Concerning rupture of the biceps brachii, which is not true?
    a. Most commonly the long head is involved.
    b. All except those occurring in young people   **Ref. 43, p. 1490**
       should be repaired.
    c. This injury has been shown to result in
       about 20% flexor power loss early after
       injury.
    d. The weight necessary to produce this injury
       is usually greater than 150 pounds.
    e. It is often associated with rotator cuff tears.

64. Decompression laminectomy is not indicated in which of the following?
    a. Increasing neurologic deficit during the
       first 24 hours after injury
    b. No improvement in an incomplete paralysis   **Ref. 43, p. 609**
       despite realignment of the vertebras
    c. Lesions of the cauda equina
    d. Vertebral malalignment, with a negative
       manometric examination
    e. Such severe deformity that weight bearing
       will be impossible later

65. In fractures of the middle three fifths of the femoral shaft, the proximal fragment generally is pulled into:
    a. Flexion
    b. Extension   **Ref. 26, p. 130**
    c. Adduction
    d. Abduction
    e. External rotation

66. Which of the following is *not* true?
    a. Primary closure of wounds occurs most
       commonly in civilian trauma.
    b. Gas gangrene can and does occur in   **Ref. 127, 56-A:1445, 1974**
       wounds closed primarily.
    c. Gas gangrene in war wounds has signifi-
       cantly decreased with adequate débride-
       ment and delayed closure.
    d. The use of delayed closure following dé-
       bridement allows the periosteum to die
       and increases the complication rate.
    e. The principles of débridement and delayed
       closure decrease the incidence of all types
       of infections in contaminated wounds.
67. The fracture described by Abraham Colles in 1814 was in what bone at
    what level?
    a. Radial head
    b. Distal radial epiphysis   **Ref. 36, p. 358**
    c. 1 cm from the base of the radius and the
       ulnar styloid
    d. 4 cm from the base of the radius
    e. Middle one third shaft of the radius
68. In a patient with a supracondylar fracture of the humerus the most im-
    portant early sign of impending Volkmann's ischemic contracture is:
    a. Pallor
    b. Coolness   **Ref. 26, p. 29**
    c. Swelling
    d. Numbness
    e. Pain
69. Considering Aitken's classification of epiphyseal fractures, in which type
    is disturbance of growth most likely to occur?
    a. Type I
    b. Type II   **Ref. 36, p. 628**
    c. Type III
70. Following Colles' fracture, what tendon will most likely rupture?
    a. Extensor pollicis longus
    b. Abductor pollicis longus   **Ref. 36, p. 375**
    c. Extensor carpi radialis indicis   **Ref. 42, p. 615**
    d. Palmaris longus
    e. Flexor carpi radialis
71. Which of the following usually does not cause ligamentous injury to the
    knee?
    a. Hyperextension
    b. Hyperflexion   **Ref. 127, 26:503, 1944**
    c. Valgus motion, flexion, and internal rotation
    d. Varus motion, flexion, and external rotation
    e. Anterior or posterior displacement of the
       tibia on the femur

72. Of the five types of knee dislocation, which is the most common?
    a. Anterior
    b. Posterior   **Ref. 127, 45-A:892, 1963**
    c. Medial
    d. Lateral
    e. Rotatory

73. Dipping a dry plaster roll into water causes which change in chemical state?
    a. $2CaSO_4 \cdot 2H_2O \longrightarrow (CaSO_4)_2 \cdot H_2O + 3H_2O$
    b. $(CaSO_4)_2 \cdot H_2O + 3H_2O \longrightarrow 2CaSO_4 \cdot 2H_2O$ **Insert in plaster**
    c. $Ca(OH)_2 \, 2 \cdot H_2O + 3H_2O \longrightarrow 2Ca\,(OH)_2 \cdot 2H_2O$ **roll**
    d. $Ca_3(PO_4)_2 + 2H_2O \longrightarrow 2Ca_3(PO_4)_2 \cdot 2H_2O$
    e. $Ca_3(PO_4)_2 + 4H_2O \longrightarrow Ca_3(PO_4)_2 \cdot 4H_2O$

74. Vitallium is an alloy composed of which of the following?
    a. Cobalt, chromium, and molybdenum
    b. Cobalt, nickel, and molybdenum   **Ref. 43, p. 33**
    c. Chromium, tantalum, and nickel
    d. Cadmium, nickel, and molybdenum
    e. Chromium, cadmium, and boron

75. Of the following, which is least likely to occur in a 16-year-old as the result of blunt trauma to the abdomen sustained while playing football?
    a. Splenic rupture
    b. Pancreatic tear   **Ref. 84, p. 327**
    c. Hepatic tear
    d. Ruptured viscus

MULTIPLE CHOICE, MULTIPLE ANSWERS (answers on pp. 290-291)

Select one or more answers that will best complete or answer each of the following statements or questions.

76. Dislocation of the distal tibiofibular joint is commonly accompanied by which of the following?
    a. Fracture of the lateral malleolus
    b. Fracture of the medial malleolus   **Ref. 43, p. 944**
    c. Rupture of the fibulocalcaneal ligament
    d. Rupture of the deltoid ligament

77. Fractures of the medial tibial plateau occur _____ frequently than do those of the lateral plateau and are _____ associated with ligamentous injury.
    a. More
    b. Less   **Ref. 96, pp. 296, 306**
    c. Commonly
    d. Uncommonly

78. After proper reduction and internal fixation of a fracture of the femoral neck, union may be expected in about _____ of cases; however, aseptic necrosis may be expected in approximately _____ of these cases.

a. 30%
b. 40%   Ref. 42, p. 825
c. 50%   Ref. 43, p. 590
d. 70%
e. 80%

79. Minimally displaced fractures of the lateral condylar epiphysis cause
_____ late deformity and nonunion of the elbow and are best
treated by _____.
a. Less
b. More   Ref. 127, 53-A:1096, 1974
c. Open reduction, internal fixation, and cast
protection
d. Ulnar traction
e. Cast immobilization in the position of
maximum stability

80. In congenital bipartite patella the secondary center of ossification is usually in the _____ quadrant of the patella and usually _____
bilateral.
a. Upper outer
b. Lower outer   Ref. 86, p. 68
c. Is   Ref. 89, p. 46
d. Is not   Ref. 107, p. 789

81. In transection of the spinal cord, which of the following appear early
following the injury?
a. Babinski's sign
b. Increased deep tendon reflexes   Ref. 107, p. 991
c. Glans-bulbar reflex
d. Clonus
e. Anal reflex

82. Avascular necrosis is fairly _____ in treated type I fractures of the
femoral neck, and nonunion may be expected in about _____ of
treated type III fractures.
a. Common
b. Uncommon   Ref. 77, p. 431
c. 20%
d. 50%
e. 70%

83. In the carpal tunnel syndrome, which of the following are true?
a. It frequently is a complication of carpal
fractures.
b. It is seen frequently in patients with   Ref. 127, 41-A:626, 1959
acromegaly.   Ref. 127, 48-A:211, 1966
c. Menopausal women have an increased incidence of the disease.
d. There may be an hereditary predisposition
to the lesion.
e. None of the above.

84. Separation of the proximal radial epiphysis generally results in a decreased ability to _____ the forearm, and fusion of the epiphysis results in a _____ deformity.
    a. Pronate
    b. Supinate   Ref. 36, p. 332
    c. Varus
    d. Valgus
    e. Flexion

85. Fractures of the scapula are most often seen in the _____ third of the bone, and here nonunion is _____.
    a. Upper
    b. Middle   Ref. 36, pp. 48, 254
    c. Lower
    d. Common
    e. Uncommon

86. Generally, the postoperative position recommended for a trimalleolar fracture is:
    a. Inversion
    b. Eversion   Ref. 43, p. 515
    c. Equinus
    d. Calcaneus

87. Perilunar dislocations are _____ frequent than are dislocations of the lunate, and the incidence of fractures of the scaphoid associated with this lesion is _____ than that seen in simple dislocations of the lunate.
    a. More
    b. Less   Ref. 42, p. 657
    c. Higher
    d. Lower

88. Fracture of the pubis may cause rupture of the bladder that generally is _____ in nature and _____ been associated with osteitis pubis.
    a. Intraperitoneal
    b. Extraperitoneal   Ref. 42, p. 720
    c. Has   Ref. 127, 35-A:685, 1953
    d. Has not

89. Which are true regarding postirradiation fractures of the femur?
    a. Pain is often a symptom that precedes the
       fracture by months.
    b. An irregular transverse line of increased   Ref. 127, 38-B:830, 1956
       density in the femoral neck often precedes
       the fracture.
    c. Coxa vara without lateral angulation of
       the femoral head is often present.
    d. Healing of the fracture is different radio-
       logically from that of an ordinary fracture.

90. Fractures of the hip in children are complicated by aseptic necrosis _____ commonly than in adults, and when this does occur, it may resemble _____ in radiographic appearance.
    a. More
    b. Less   Ref. 127, 43-B:16, 1961
    c. Gaucher's disease
    d. Caisson's disease
    e. Legg-Perthes disease
91. Fracture of the thyroid cartilage is most common in _____ and has been associated with a mortality rate of about _____.
    a. Males
    b. Females   Ref. 107, p. 929
    c. 20%
    d. 50%
    e. 70%
92. Fractures of the os calcis comprise _____ than 50% of all tarsal fractures, and the fracture usually is _____ .
    a. Greater
    b. Less   Ref. 42, p. 1086
    c. An avulsion of the tuberosity or an epiphy-
       seal separation
    d. An isolated injury to the sustentaculum tali
    e. Of the body of the bone
93. Fractures of the malar-maxillary unit of the face include injuries to which of the following?
    a. Nasal bones
    b. Maxilla   Ref. 107, p. 923
    c. Palate
    d. Zygoma
    e. All of the above
94. Anterior dislocation of the lunate should be treated surgically when _____, and the approach should be made on the _____ surface.
    a. The affected joints or the median nerve
       are severely damaged
    b. Closed reduction has been unsuccessful   Ref. 43, p. 431
    c. The dislocation is older than 2 weeks   Ref. 127, 47-A:915, 1965
    d. Dorsal
    e. Volar
95. Early active exercise without weight bearing after either open or closed reduction of a traumatic hip dislocation or fracture dislocation will cause _____ incidence of myositis ossificans and will yield a _____ result than will immobilization.
    a. Increased
    b. No difference in the   Ref. 127, 36-A:327, 1954
    c. Decreased
    d. Better
    e. Worse

96. About _____ of all fractures of the hip occur in patients older than 60 years of age, with _____ being affected most commonly.
    a. 50%
    b. 70%   **Ref. 43, p. 572**
    c. 80%
    d. Males
    e. Females

97. Epiphyseal fractures of the upper humerus, with displacement of the proximal fragment, generally _____ require open reduction with or without internal fixation and should be immobilized in a _____ cast.
    a. Do
    b. Do not   **Ref. 42, p. 427**
    c. Hanging
    d. Shoulder spica

98. Which of the following have been indicated as factors predisposing to injury of the menisci?
    a. Poor mechanics of the knee
    b. Degenerative changes in the menisci   **Ref. 43, p. 907**
    c. Inadequate muscular support of the joint
    d. Knee effusion
    e. Chondromalacia of the patella

99. A 3-month-old untreated traumatic posterior dislocation of the hip in a 10-year-old boy is best treated by:
    a. Arthrodesis
    b. Open reduction of the hip, followed by   **Ref. 7, 9:1, 1952**
       physical therapy
    c. Angulation osteotomy
    d. Reduction and cup arthroplasty
    e. Range of motion exercises and no surgery

100. Pauwels' classification of fractures of the proximal femur is related to the _____, type III being the _____ stable.
    a. Angle of the fracture line
    b. Number of fragments   **Ref. 43, p. 590**
    c. Femoral head diameter in relation to that
       of the neck
    d. Most
    e. Least

101. The casted position of a fracture of both bones of the distal forearm should be in _____ so as to relax the _____ muscle.
    a. Pronation
    b. Supination   **Ref. 26, p. 78**
    c. Pronator teres
    d. Pronator quadratus
    e. Supinator

102. In a fracture of the proximal radius the arm is usually casted in
_____ to align the distal and proximal fragments, the latter being
controlled by the _____ muscle.
a. Pronation
b. Supination   **Ref. 26, p. 93**
c. Anconeus
d. Supinator
e. Pronator quadratus

103. In displaced fractures of the femur in children the average amount of
longitudinal overgrowth seen is:
a. 0 cm
b. 0.5 cm   **Ref. 115, 49:147, 1940**
c. 1 cm
d. 1.5 cm

104. Which of the following have been noted in adults in whom the radial
head has been excised during childhood?
a. Shortening of the forearm
b. Valgus deformity of the elbow   **Ref. 26, p. 67**
c. Motor weakness in the forearm and hand   **Ref. 141, 64:1079, 1937**
d. Radial deviation of the hand
e. Sensory changes

105. Which of the following are true regarding Köhler's disease and Freiberg's disease?
a. Both should be treated with nonweight-
bearing plaster immobilization initially.
b. Köhler's disease frequently results in   **Ref. 26, p. 196**
permanent deformity.
c. Freiberg's disease is most common in girls.
d. Shoes that are too tight or cramped have
been implicated as a caused of Freiberg's
disease.
e. Permanent loss of motion of the involved
joints is likely with Freiberg's disease.

106. In fractures of the proximal femur in children the poorest results are
usually seen in:
a. Transepiphyseal fractures
b. Transcervical fractures   **Ref. 43, p. 606**
c. Fractures at the base of the neck
d. Intertrochanteric fractures
e. None of the above

107. Fractures of the neck of the femur occur in a(an) _____ age group
than do intertrochanteric fractures and are seen somewhat more commonly in _____ .
a. Younger
b. Older   **Ref. 42, p. 794**
c. Males   **Ref. 43, pp. 572-576**
d. Females

108. Open reduction of the clavicle should be instituted in which circumstances?
    a. An undesirable cosmetic effect of a bony
       prominence
    b. A fracture of the distal third, with   **Ref. 43, p. 631**
       disruption of the corracoclavicular
       ligaments
    c. Pressure on the brachial plexus
    d. Persistent wide separation of the
       fragments
    e. In patients with a history of nonunion in
       other fractures or poor healing of soft
       tissue wounds

109. Myositis ossificans occurs _____ frequently in the upper than in
    the lower extremity and is _____ intimately associated with bone.
    a. More
    b. Less   **Ref. 127, 40-A:279, 1958**
    c. Always
    d. Not always

110. O'Donoghue's triad consists of rupture or damage to which of the
    following?
    a. Anterior cruciate ligament
    b. Posterior cruciate ligament   **Ref. 43, p. 927**
    c. Tibial collateral ligament
    d. Fibular collateral ligament
    e. Medial meniscus

111. Causalgia results from injuries to the _____ and _____ nerves
    considerably more frequently than from injuries to other peripheral
    nerves.
    a. Radial
    b. Peroneal   **Ref. 43, p. 1746**
    c. Median
    d. Tibial
    e. Ulnar

112. After reduction of a supracondylar fracture of the humerus the arm
    is immobilized in a long-arm plaster cast, with the elbow beyond
    90° of flexion because:
    a. The incidence of Volkmann's ischemic
       contracture is thereby decreased
    b. Then the cast will not act as a lever against   **Ref. 42, p. 483**
       the proximal fragment when hanging
       at the patient's side
    c. Such a position controls rotation most
       efficiently
    d. Full flexion of the joints is thereby
       maintained
    e. This position relaxes the elbow flexors

113. The immediate treatment of wringer injuries of the arm should include which of the following?
    a. Compression bandages
    b. Local heat to increase circulation   Ref. 26, p. 95
    c. Loose closure of any lacerations with   Ref. 51, p. 378
       sutures
    d. Systemic antibiotics in all cases
    e. Plaster immobilization of fractures only
114. A patient in traumatic shock may be expected to have an increase in which of the following laboratory values?
    a. Serum sodium
    b. Serum potassium   Ref. 107, p. 228
    c. Serum chloride
    d. Blood pH
    e. Serum alkaline phosphatase
115. Fatigue fractures occur most frequently in which of the following?
    a. Distal fibula
    b. Proximal tibia   Ref. 107, p. 348
    c. Distal femur
    d. First metatarsal
    e. Clavicle

SITUATION AND PROGRESSIVE THOUGHT (answers on p. 291)

Select the answer or answers that best apply in accordance with the information given in the following statements.

116. A 25-year-old black man complains of pain in his right wrist after a fall on his outstretched hand that afternoon. Physical examination reveals tenderness over the dorsal and volar aspects of the wrist, with pain on palpation over the "snuffbox." X-ray films in the anteroposterior and lateral views reveal no fracture. You should:
    a. Start hot soaks
    b. Reassure the patient that no fracture   Ref. 42, p. 643
       has been sustained
    c. Obtain x-ray films in the oblique position
       and with the hand in ulnar deviation
    d. Apply a short-arm cast
    e. Wrap the hand and wrist with elastic
       bandage
117. The patient should be instructed to:
    a. Return for repeat x-ray examinations in
       a week
    b. Call or return for a cast check in 24 hours   Ref. 42, p. 644
    c. Start active and passive exercises
    d. Continue the elastic wrap until all
       pain has disappeared
    e. Return in 3 weeks for cast removal and
       repeat x-ray examination

118. Assume that the initial x-ray films showed a fracture of the navicular bone through its waist. You can predict that delayed or nonunion will occur in _____ of cases.
    a. One fourth
    b. One third   Ref. 127, 20:424, 1938
    c. One half
    d. Two thirds

119. Assuming that a fracture of the navicular bone is present, the casted position of the wrist should be 30° of:
    a. Volar flexion and slight ulnar deviation
    b. Dorsiflexion and slight ulnar deviation   Ref. 115, 78:379, 1949
    c. Volar flexion and slight radial deviation
    d. Dorsiflexion and slight radial deviation

120. Had the patient having had no previous treatment come to you five months after injury with a fracture of the navicular bone, you should have:
    a. Done nothing and waited to see if a
       degenerative arthritis developed
    b. Immobilized the fracture in a short-arm   Ref. 119, 53:164, 1946
       cast
    c. Excised the distal fragment
    d. Planned to fuse the wrist
    e. Done a bone graft of the fracture site

121. A 45-year-old white woman is brought to the emergency room unconscious after having been thrown from a pickup truck in which she was a passenger. Physical examination reveals a blood pressure of 60/0, pulse 160, respiration 60 and unobstructed, and temperature 98.8° F. There is a 6 cm laceration over the right frontal area of the skull, a large area of contusion, and abrasion over the left anterolateral chest, with crepitus on palpation anteriorly and laterally over a 12 cm area, and a flexed and adducted left thigh. The left pupil is slightly larger than the right but reacts to light slowly. The abdomen is moderately tense; however, no skin lesions are noted. Bowel sounds are absent. Immediately you should:
    a. Start intravenous vasopressors
    b. Obtain a base-line hematocrit study   Ref. 36, p. 197
    c. Splint the chest wall
    d. Do an x-ray examination of the skull
    e. Tap the peritoneal cavity

122. Of the following, which is the most important x-ray examination to be obtained early in the care of this patient?
    a. Skull series
    b. Anteroposterior chest x-ray films   Ref. 36, p. 97
    c. Anteroposterior x-ray films of the pelvis
    d. Abdominal flat plate films
    e. Anteroposterior upright x-ray films of the
       abdomen

123. The pupillary findings may be indicative of:
    a. Right cerebral damage
    b. Left cerebral damage   Ref. 109, p. 108
    c. Argyll Robinson pupil
    d. Tonic pupil of Adie

124. X-ray examination of the pelvis reveals a fracture-dislocation of the left
    hip, with a small chip off the posterior acetabulum without a fracture
    of the head of the femur. This should be classified as a type _____
    fracture-dislocation.
    a. I
    b. II   Ref. 43, p. 415
    c. III
    d. IV

125. An incidental finding on x-ray examination of the pelvis is a mass
    approximately 8 cm in diameter over the right buttock that seems to
    have bony attachment and contains speckled areas of calcification.
    Treatment of this lesion at a later date should include:
    a. Needle biopsy
    b. Open biopsy   Ref. 1, p. 1054
    c. Wide local excision followed by   Ref. 2, pp. 22, 60, 66
       irradiation
    d. Wide local excision
    e. Irradiation

126. On the third postoperative day the patient is noted to be vomiting dark,
    foul-smelling fluid in small amounts. She complains of severe thirst.
    Pain status is equivocal, since the operative site on the left hip is bother-
    ing her. Vital signs are blood pressure 90/60, pulse 120, respiration
    36 and shallow, and temperature 99.4° F. You should:
    a. Allow clear liquids in small amounts as
       tolerated
    b. Order antiemetic drugs   Ref. 6, p. 308
    c. Pass a nasogastric tube and continue
       small amounts of clear liquids
    d. Pass a nasogastric tube and irrigate it until
       return is noted
    e. Start intravenous replacement therapy

127. Four days postoperatively the patient has begun to confabulate and has
    intermittent periods of delirium. Neurologic examination is within nor-
    mal limits except for bilaterally hyperactive deep tendon reflexes. Bowel
    sounds are decreased. The vital signs are normal. Which of the follow-
    ing is most likely abnormal?
    a. Serum sodium
    b. Serum calcium   Ref. 6, p. 312
    c. Serum potassium
    d. Blood CO_2
    e. Urine fat stain

128. Five days after reduction of the hip the patient's temperature rises to 103° F and she complains of leg cramps. Calf tenderness is noted on the left, but Homan's sign is negative. You should:
    a. Start active and passive exercises
    b. Heparinize the patient   Ref. 6, p. 303
    c. Wrap the legs with elastic bandages
    d. Employ ice packs
    e. Consider and schedule the patient for
       vena cava ligation

129. A track star notes severe pain in his anterior lower leg several hours after his first day of spring training. The pain is severe; however, muscle function is normal and there are palpable dorsal pedal and posterior tibial pulses. You should:
    a. Have him go home and soak in a hot tub,
       since this will relieve the muscle spasm
    b. Have him elevate the leg and apply ice   Ref. 43, p. 1462
       bags that night while studying
    c. Hospitalize him for observation after
       putting on a long-leg cast to immobilize
       the muscles
    d. Hospitalize the patient and prepare for
       a fasciotomy of the leg
    e. Do nothing since he probably only has
       severe "shin splints"

130. A 30-year-old previously healthy patient with a history of blunt trauma to the anterior chest without fracture and with a closed fracture of the tibia is admitted for observation. Because of a "queer feeling" in his chest several days after the accident, an EKG is obtained that demonstrates "arrhythmia" according to the house officer. This is most likely due to:
    a. Acute myocardial infarction
    b. Acute pulmonary infarction   Ref. 43, p. 2
    c. Cardiac tamponade
    d. Pulmonary contusion
    e. Myocardial contusion

131. A 30-year-old man is brought to the emergency room having sustained a gunshot wound of the thigh, with a comminuted fracture of the midshaft femur. There are no palpable pulses distal to the wound. Inspection reveals a dirty wound full of torn clothing, wadding, shot, soil, and leaves and a shredded profunda femoris over 8 cm in length. After evaluation and stabilization, the treatment should be:
    a. Packing the limb in ice because it will
       have to be amputated and this will
       decrease the amount of circulating toxins
    b. Internal fixation of the fracture and   Ref. 42, p. 124
       grafting of the vessel through a second
       incision if possible, thus allowing the

gunshot wound to be packed open with
gauze

c. Repair of the vessel and skeletal traction
through the proximal tibia

d. Débridement of the wound and ligature
of the vessel, since adequate collateral
circulation exists to allow the distal
limb to survive

e. Débridement of the wound, repair of the
vessel, and bone grafting

132. A 25-year-old man is brought to the emergency room after having been
struck by an auto below his right knee approximately 6 hours before.
There is an 8 cm laceration over the anterolateral aspect of the tibia,
extending in one area down to the bone without apparent involvement
of the knee joint. The wound edges are slightly dark, and there is some
foreign material in the wound. X-ray examination reveals a depressed
fracture of the lateral tibial plateau as well as a fracture of the fibula.
You should prepare and irrigate the wound and:

a. Excise the wound edges and close the
defect in layers

b. Excise the wound edges and close the
lesion in one layer, with drains in the
depth of the wound

        Ref. 42, p. 166
        Ref. 77, p. 65
        Ref. 107, p. 269

c. Perform an en bloc excision of the wound
and apply a split-thickness skin graft

d. Excise the wound edges and pack the
defect open, planning on either delayed
or secondary closure

133. The most significant injury likely in this patient is to the:
a. Anterior tibial artery
b. Circumflex fibular artery   Ref. 96, p. 153
c. Anterior tibial recurrent artery
d. Posterior tibial recurrent artery
e. Descending branch of the lateral femoral
circumflex artery

134. Anteroposterior x-ray views are taken of both knees during application
of abduction stress and demonstrate a 1.5 cm widening of the medial
joint space on the right by comparison with the same area on the left.
This is presumptive evidence of:
a. Crush injury of the medial meniscus
b. Tear of the anterior cruciate ligament   Ref. 127, 42-A:13, 1960
c. Tear of the posterior cruciate ligament
d. Tear of the medial collateral ligament

135. Concerning treatment of this fracture, which are true?
a. The meniscus should always be removed so
that visualization of the joint surface
will allow accurate reduction.

b. The area below the fracture should
   always be grafted with cancellous bone.   Ref. 43, p. 531
c. Internal fixation may not be necessary.
   unless there is gross comminution.
d. Passive motion of the knee should be
   started at least 3 weeks after operation.

TRUE OR FALSE (answers on p. 291)

136. Intramedullary nailing of the femur in the treatment of fractures does
     little if any damage to the cortical blood supply of the bone.
     (T) (F)   Ref. 127, 37-B:492, 1955
137. Because of its blood supply, aseptic necrosis is common following dis-
     location of the lunate, and therefore late reduction will generally result
     in poor function.   Ref. 36, p. 389
     (T) (F)   Ref. 127, 46-B:55, 1964
138. Despite anatomic differences in blood supply, carpal navicular fractures
     may be expected to heal in more than 90% of cases merely by cast im-
     mobilization.   Ref. 127, 36-A:998, 1954
     (T) (F)
139. Because of the obliquity of the spinous processes and the vertical align-
     ment of the facets, fracture-dislocations of the vertebral bodies with dis-
     placement is most common in the lower dorsal area.
     (T) (F)   Ref. 127, 29:107, 1947
140. Central injuries to the epiphysis tend to cause less deformity but more
     interference with growth than do peripheral epiphyseal injuries.
     (T) (F)   Ref. 127, 38-A:84, 1956
141. Fracture of the tibial spine is most comonly seen in adults, whereas rup-
     ture of the anterior cruciate ligament is noted generally in adolescents
     and young adults.   Ref. 107, p. 759
     (T) (F)
142. Priapism is often a characteristic finding in traumatic lesions of the
     cervical area of the spinal cord.   Ref. 65, p. 295
     (T) (F)
143. If after intramedullary nailing of a femoral shaft fracture, an infection
     develops along the course of the nail, the nail should be removed and
     the patient treated with traction and plaster immobilization.
     (T) (F)   Ref. 43, p. 565
144. The incidence of infection after open reduction of a femoral fracture is
     about twice that seen in all other bones.   Ref. 43, p. 555
     (T) (F)
145. Generally speaking, fractures of the tibial plateaus treated by surgery,
     regardless of the method, should be kept immobilized until sufficient
     healing has occurred to allow weight bearing.   Ref. 43, p. 534
     (T) (F)
146. Motion at a fracture site, whether side to side, rotatory, or shearing in
     nature, stimulates abundant callous formation but interferes with final
     bridging of the fractures.   Ref. 43, p. 485
     (T) (F)

147. Spastic paraplegia would not develop following a complete interruption of the spinal cord at the level of T-10. **Ref. 9, p. 515**
(T) (F)

148. Delay in reduction of a traumatic posterior hip dislocation of 24 hours almost always will result in poor hip function. **Ref. 127, 36-A:323, 1954**
(T) (F)

149. After an injury to the popliteal artery, as in a traumatic dislocation of the knee, the skin on the dorsum of the foot may remain warm to touch despite arterial thrombus formation. **Ref. 127, 45-A:897, 1963**
(T) (F)

150. Conservative treatment of the ruptured Achilles tendon in a young athlete may be contraindicated because of failure of significant contact between the tendon fragments. **Ref. 127, 56-A:174, 1974**
(T) (F)

151. Primary total hip arthroplasty is never indicated in an acute fracture dislocation of the hip. **Ref. 127, 56-A:1134, 1974**
(T) (F)

152. In a young person, rupture of a muscle due to stress is less common than rupture of the tendon. **Ref. 43, p. 1464**
(T) (F)

153. A defect in the posterior humeral head due to recurrent dislocation of the shoulder is called a Bankart defect. **Ref. 43, p. 456**
(T) (F)

154. In treating a fresh fracture of the femoral head, it is usually best to remove the fragments without attempting reduction. **Ref. 43, p. 419**
(T) (F)

155. Fractures of either the greater or the lesser trochanter may be realistically treated by plaster immobilization. **Ref. 42, p. 790**
(T) (F)

156. Elevated temperature, odor, and pain are the symptoms that are usually seen with infection, whereas the order of those symptoms is reversed in the presence of gangrene. **Ref. 26, p. 123**
(T) (F)

157. Leadbetter's heel-palm test is utilized to test the stability of a reduced fracture of the femoral neck. **Ref. 42, p. 810**
(T) (F)

158. In children the coxa vara deformity resulting from a fracture of the proximal femur due to trauma will usually remodel, whereas such is not the case when the defect is caused by a slipped capital femoral epiphysis.
(T) (F) **Ref. 26, p. 152**

159. Bayonet apposition of a fracture in a child generally results in solid healing in less time than that required when there is end-to-end apposition. **Ref. 26, p. 78**
(T) (F)

160. Delayed ulnar nerve palsy is frequently seen after unreduced fractures of the lateral condyle of the humerus **Ref. 26, p. 45**
(T) (F)

161. In children a displaced fracture of the lateral condyle of the humerus can usually be reduced by closed methods. **Ref. 26, p. 43**
   (T) (F)

162. In midshaft fractures of the humerus in children, radial nerve damage is a far less common complication than in adults. **Ref. 26, p. 22**
   (T) (F)

163. In children, displaced flake fractures of the superior articular surface of the talus should be removed, since they will not heal adequately. **Ref. 26, p. 196**
   (T) (F)

164. Displaced transcervical and cervicotrochanteric femoral fractures in children, treated with the best of methods available, have a subsequent complication rate of about 60%. **Ref. 132, 3-1:1675, 1972**
   (T) (F)

165. Contraction of a patient's extracellular fluid volume will not effect his tolerance to either general or spinal anesthesia. **Ref. 42, p. 85**
   (T) (F)

LIST (answers on pp. 291-293)

166. List five surgical procedures that may be recommended for the treatment of a malunited fracture of the ankle. **Ref. 43, p. 700**

167. List six injuries interrupting the extensor mechanism of the knee and state in which age group each is most commonly seen. **Ref. 36, p. 523**
   Ref. 42, pp. 919, 971
   Ref. 96, p. 245

168. List six osseous and soft tissue lesions that may accompany Colles' fracture. **Ref. 36, p. 361**

169. List five conditions that must be met before osteosynthesis should be attempted in treating nonunion of a femoral neck fracture.
   Ref. 43, p. 783

170. List seven causes contributing to nonunion of a fracture. **Ref. 43, p. 750**

171. List in order the four events that occur in producing a complete acromioclavicular separation. **Ref. 127, 36-B:194, 1954**

172. List the three classic signs of hemopericardium. **Ref. 6, p. 1233**
   Ref. 141, 74:406, 1942

173. List four procedures recommended for the treatment of nonunion of the carpal navicular. **Ref. 42, p. 648**

174. List five visceral complications of chest injuries. **Ref. 107, p. 929**

175. List five complications of a septic arthritis involving the hip.
   Ref. 42, p. 843

176. List the four most common obstacles to closed reduction of a displaced fracture of the surgical neck of the humerus. **Ref. 115, 91:627, 1956**

177. List six indications for amputation. **Ref. 97, p. 3**

178. List five indications for the surgical treatment of scars on an extremity.
   Ref. 43, p. 213

179. List four indications for open reduction of an acetabular fracture.
   Ref. 43, p. 419

180. List five methods in addition to fascial grafts and primary ligament repair that have been recommended for treating acromioclavicular joint separations. **Ref. 43, p. 424**
Ref. 115, 85:760, 1953
Ref. 141, 73:866, 1941

181. List four methods of repairing an old tear of the tibial collateral ligament. **Ref. 43, p. 934**

182. List three important factors that influence the recurrence of a shoulder dislocation. **Ref. 42, p. 408**
Ref. 127, 38-A:957, 1956

183. List five common complications that occur late following a fracture of the distal radius with dorsal displacement, that is, Colles' fracture.
Ref. 36, p. 373
Ref. 42, p. 614

184. List three commonly employed methods of reducing a posterior hip dislocation. **Ref. 42, p. 757**

185. List four methods of reducing a dislocated shoulder. **Ref. 42, p. 391**

186. List the steps utilized in performing Kocher's method of reducing a shoulder dislocation. **Ref. 42, p. 391**

187. List six causes of inability to reduce and maintain reduction in fractures of the femoral neck. **Ref. 127, 47-A:819, 1965**

188. List six complications of surgical amputation. **Ref. 127, 35-A:661, 1953**

189. List five derangements of the distal radioulnar joint that may produce pain, clicking on supination or pronation, or weakness of grip.
Ref. 43, p. 947

190. List five indications for prosthetic replacement of the femoral head in fresh fractures of the neck of the femur. **Ref. 43, p. 603**

191. List five factors that lead to consideration of a battered child syndrome.
Ref. 125, 181:17-24, 1962

References and Answers

References

1. Ackerman, L. V., and Rosai, J.: Surgical pathology, ed. 5, St. Louis, 1974, The C. V. Mosby Co.
2. Ackerman, L. V., and Spjut, H. J.: Tumors of bone and cartilage, fasc. 4, Washington, D.C., 1962, Armed Forces Institute of Pathology.
3. Ackerman, L. V., Spjut, H. J., Dorfman, H. D., and Fechner, R. E.: Tumors of bone and cartilage, fasc. 5, series 2, Washington, D.C., 1971, Armed Forces Institute of Pathology.
4. Adams, R. D., Denny-Brown, D., and Pearson, C. M.: Diseases of muscle, ed. 3, New York, 1975, Harper & Row, Publishers.
5. Aegerter, E., and Kirkpatrick, J. A., Jr.: Orthopedic diseases, ed. 3, Philadelphia, 1968, W. B. Saunders Co.
6. Allen, J. G., Harkins, H. N., Moyer, C. A., and Rhodes, J. E.: Surgery—principles and practice, ed. 3, Philadelphia, 1965, J. B. Lippincott Co.
7. American Academy of Orthopaedic Surgeons: Instructional course lectures; vols. 1-15, Ann Arbor, J. W. Edwards, Publisher, Inc.; vols. 16-18, St. Louis, The C. V. Mosby Co.
8. American Academy of Orthopaedic Surgeons: Instructional course lectures, vols. 19-23, St. Louis, 1970-1974, The C. V. Mosby Co.
9. American Academy of Orthopaedic Surgeons: Orthopaedic appliances atlas, vol. 1, Ann Arbor, 1952, J. W. Edwards, Publisher, Inc.
10. American Academy of Orthopaedic Surgeons: Orthopaedic appliances atlas, vol. 2, Ann Arbor, 1960, J. W. Edwards, Publisher, Inc.
11. American Academy of Orthopaedic Surgeons: Symposium on the spine, St. Louis, 1969, The C. V. Mosby Co.
12. American Academy of Orthopaedic Surgeons: Symposium on sports medicine, St. Louis, 1969, The C. V. Mosby Co.
13. American Congress of Physical Medicine and Rehabilitation, American Academy of Physical Medicine and Rehabilitation (sponsors): Third International Congress of Physical Medicine, Chicago, 1963, Westlake Press, Inc.
14. Anderson, M. H.: Functional bracing of the upper extremities, Springfield, Ill., 1958, Charles C Thomas, Publisher.
15. Anderson, M. H., Bechtol, C. O., and Sollars, R. E.: Clinical prosthetics for physicians and therapists, Springfield, Ill., 1959, Charles C Thomas, Publisher.

16. Anderson, M. H., Bray, J. J., Hennessy, C. A., and Sollars, R. E.: Prosthetic principles—above the knee amputation, Springfield, Ill., 1960, Charles C Thomas, Publisher.

17. Anson, Barry J., editor: Morris' human anatomy, ed. 12, New York, 1966, McGraw-Hill Book Co.

18. Barnett, C. H., Davies, D. V., and MacConaill, M. A.: Synovial joints—their structure and mechanics, Springfield, Ill., 1961, Charles C Thomas, Publisher.

19. Basmajian, J.: Muscles alive, ed. 3, Baltimore, 1974, The Williams & Wilkins Co.

20. Basmajian, J. V.: Grant's method of anatomy, ed. 9, Baltimore, 1975, The Williams & Wilkins Co.

21. Bechtol, C., Ferguson, A., and Laing, P.: Metals and engineering in bone and joint surgery, Baltimore, 1959, The Williams & Wilkins Co.

22. Beeson, P. B., and McDermott, W., editors: Cecil-Loeb textbook of medicine, ed. 13, Philadelphia, 1971, W. B. Saunders Co.

23. Bender, L.: Prostheses and rehabilitation after arm amputation, Springfield, Ill., 1974, Charles C Thomas, Publisher.

24. Blakeslee, B., editor: The limb-deficient child, Berkeley, 1963, University of California Press.

25. Bloom, W., and Fawcett, D. W.: A textbook of histology, ed. 9, Philadelphia, 1968, W. B. Saunders Co.

26. Blount, W. P.. Fractures in children, Baltimore, 1955, The Williams & Wilkins Co.

27. Blount, W. P., and Moe, J. H.: The Milwaukee brace, Baltimore, 1973, The Williams & Wilkins Co.

28. Bourne, G. H., editor: The biochemistry and physiology of bone, New York, 1956, Academic Press, Inc.

29. Bourne, G. H., and Golarz, M. N., editors: Muscular dystrophy in man and animals, New York, 1963, Hafner Publishing Co., Inc.

30. Boyes, H.: Bunnell's surgery of the hand, ed. 4, Philadelphia, 1964, J. B. Lippincott Co.

31. Boyes, J. H.: Bunnell's surgery of the hand, ed. 5, Philadelphia, 1970, J. B. Lippincott Co.

32. Bunnell, S.: Surgery of the hand, ed. 2, Philadelphia, 1944, J. B. Lippincott Co.

33. Burgess, E. M., Traub, J. E., and Wilson, A. B.: Immediate post-surgical prosthetics in the management of lower extremity amputees, TR 10-5, Veterans Administration, 1967, Washington, D.C.

34. Caffey, J.: Pediatric x-ray diagnosis, ed. 6, Chicago, 1972, Year Book Medical Publishers, Inc.

35. Cailliet, R.: Low back pain syndrome, Philadelphia, 1962, F. A. Davis Co.

36. Cave, E. F., editor: Fractures and other injuries, Chicago, 1958, Year Book Medical Publishers, Inc.

37. Charnley, J.: The closed treatment of common fractures, ed. 3, Baltimore, 1963, The Williams & Wilkins Co.

38. Close, J. R.: Motor function in the lower extremities, Springfield, Ill., 1964, Charles C Thomas, Publisher.

39. Committee of the American Rheumatism Association Section of the Arthritis Foundation: Primer on the rheumatoid diseases, ed. 7, J.A.M.A. (suppl. 5) **224**, 1973.

40. Committee on Prosthetic, Orthotic Education: Gait analysis, Chicago, Northwestern University Medical School.

41. Converse, J. M., and Littler, J. W.: Reconstructive plastic surgery. The hand and upper and lower extremities, vol. 4, Philadelphia, 1964, W. B. Saunders Co.

42. Conwell, H. E., and Reynolds, F. C.: Key and Conwell's Management of fractures, dislocations, and sprains, ed. 7, St. Louis, 1961, The C. V. Mosby Co.

43. Crenshaw, A. H., editor: Campbell's operative orthopaedics, ed. 5, St. Louis, 1971, The C. V. Mosby Co.

44. Davenport, H. W.: The ABC of acid-base chemistry, ed. 6, Chicago, 1974, University of Chicago Press.

45. DePalma, A. F., editor-in-chief: Clinical orthopaedics and related research, Philadelphia, J. B. Lippincott Co.

46. Department of Medicine and Surgery, Veterans Administration: Bulletin of Prosthetics Research, vol. 10(1), Washington, D.C., 1964.

47. Department of Medicine and Surgery, Veterans Administration: Bulletin of Prosthetics Research, vol. 10(2), Washington, D.C., 1964.

48. Downey, J. A., and Darling, R. C.: Physiological basics of rehabilitation medicine, Philadelphia, 1971, W. B. Saunders Co.

49. Edeiken, J., and Hodes, P. J.: Roentgen diagnosis of disease of bone, ed. 2, vols. I and II, Baltimore, 1973, The Williams & Wilkins Co.

50. Evans, F. G., editor: Biomechanical studies of the musculoskeletal system, Springfield, Ill., 1961, Charles C Thomas, Publisher.

51. Ferguson, A. B., Jr.: Orthopedic surgery in infancy and childhood, ed. 3, Baltimore, 1968, The Williams & Wilkins Co.

52. Flatt, A. E.: The care of minor hand injuries, ed. 2, St. Louis, 1963, The C. V. Mosby Co.

53. Frankel, V. H., and Burstein, A. H.: Orthopaedic biomechanics, Philadelphia, 1970, Lea & Febiger.

54. Frost, H. M., editor: Bone biodynamics, Henry Ford Hospital International Symposium, Boston, 1963, Little, Brown & Co.

55. Frost, H. M.: Bone remodeling dynamics, Springfield, Ill., 1963, Charles C Thomas, Publisher.

56. Frost, H. M.: Orthopaedic biomechanics, Springfield, Ill., 1973, Charles C Thomas, Publisher.

57. Ganong, W. F.: Review of medical physiology, ed. 6, Los Altos, Calif., 1973, Lange Medical Publications.

58. Gillette, H. E.: Systems of therapy in cerebral palsy, Springfield, Ill., 1973, Charles C Thomas, Publisher.

59. Goodman, L. S., and Gilman, A.: The pharmacological basis of therapeutics, ed. 4, New York, 1970, The Macmillan Co.

60. Goss, C. M., editor: Gray's anatomy of the human body, ed. 29, Philadelphia, 1973, Lea & Febiger.

61. Greene, N. M.: Physiology of spinal anesthesia, ed. 2, Baltimore, 1969, The Williams & Wilkins Co.

62. Hall, M. C.: The locomotor system functional histology, Springfield, Ill., 1965, Charles C Thomas, Publisher.
63. Ham, A. W.: Histology, ed. 7, Philadelphia, 1974, J. B. Lippincott Co.
64. Hirschberg, G. G., Lewis, L., and Thomas, D.: Rehabilitation, Philadelphia, 1964, J. B. Lippincott Co.
65. Howorth, M. B., and Petrie, J. G.: Injuries of the spine, Baltimore, 1964, The Williams & Wilkins Co.
66. Hueston, J. T.: Dupuytren's contracture, Baltimore, 1963, The Williams & Wilkins Co.
67. Interdisciplinary clinical, educational, and research aspects of a regional center for the rehabilitation of spinal cord injured persons—a final report, Sept. 1969, SRS Grant RD-2114M-68-C2, Attending Staff Association of the Rancho Los Amigos Hospital, Downey, Calif.
68. Jaffe, H. L.: Tumors and tumorous conditions of the bones and joints, Philadelphia, 1958, Lea & Febiger.
69. Jaffe, H. L.: Metabolic, degenerative, and inflammatory diseases of bones and joints, Philadelphia, 1972, Lea & Febiger.
70. Jorden, H.: Orthopaedic appliances, New York, 1939, Oxford University Press.
71. Kanavel, A. B.: Infections of the hand, ed. 7, Philadelphia, 1939, Lea & Febiger.
71a. Keim, H.: The adolescent spine, New York, 1976, Grune & Stratton, Inc.
72. Klopsteg, E., and Wilson, D.: Human limbs and their substitutes, New York, 1954, McGraw-Hill Book Co., Inc.
73. Koehler, A., and Zimmer, E. A.: Borderlands of the normal and early pathologic in skeletal roentgenology, translated by Stefen P. Wilk, ed. 11, New York, 1968, Grune & Stratton, Inc.
74. Krusen, F. H., Kottke, F. V., and Ellwood, P. M.: Handbook of physical medicine and rehabilitation, ed. 2, Philadelphia, 1971, W. B. Saunders Co.
75. Licht, Sidney, editor: Therapeutic exercise, Baltimore, 1961, Licht.
76. Licht, S.: Orthotics etcetera, Baltimore, 1966, Waverly Press, Inc.
77. McLaughlin, H. L.: Trauma, Philadelphia, 1959, W. B. Saunders Co.
78. Mereday, C., Dolan, C., and Lusskin, R.: Evaluation of the UC-BL shoe insert in "flexible" pes planus, Prosthetics and Orthotics, New York University, Sept., 1969.
79. Mital, M., and Pierce, D.: Amputees and their prostheses, Boston, 1971, Little, Brown & Co.
80. Moore, D. C.: Regional block, ed. 4, Springfield, Ill., 1965, Charles C Thomas, Publisher.
81. Mountcastle, V. B., editor: Medical physiology, ed. 12, St. Louis, 1968, The C. V. Mosby Co.
82. National Academy of Sciences—National Research Council, Committee on Prosthetics Research and Development: The geriatric amputee, publ. 919, Washington, D.C., 1961, National Academy of Sciences—National Research Council.
83. Nelson, W. E.: Textbook of pediatrics, ed. 9, Philadelphia, 1969, W. B. Saunders Co.

84. O'Donoghue, D. H.: Treatment of injuries to athletes, Philadelphia, 1962, W. B. Saunders Co.

85. Ontario Crippled Children's Centre: Rehabilitation engineering, research report, 1971.

86. Paul, L. W., and Juhl, J. H.: The essentials of roentgen interpretation, ed. 3, New York, 1972, Harper & Row.

87. Physician's desk reference, ed. 30, Oradell, N.J., 1976, Medical Economics Co.

88. Proceedings, Sixteenth Annual Clinical Spinal Cord Injury Conference, Veterans Administration Hospital, Long Beach, Calif., Sept. 1967, Publication SCIC 10-68-1, Veterans Administration, Washington, D.C.

89. Raney, R. B., and Brashear, H. R.: Shands' handbook of orthopaedic surgery, ed. 8, St. Louis, 1971, The C. V. Mosby Co.

90. Ropes, M. W., and Bauer, W.: Synovial fluid changes in joint disease, Cambridge, Mass., 1953, Harvard University Press.

91. Rusk, H. W.: Rehabilitation medicine, ed. 3, St. Louis, 1971, The C. V. Mosby Co.

92. Sabiston, D. C., Jr., editor: Davis-Christopher textbook of surgery, ed. 10, Philadelphia, 1972, W. B. Saunders Co.

93. Schaffer, J. P., editor: Morris' human anatomy, ed. 11, New York, 1953, McGraw-Hill Book Co., Inc.

94. Sharrard, W. J. W.: Paediatric orthopaedics and fractures, Oxford, England and Edinburgh, Scotland, 1971, Blackwell Scientific Publications.

95. Simon, G.: Principles of bone x-ray diagnosis, Washington, D.C., 1965, Butterworth Inc.

96. Slocum, D. B.: An atlas of amputation, St. Louis, 1949, The C. V. Mosby Co.

97. Smillie, I. S.: Injuries of the knee joint, Baltimore, 1962, The Williams & Wilkins Co.

98. Sobotta, J., and Uhlenhuth, E.: Atlas of descriptive anatomy, New York, 1957, Hafner Publishing Co.

99. Staff of the Prosthetics Research Group Biomechanics Laboratory: Manual of below knee prosthetics, University of California, 1959.

100. Steindler, A.: Kinesiology, Springfield, Ill., 1973, Charles C Thomas, Publisher.

101. Stout, A. P., and Lattes, R.: Tumors of the soft tissues, fasc. 1, series 2, Washington, D.C., 1967, Armed Forces Institute of Pathology.

102. Stryer, L.: Biochemistry, San Francisco, 1975, W. H. Freeman & Co.

103. Tachdjian, M. O.: Pediatric orthopedics, vols. 1 and 2, Philadelphia, 1972, W. B. Saunders Co.

104. Talbott, J. H., and Seegmiller, J. E.: Gout, ed. 3, New York, 1967, Grune & Stratton, Inc.

105. Turek, S. L.: Orthopaedics: principles and their application, ed. 2, Philadelphia, 1967, J. B. Lippincott Co.

106. Urist, Marshall, editor-in-chief: Clinical orthopaedics and related research, Philadelphia, J. B. Lippincott Co.

107. Watson-Jones, R.: Fractures and joint injuries, ed. 2, Baltimore, 1962, The Williams & Wilkins Co.

108. Wilson, A. B., Jr.: Limb prosthetics, Huntington, N.Y., 1972, Robert E. Krieger, Publisher.

109. Wintrobe et al., editors: Harrison's principles of internal medicine, ed. 7, New York, 1974, McGraw-Hill Book Co., Inc.

110. Woodburne, R. T.: Essentials of human anatomy, ed. 5, New York, 1973, Oxford University Press.

111. Yearbook of orthopedic and traumatic surgery, Chicago, Yearbook Medical Publishers.

112. Zancolli, E.: Structural and dynamic bases of hand surgery, Philadelphia, 1968, J. B. Lippincott Co.

113. Acta Orthopaedica Scandinavica.

114. American Journal of Roentgenology, Radium Therapy and Nuclear Medicine.

115. American Journal of Surgery.

116. Annals of the Royal College of Surgeons, England.

117. Annals of Surgery.

118. Archives of Physical Medicine and Rehabilitation.

119. Archives of Surgery.

120. Artificial Limbs.

121. British Journal of Surgery.

122. Bulletin of Prosthetics Research.

123. Canadian Medical Association Journal.

124. Inter-clinic Information Bulletin, New York University.

125. Journal of the American Medical Association.

126. Journal of the American Medical Association: Primer on rheumatoid diseases 171:1205-1220, 1345-1356, 1680-1691, 1959.

127. Journal of Bone and Joint Surgery.

127a. Journal of Hand Surgery.

128. Journal of Neurosurgery.

129. Missouri Medicine.

130. New England Journal of Medicine.

131. Ortho-Pros. The Canadian Association of Prosthetics and Orthotists Publishers.

132. Orthopaedic Clinics of North America.

133. Orthopaedic and Prosthetic Appliance Journal.

134. Orthotics and Prosthetics.

135. Pediatrics.

136. Physical Therapy Review.

137. Plastic and Reconstructive Surgery.

138. Radiology.

139. Southern Medical Journal.

140. Surgery.

141. Surgery, Gynecology and Obstetrics.

142. Surgical Clinics of North America.

Answers

SECTION 1—ADULT ORTHOPAEDICS
Multiple choice, single answer
(pp. 1-12)

1. b	32. d
2. d	33. d
3. a	34. c
4. d	35. d
5. c	36. c
6. d	37. a
7. b	38. c
8. d	39. b
9. b	40. e
10. c	41. e
11. b	42. a
12. c	43. b
13. e	44. c
14. d	45. b
15. a	46. d
16. d	47. c
17. b	48. c
18. b	49. b
19. d	50. d
20. d	51. d
21. e	52. a
22. e	53. c
23. a	54. e
24. e	55. d
25. e	56. d
26. a	57. e
27. a	58. c
28. e	59. b
29. d	60. a
30. c	61. a
31. a	62. c
	63. a
	64. d
	65. d
	66. e

67. b
68. a
69. b
70. c

Multiple choice, multiple answers
(pp. 12-18)

71. c, d
72. b, d
73. a, c, e
74. b, d
75. b, c
76. a, c, e
77. f
78. c, d
79. a, c, e
80. a, b, e
81. a, b, c
82. a, b, d, e
83. b, c, d
84. a, b, e
85. a, b, e
86. a, c, d, b
87. a, c, e
88. b, c
89. c, d, e
90. a, b, e
91. a, c, d
92. b, d
93. a, c, d
94. a, b, d
95. c, e
96. a, b, c
97. a, b, c, d, e

Situation and progressive thought
(pp. 18-21)

98. d
99. d
100. c
101. c
102. d
103. c
104. b
105. e
106. c
107. a
108. e

109. e
110. d
111. d
112. c
113. b

True or false (pp. 21-23)

114. T
115. T
116. T
117. T
118. F
119. F
120. T
121. F
122. T
123. T
124. T
125. F
126. T
127. F
128. F
129. T
130. T
131. T
132. F
133. F
134. F
135. F
136. F
137. T
138. T
139. F
140. T
141. T
142. F
143. F
144. T
145. T
146. T
147. F
148. T
149. T
150. T
151. T
152. T
153. F
154. T

155. a. Acute traumatic bursitis
    b. Chronic traumatic bursitis
    c. Acute infectious bursitis
    d. Chronic infectious bursitis
    e. Gouty bursitis
    f. Bursitis associated with arthritis
    g. Neoplasms of bursa, osteo-chondromatosis, villonodular synovitis, xanthomatosis, and synovioma
    h. Calcified bursitis
156. a. First metatarsophalangeal joint severely arthritic
    b. When valgus of the great toe exceeds 50°
    c. When circulation in the foot is impaired
    d. When the great toe laps under or over the second toe
157. a. Ligamentous
    b. Muscular
    c. Neuritic
    d. Arthritic
    e. Traumatic
    f. Mechanical
    g. Circulatory
    h. Metabolic
    i. Infectious
    j. Osteochondrosis of the metatarsal head
158. a. Poor mechanics of the knee
    b. Degenerative changes or con-genital anomalies of the meniscus
    c. Inadequate muscular control of the joint
159. a. Bucket-handle tear of the meniscus
    b. Intra-articular tumors
    c. Pedunculated flap of fat
    d. Loose body
160. a. Positive McMurray's sign
    b. Positive grinding test of Apley
    c. Positive squat test
161. *Advantages:*
    a. The operation is smaller and less traumatic.

b. The surgery is done through an avascular plane.
    c. Convalescence is rapid.
Disadvantage:
    a. The chief disadvantage is that a further tear may be present at a later date secondary to undetected degenerative changes of the meniscus.
162. a. An anteroposterior ridge pro-jecting distally from the margin of the femoral con-dyle
    b. Flattening of the peripheral half of the articular surface of the condyle
    c. Flattening of the joint space
163. a. Osseous
    b. Ligamentous
    c. Muscle imbalance
    d. Postural or static
    e. Arthritic
164. a. Osteochondritis dissecans
    b. Synovial chondromatosis
    c. Osteophytes
    d. Fracture articular surfaces
    e. Damaged menisci
165. a. Traumatic arthritis
    b. Loose bodies frequently in the olecranon fossa
    c. Chip fractures or ectopic bone in the common origin of the flexor muscles
166. a. Bilateral crossing of the teardrop
    b. Intertuberous distance less than normal
    c. Shenton's line intact bilaterally
    d. Greater than normal C-E angle bilaterally
167. a. Disabling pain and failure of efficient conservative treatment
    b. When flexing the knee at least 90° is possible
    c. When the x-ray films show only mild or moderate degenerative arthritis
    d. When the patient is muscular and sufficiently motivated to

carry out an effective program of rehabilitation

168. a. Profuse but controlled hemorrhage after injury
b. A thrill or bruit
c. Venous insufficiency
d. Gangrene
e. Increase in length of limb
f. Increased skin temperature
g. Cardiac enlargement
h. Increased oxygenation of venous blood
i. Branham's sign

169. a. To improve function of joints impaired by pain or mechanical derangement
b. To prevent impending ulceration
c. To make the wearing of gloves or shoes possible
d. To improve appearance
e. To stop drainage caused by secondary infection of tophus

170. a. Tabes dorsalis
b. Syringomyelia
c. Diabetic neuropathy
d. Alcoholism
e. Leprosy
f. Spinal cord tumors
g. Injury to the central or peripheral nervous system
h. Congenital indifference to pain

171. a. Congenital
b. Traumatic
c. Myositis or fibromatosis
d. Spasmodic
e. Neuritis of the spinal accessory nerve
f. Infections of the cervical spine

172. a. Infections of the genito-urinary tract
b. Pelvic or perineal surgery
c. Pregnancy
d. Degenerative or rheumatoid arthritis
e. Unknown causes

173. *Cervical spine:*
a. The abscess may present retropharyngeally in the posterior triangle of the neck, or in the supraclavicular area, or as a medial spinal abscess.
Lumbar spine and hip:
a. This may present as an iliac abscess that presents just above Poupart's ligament or less frequently in Petit's triangle, or on the anterior surface of the adductor region of the thigh, or in the gluteal region.

174. a. Hypervitaminosis A
b. Scurvy
c. Osteomyelitis
d. Malignant tumor

175. *Intra-articular:*
a. Acute infectious arthritis
b. Penetrating wounds
c. Low-grade infections such as tuberculosis or syphilis
d. Rheumatoid arthritis or osteoarthritis
e. Comminuted fractures causing irregularities that block joint motion
Extra-articular:
a. Contractures of the periarticular structure secondary to disease of the joint
b. Pyogenic infections of soft tissues alone
c. Pyogenic infections of soft tissues secondary to osteomyelitis
d. Crushing or laceration of soft tissues by open or closed fractures
e. Contractures of overactive or unopposed muscle groups as in poliomyelitis or spastic paralysis

176. a. Loss of protective joint sensibility
b. Relaxation of the lateral

ligaments with consequent
minor marginal joint
fractures

c. Destruction of the articular
cartilage and the intra-
articular ligaments

d. Sclerosis of the bone ends
denuded of cartilage

e. Periarticular and parosteal
bone production

f. Continued erosion and fracture of articulating ends
of bone

g. Atrophy of the surrounding
musculature

177. a. Rest in bed with protective
splints

b. Elevation of the infected part
and application of warm
moist soaks

c. Systemic treatment including
blood transfusions when
necessary

d. Appropriate antibiotics

e. Properly timed surgery
when indicated

178. a. When the infection is so
extensive that it cannot be
cured by antibiotics and
surgery

b. When resecting the diseased
bone is possible but so
disabling that function would
be better after a satisfactory
amputation or prosthesis

c. Before the patient's life is
endangered by infection

179. a. Symptoms and signs of
neurovascular disturbance

b. Shoulder held downward
and backward by traction
maintained for prolonged
periods

c. Symptoms reproduced and
radial pulse obliterated by
forcibly pulling the arm
downward and backward

d. Thoracic outlet narrowed by

cervical rib or deformed first
thoracic rib

e. Relief by corrective posture

180. a. Unrestricted passive motion
of the shoulder joint

b. Selective atrophy of the
supraspinatus and infra-
spinatus muscles that
develops within 2 weeks
after rupture

c. Absence of calcific deposits
on x-ray films

d. Palpable defect in the cuff

e. Soft crepitation when the
retracted tendon stump is
rolled between the examiner's
fingers in the humeral
head

f. Marked weakness of abduction or inability to maintain
abduction at 90° against
gravity or light resistance

181. a. The muscle should be large
enough and strong enough.

b. The musculocutaneous unit
should work in a straight line.

c. Essential body mechanics
should not be hindered by
loss of function from the
transplanted muscle.

d. The transplanted muscle
should be securely attached.

e. Each transplantation requires
specific care and fixation
after surgery.

f. The musculotendinous unit
must be placed under
sufficient tension.

g. The muscle chosen for
transplantation should have
sufficient length to permit
desirable range of motion.

h. The neurovascular bundle
must not be damaged by
kinking or stretching.

i. The muscle should never be
expected to perform two
separate functions.

182. a. Subperiosteal cortical bone erosion
  b. Generalized deossification
  c. Local destructive bone lesions (brown tumor)
  d. Calcification of the soft tissues

SECTION 2—ANATOMY
Multiple choice, single answer
(pp. 25-38)

1. a
2. e
3. b
4. a
5. d
6. b
7. a
8. e
9. b
10. c
11. c
12. c
13. d
14. c
15. b
16. d
17. b
18. b
19. b
20. d
21. d
22. a
23. c
24. d
25. c
26. b
27. d
28. b
29. a
30. b
31. b
32. c
33. e
34. d
35. b
36. b
37. e
38. c
39. d
40. e
41. c
42. b
43. d
44. d
45. d
46. a
47. d
48. b
49. a
50. c
51. b
52. e
53. a
54. c
55. a
56. d
57. d
58. a
59. d
60. b
61. c
62. a
63. a
64. e
65. a
66. a
67. a
68. b
69. c
70. a
71. d
72. c
73. a
74. c
75. b
76. d
77. b
78. b
79. e
80. b

Multiple choice, multiple answers
(pp. 38-42)

81. a, c, d
82. c, e

83. a, b, c, d, e
84. d
85. a, b, d, e
86. a, e
87. a, b
88. b, d, e
89. b, d, e
90. c, e
91. b, d, e
92. d, e
93. a, b, c, d, e
94. b, d
95. d
96. c, d
97. a, c, d
98. b, d
99. b, c
100. a, d, e, b, c
101. c, e
102. c
103. d, e
104. a, c
105. a, c
106. c, e
107. b, d
108. a, d, e
109. a, b, c
110. c

Situation and progressive thought
(pp. 42-44)

111. e
112. b, c
113. d
114. a, b, c
115. d
116. d
117. c, d
118. e
119. a, b, e
120. a
121. b
122. c
123. a, c
124. b, c
125. c

True or false (pp. 45-46)

126. F
127. F
128. F
129. F
130. T
131. T
132. F
133. F
134. T
135. T
136. F
137. F
138. F
139. T
140. T

List (p. 46)

141. a. Syndemosis; dense connective tissue
     b. Synchondrosis; cartilage
     c. Synostosis (sutura); bone
142. a. Tibialis posterior
     b. Flexor digitorum longus
     c. Venae comitantes
     d. Posterior tibial artery
     e. Venae comitantes
     f. Tibial nerve
143. a. Coracoacromial ligament
     b. Coracohumeral ligament
     c. Conoid ligament
     d. Trapezoid ligament
     e. Superior transverse ligament
     f. Inferior transverse ligament
144. a. Anterior tibial tendon
     b. Extensor hallucis longus tendon
     c. Anterior tibial artery
     d. Deep peroneal nerve
     e. Extensor digitorum longus tendon
     f. Peroneus tertius tendon
145. a. Articular branch of the nerve to the rectus femoris (femoral)
     b. Articular branch of obturator

c. Articular branch of the nerve to the quadratus femoris
d. Articular branch of sciatic
e. Articular branch of the superior gluteal
146. a. Capital femoral; 15%
b. Distal femoral; 35%
c. Proximal tibial; 30%
d. Distal tibial; 20%
147. a. Calcified cartilage stratum
b. Superficial or tangential stratum
c. Intermediate stratum
d. Radiate stratum
148. a. Deltoid muscle
b. Cutaneous structures over the deltoid insertion
c. Teres minor
d. Shoulder joint
149. a. Iliacus
b. Psoas major
c. Pectineus
d. Sometimes a portion of the adductor brevis
150. a. Ligamentum teres vessels; during childhood before closure of the epiphyseal plate
b. Retinacular vessels; at all ages
c. Nutrient vessels; during young adulthood while the femoral neck still contains cancellous bone but after the epiphyseal plate has closed

SECTION 3—BIOMECHANICS
Multiple choice, single answer
(pp. 47-52)

1. d
2. a
3. b
4. d
5. c
6. b
7. c
8. b
9. b
10. a
11. a
12. a
13. d
14. b
15. a
16. b
17. c
18. d
19. a
20. d
21. c
22. b
23. b
24. a
25. d
26. d
27. b
28. b
29. a
30. d

Multiple choice, multiple answers
(pp. 52-57)

31. b, d
32. c
33. b, d
34. b, d
35. a, c
36. b, c
37. c, d
38. b, c
39. a, d
40. a, d
41. a, b, d
42. a, b, d
43. b, c, d
44. a, b, c
45. a, c
46. b, c
47. a, c, d
48. b, d
49. a, b, c, d
50. a, b, d
51. a, c

52. a, b, c
53. a, c, d
54. a, c, d
55. c, d
56. a, c
57. a, b, c, d
58. b, d
59. b, d
60. a, b, c

Situation and progressive thought
(pp. 58-59)

61. a
62. d
63. a
64. d
65. a
66. d
67. d
68. a
69. a
70. c

True or false (pp. 59-60)

71. T
72. T
73. T
74. F
75. F
76. F
77. T
78. F
79. T
80. F
81. T
82. T
83. F
84. T
85. F

List (p. 61)

86. a. Pelvic rotation
    b. Pelvic tilt
    c. Knee flexion in stance phase
    d. Foot and ankle motion
    e. Knee flexion after "heel strike"
    f. Lateral motion of the pelvis

87. a. Electrolytic dissolution or corrosion of metal
    b. Electrolytic dissolution of the bone
    c. Improper drill size
    d. Improper technical placement causing microfracture of bone, stripping of threads, etc.
88. a. Beam
    b. Arch
    c. Muscle mechanism
89. a. Chemical composition of the components
    b. Surface abrasions
    c. Cold welding
    d. Mechanical distortion
    e. Differential oxygenation
90. a. Canaliculi
    b. Lacunae
    c. Haversian canals
    d. Volkmann's canals
    e. Primary longitudinal canals
    f. Medullary spaces
91. a. Torque
    b. Compression
    c. Tension
    d. Shear
    e. Flexure
92. a. Direct measurement
    b. Strain gauge
    c. Stress coat
    d. Photoelasticity
93. a. Elasticity—ability to return to original dimensions
    b. Resilience—ability to return energy from a deforming force
    c. Damping—ability to dissipate energy from a deforming force
    d. Fragility—resistance to fracture
    e. Brittleness—breakage related to strain
    f. Ductibility—ability to deform under tension without fracture
    g. Malleability—ability to deform under compression without fracture

h. Compliance—readiness to
  deform under load
i. Hardness—resistance to
  penetration
94. a. Muscles of lower limb
  b. Muscles of upper limb
  c. Elastic strain soft tissues
    upper and lower limbs
  d. Elastic strain skeletal members
    upper and lower limbs
  e. Plastic strain skeletal members
    upper and lower limbs
95. a. Fatigue or mechanical failure
    in the device or bone
  b. Failure of bone to support
    stress of implanted device
  c. Continued pain
  d. Tissue reaction
  e. Infection

SECTION 4—CHILDREN'S ORTHOPAEDICS
Multiple choice, single answer
(pp. 62-75)

1. e
2. e
3. e
4. a
5. b
6. b
7. c
8. c
9. d
10. c
11. a
12. c
13. b
14. d
15. d
16. e
17. a
18. e
19. d
20. d
21. c
22. c
23. e
24. d
25. a
26. e
27. d
28. b
29. b
30. d
31. c
32. a
33. a
34. c
35. e
36. b
37. d
38. e
39. a
40. d
41. a
42. c
43. d
44. b
45. d
46. b
47. e
48. a
49. d
50. d
51. d
52. b
53. e
54. d
55. b
56. b
57. c
58. c
59. c
60. e
61. e
62. a
63. b
64. c
65. b
66. c
67. c
68. d
69. b
70. d

71. c
72. e
73. c
74. b
75. b
76. b
77. d
78. e
79. b
80. c

Multiple choice, multiple answers
(pp. 75-83)

81. a
82. a, e, c, f, b, d
83. a, b, c, d
84. a, b, c, e
85. a
86. a, b, d
87. a, d
88. c, e
89. a, b, d, e
90. b, c, d
91. a, b, c
92. b, c
93. a, b, c, d, e
94. b, c, d
95. a, b, c, d, e
96. a, b, c, e
97. b, d
98. a, b, c, e
99. a, b, c, d
100. a, c
101. a, d
102. a, e
103. a, b, c, d
104. a, e
105. a, b, c, e
106. c, e
107. b, c, e
108. a, b, c, e
109. d, e
110. a, c, d
111. b, d
112. a, b, e
113. a, b, d
114. b, c, e
115. b, d

116. a, e
117. a, b, c, d
118. a, d
119. b, c
120. a, d
121. a, d
122. a, c
123. a, e
124. b, d
125. a, b, c, e
126. a, c, d
127. b, c
128. a, c, e
129. a, b, d, e
130. b, c, d

Situation and progressive thought
(pp. 83-86)

131. c
132. b
133. d
134. b, c
135. b
136. e
137. a, c
138. c
139. a
140. d
141. c
142. b, c
143. b, c
144. a, e
145. b, d

True or false (pp. 86-89)

146. F
147. F
148. F
149. T
150. T
151. F
152. T
153. T
154. T
155. F
156. F
157. T
158. T

159. F
160. F
161. F
162. F
163. F
164. F
165. T
166. T
167. T
168. F
169. F
170. F
171. T
172. F
173. T
174. F
175. T
176. T
177. T
178. F
179. F
180. F

List (pp. 89-90)

181. a. Forefoot adduction or varus; occurring primarily at the talonavicular and calcanio-cuboid joints
   b. Inversion or hindfoot varus; occurring at the subtalar joint
   c. Equinus; occurring at the ankle joint
182. a. Anterior poliomyelitis
   b. A degenerative neurologic disease such as Friedreich's ataxia
   c. Anomalies of the lumbo-sacral plexus with secondary muscle imbalance
183. a. Separate ossification centers
   b. Birth, neonatal, or stress fractures
   c. Increased lumbar lordosis
   d. Impingement of the articular process on the pars interarticularis

e. Pathologic change in the pars interarticularis
184. a. Grice extra-articular subtalar arthrodesis
   b. Osmond-Clark transfer of the peroneus brevis to the lateral aspect of the talus
   c. Hark procedure
185. a. Varus osteotomy
   b. Pelvic support osteotomy
   c. Arthrodesis
   d. Osteotomy of the ilium (Pemberton)
   e. Osteotomy of the innominate bone (Salter)
   f. Muscle transfer (Mustard, Sharrard)
186. a. Triple arthrodesis
   b. Pantalar arthrodesis
   c. Ankle arthrodesis
   d. Lambrinudi arthrodesis
   e. Posterior ankle bone block
187. a. Tarsometatarsal capsulotomy (Heyman procedure)
   b. Excision of the abductor hallucis longus muscle and possibly removal of the flexor hallucis brevis division of the adductor hallucis
188. a. Anoxia
   b. Birth trauma
   c. Prematurity
   d. Congenital anomaly
   e. Postnatal trauma
189. a. Steindler flexorplasty
   b. Anterior transfer of the triceps brachii
   c. Transfer of part of the pec-toralis major to the arm
   d. Transfer of the pectoralis major tendon
   e. Transfer of the sternocleido-mastoid
   f. Transfer of the pectoralis minor to the arm
190. a. Hemangioma
   b. Arteriovenous fistula
   c. Neurofibromas

274

d. Lymphangioma
e. Infection
191. a. Triple arthrodesis
b. Pantalar arthrodesis
c. Ankle arthrodesis
d. Lambrinudi arthrodesis
e. Posterior bone block
192. a. Eosinophilic granuloma
b. Hand-Schüller-Christian disease
c. Gaucher's disease
d. Niemann-Pick disease
e. Letterer-Siwe disease
193. a. Cervical, pointing into the mediastinum
b. Dorsal, pointing along the ribs
c. Lumbar, pointing to the lumbar triangle posteriorly or beneath the inguinal ligament anteriorly
194. a. Spastic
b. Athetotic
c. Ataxia
d. Rigid
e. Tension athetoid or tremor
195. a. Poliomyelitis
b. Marfan's syndrome
c. Neurofibromatosis
d. Friedreich's ataxia
e. Sprengel's deformity
196. a. Rickets
b. Advanced tuberculosis affecting the knee joint
c. Trauma with scarring of the lateral soft tissues or damage to the lateral portion of the epiphysis
d. Postpoliomyelitis
e. Growth disturbance such as achondroplasia or Ollier's disease
197. a. Caffey's disease
b. Scurvy
c. Battered-child syndrome
d. Sickle cell anemia
e. Osteomyelitis
f. Hypervitaminosis A

198. a. Genu valgum
b. Relaxation of the medial patellar retinaculum
c. Abnormal insertion of the ligamentum patella
d. Flatness of the lateral femoral condyle
e. Abnormality of the quadriceps mechanism with a high-riding patella
199. a. Baker's cyst
b. Lipoma
c. Arterial aneurysm
d. Xanthoma
e. Malignant neoplasm
200. a. Interference with joint function
b. Repeated painful bursitis
c. Fracture of the tumor with symptoms
d. Suspicion of malignancy

SECTION 5—HAND SURGERY
Multiple choice, single answer
(pp. 91-99)

1. c
2. e
3. d
4. a
5. c
6. c
7. d
8. a
9. c
10. d
11. d
12. b
13. c
14. c
15. c
16. b
17. c
18. a
19. b
20. a
21. b
22. b
23. a

24. a
25. a
26. d
27. a
28. d
29. c
30. b
31. b
32. b
33. c
34. c
35. a
36. a
37. c
38. a
39. c
40. d
41. c
42. d
43. d
44. b
45. d
46. c
47. b
48. c
49. c
50. c

Multiple choice, multiple answers
(pp. 99-106)

51. b, c
52. a, b, c, e
53. a, b
54. a, b, d
55. a, b, c, d
56. a, d
57. b, c
58. a, d
59. c, d
60. a, b
61. b, c, d
62. a
63. a, b, c, d, e
64. a, e
65. b, d
66. b, d
67. a, c, d
68. a, b, d

69. a, b, c
70. a, b
71. a, c, d
72. b, c
73. a, b, c
74. a
75. a, d
76. d
77. b, c
78. a, d
79. b, d
80. a, d
81. a, b, c, d, e
82. a, c, d
83. a, b, c
84. b, d
85. a, c

Situation and progressive thought
(pp. 106-110)

86. c, d
87. d
88. c, d
89. c
90. d
91. b, c
92. d
93. c
94. b, d
95. c
96. d
97. a, d
98. a
99. b
100. a, b, d

True or false (pp. 110-111)

101. T
102. F
103. F
104. F
105. F
106. T
107. F
108. T
109. F
110. F
111. T

112. T
113. F
114. F
115. T
116. T
117. T
118. T
119. T
120. T

List (pp. 112-113)

121. a. Sublimis tendon transfer—Stiles-Bunnell
     b. Capsulorrhaphy or volar skin excision—Zancolli
     c. Extensor tenodesis transfer—Fowler
     d. Active wrist motor transfers—Riordan, Brand, Fowler, and Boyes
122. a. Inability to cooperate or poor motivation
     b. Severe athetosis
     c. Complete sensory loss or alienation of the part
     d. Inability to control the shoulder or elbow
123. a. Erosion of joint surface and supporting bony architecture
     b. Stretching of collateral ligaments
     c. Stretching of the supporting ligaments to the flexor sheath, allowing volar and ulnar displacement of the flexor tendons
     d. Ulnar subluxation of the extensor hood
     e. Interosseous muscle contracture
124. a. Bilateral triangular flap advancement (Kutler)
     b. Volar triangular flap advancement
     c. Wolf graft
     d. Palmar pedicle graft or free full-thickness graft

125. a. Matti-Russi (bone graft—volar approach)
     b. Murray (bone graft—blind approach)
     c. Bentzon (interposition membrane)
     d. Barnard and Stubbins (resection of radial styloid)
126. a. Joint contractures must be corrected first.
     b. Adequate power must be present in the muscle to be transferred.
     c. Maintenance of integrity of the muscle function is necessary when possible.
     d. Transfers must be in straight lines when possible.
     e. Adequate amplitude of action must be present in the muscle to be transferred.
127. a. Severed or avulsed tendon
     b. Adherent tendons
     c. Muscle paralysis
     d. Muscle contracture
     e. Skin contracture
     f. Joint contracture
128. a. Use separate incisions when operating on both bones of the forearm in the same area.
     b. Put fractures of the forearm up in supination when there are no contraindications.
     c. Perform a thorough excision of the synostosis.
     d. Cover the common surface of the bones with polyethylene after resection of synostosis.
129. a. Conservative casting for six months
     b. Multiple drill holes in the bone
     c. Removal
     d. Prosthetic replacement
     e. Curettement and bone graft

130. a. Tenotomy of the lateral bands
b. Stripping of the muscles
c. Removal and advancement of scarred and damaged muscle
d. Nerve transfer
e. Bone block and shortening procedures
f. Tendon transfers

131. a. Ulnar deviation of the wrist
b. Flexion of the distal phalanx of the small finger
c. Finger abduction and adduction
d. Digital balance of the ring and small fingers
e. Sensation over the ulnar one third of the hand

132. a. Supracondylar process of the humerus
b. Cervical rib
c. Cervical disc
d. Median nerve compression between the heads of the pronator teres

133. a. Sacrifice the finger and resect the metacarpal at its base.
b. Bone graft the metacarpal head or metacarpophalangeal joint.
c. Perform arthroplasty.
d. Fuse the proximal phalanx to the metacarpal.

134. a. Meissner's corpuscle
b. Ruffini
c. Krause
d. Pacinian corpuscle

135. a. Glomus tumor
b. Neurofibroma
c. Neurolemmoma
d. Lipoma
e. Giant cell tumor of tendon sheath
f. Fibroma

136. a. Loss of extension of the interphalangeal joints
b. Hyperextension of the metacarpophalangeal joints
c. Loss of finger abduction and adduction power
d. Excessive initial flexion of the terminal joint during grasp
e. Decreased pinch and grasp strength

137. a. Excision of the trapezium
b. Fusion of the carpometacarpal joint
c. Ligamentous reconstruction
d. Prosthetic replacement of the trapezium

138. a. Trauma
b. Rheumatoid arthritis
c. Diabetes
d. Nonspecific synovitis
e. Myxedema (hypothyroidism)
f. Acromegaly

139. a. Regional IV anesthesia
b. Corollary nerve block
c. Brachial plexus (cervical) block
d. Selective peripheral nerve blocks
e. Local infiltrative field blocks

140. a. Phenol injections of the appropriate nerves
b. Flexor origin release
c. Selective tendon lengthening
d. Transfer of sublimus to profundus tendons in distal forearm
e. Release of intrinsic muscles of the thumb
f. Pronator terres release or transfer

SECTION 6—PATHOLOGY
Multiple choice, single answer
(pp. 114-126)

1. b
2. a
3. d
4. c
5. b

6. b
7. c
8. d
9. c
10. b
11. c
12. b
13. b
14. b
15. c
16. b
17. e
18. b
19. d
20. c
21. b
22. b
23. c
24. e
25. c
26. d
27. c
28. c
29. d
30. d
31. c
32. b
33. b
34. c
35. b
36. c
37. a
38. a
39. a
40. a
41. b
42. d
43. a
44. c
45. a
46. a
47. d
48. d
49. d
50. b
51. c
52. c
53. d

54. b
55. c
56. a
57. a
58. b
59. a
60. c
61. d
62. a
63. d
64. b
65. a
66. d
67. d
68. e
69. d
70. c
71. c
72. c
73. c
74. b
75. b
76. a
77. d
78. d
79. c
80. b

Multiple choice, multiple answers
(pp. 126-135)

81. a, c
82. b, c, e
83. a, d
84. a, b, c, d
85. b, d
86. b, c, d
87. b, c
88. a, b, c, e
89. a, d
90. c, d
91. b, d
92. a, c
93. a, c
94. a, d
95. b, d
96. b, d
97. a, d
98. b, d

99. a, b, c
100. a, b
101. a, d
102. a, b, c, d, e
103. a, b
104. b, c
105. b, d
106. a, b, c
107. b, c
108. c, d
109. b, d
110. a, d
111. b, d, e
112. a, b, c, d
113. a, b, c, d
114. a, b, c, d
115. a, b, c, d
116. a, b, c, d
117. a, b, c, d, e
118. a, b, d, e
119. b, c, d, e
120. a, b, c, d
121. a, b, c, d
122. a, b, c, d
123. a, b, c
124. a, b, d, e
125. a, b, c, e
126. a, c, e
127. a, d, e
128. a, b, d
129. a, b, c, d
130. a, b, c, d

Situation and progressive thought
(pp. 135-139)

131. d
132. d
133. d
134. c
135. a
136. d
137. b
138. a, b, c, d
139. c
140. c
141. d
142. d
143. b

144. b
145. d
146. c
147. a
148. a
149. b
150. c

True or false (pp. 139-142)

151. T
152. T
153. T
154. F
155. T
156. T
157. T
158. T
159. F
160. T
161. F
162. F
163. T
164. F
165. F
166. T
167. F
168. F
169. T
170. F
171. F
172. F
173. F
174. F
175. F
176. F
177. F
178. T
179. F
180. T
181. T
182. T
183. T
184. F
185. T
186. F
187. T
188. T
189. T

190. T
191. T
192. F
193. T

List (p. 142)

194. a. Breast
 b. Prostate
 c. Lung
 d. Colon
195. a. Unicameral bone cyst
 b. Fibrous dysplasia
 c. Fibrous metaphyseal defect
 d. Nonosteogenic fibroma
 e. Aneurysmal bone cyst
 f. Giant cell tumor
196. a. Eosinophilic granuloma
 b. Hand-Schüller-Christian disease
 c. Letterer-Siwe disease
 d. Niemann-Pick disease
 e. Gaucher's disease
197. a. Osteosarcoma
 b. Chondrosarcoma
 c. Fibrosarcoma
 d. Giant cell tumor
198. a. Liposarcoma
 b. Rhabdomyosarcoma
 c. Synovioma
 d. Fibrosarcoma
 e. Angiosarcoma
199. a. Paget's disease
 b. Osteochondroma
 c. Enchondroma
 d. Chondromyxoid fibroma
200. a. Café au lait spots
 b. Diffuse soft tissue hypertrophy
 c. Scoliosis
 d. Bone hypertrophy
 e. Hemangioma and venous wall thickening
201. a. Osteogenic sarcoma
 b. Fibrous dysplasia
 c. Paget's disease
202. a. Osteitis fibrosa cystica
 b. Giant cell reparative granuloma
 c. Unicameral bone cyst

 d. Fibrous dysplasia
 e. Aneurysmal bone cyst
 f. Metaphyseal fibrous defect
 g. Chondroblastoma
203. a. Hodgkin's disease
 b. Carcinoma of the prostate
 c. Carcinoma of the breast
 d. Carcinoma of the urinary bladder

SECTION 7—PHYSICAL MEDICINE AND REHABILITATION
Multiple choice, single answer
(pp. 143-147)

1. b
2. c
3. b
4. b
5. d
6. d
7. d
8. a
9. d
10. b
11. c
12. c
13. b
14. b
15. d
16. b
17. d
18. d
19. d
20. a
21. d
22. c
23. d
24. b
25. d

Multiple choice, multiple answers
(pp. 148-150)

26. a, b, c, d
27. a, b, c
28. a
29. c
30. b, c, d
31. a, b
32. a, b

33. b, c, d
34. a, b
35. a, c
36. a, b, d
37. a, b, c, d
38. a, b, d
39. c
40. b, d

Situation and progressive thought
(pp. 151-156)

41. c
42. b
43. d
44. c
45. a, b, c, d
46. c
47. b
48. b, d
49. a, b, d
50. c
51. b
52. c, d
53. d
54. c
55. b, d
56. a, c
57. d
58. d
59. c
60. b

True or false (pp. 156-157)

61. T
62. F
63. F
64. F
65. T
66. T
67. T
68. F
69. F
70. F

List (p. 157)

71. a. Passive
    b. Active
    c. Active assistive
    d. Resistive
    e. Stretching
72. a. Four-point gait
    b. Two-point gait
    c. Tripod crutch gait, alternate, and simultaneous
    d. "Swing to" and "swing through" gait
73. a. Mobility and ambulation
    b. Self-care
    c. Psychosocial adjustment to disability
    d. Prevention of secondary disability
74. a. Muscle atrophy
    b. Joint contracture
    c. Metabolic disturbance
    d. Circulatory disturbance
    e. Sphincter disturbance
    f. Psychologic deterioration
75. a. Internal and external rotation of the lower limb
    b. Flat feet
    c. Internal tibial torsion and pigeon toes
    d. Metatarsus varus
    e. Genu varum and genu valgum

SECTION 8—PHYSIOLOGY AND BIOCHEMISTRY
Multiple choice, single answer
(pp. 158-173)

1. a
2. a
3. c
4. b
5. a
6. b
7. b
8. d
9. d
10. b
11. b
12. c
13. b
14. b
15. d

16. a		65. a
17. b		66. a
18. c		67. c
19. b		68. b
20. c		69. d
21. d		70. a
22. c		71. b
23. a		72. c
24. b		73. b
25. a		74. d
26. c		75. c
27. d		76. d
28. c		77. a
29. c		78. b
30. c		79. b
31. a		80. c
32. b		81. d
33. b		82. c
34. d		83. d
35. b		84. b
36. a		85. b
37. b		86. a
38. b		87. c
39. a		88. c
40. d		89. b
41. a		90. b
42. b		91. d
43. b		92. c
44. d		93. a
45. d		94. b
46. a		95. a
47. c		96. b
48. c		97. a
49. c		98. a
50. b		99. b
51. d		100. b
52. d		101. d
53. d		102. c
54. d		103. a
55. c		104. d
56. c		
57. a		

Multiple choice, multiple answers
(pp. 173-185)

58. a	105. c, d
59. a	106. a, b, c
60. c	107. a, b, c
61. a	108. c, d
62. b	109. a, b
63. b	110. b, c, d
64. c	

111. a, c, d
112. a, c, d
113. a, b, c, d
114. a, b, c
115. a, b
116. a, c
117. a, e
118. b, d
119. a, b, c
120. d
121. d, b, c, a
122. a, c, d
123. a, d
124. c
125. a, b, c
126. a, c, d
127. a, b, c, d
128. a, b
129. a, b, d
130. a, b, c
131. b, d
132. a, b, d
133. b, c, d
134. a, d
135. b, c
136. a, d
137. a, b, d
138. a, c, d
139. b, d
140. c, d
141. a, b, c
142. c
143. a, b, d
144. d
145. d
146. c, d
147. b, c
148. a, b
149. d, c, a, b
150. b, d
151. c
152. a, b
153. c, d
154. c, d
155. a, b, c, d
156. b, d
157. a, b
158. b, c, d
159. b, d

160. a, b
161. d
162. c
163. a, b, c
164. b, d
165. d
166. d
167. b, d
168. b, d
169. b, c
170. a, b, c
171. b, d
172. a, b, d
173. a, c, d
174. a, b, c, d
175. b, c
176. b, d
177. a, c
178. c, d
179. b, c

Situation and progressive thought
(pp. 185-189)

180. d
181. b
182. a
183. b
184. c, a, b, e, d
185. b
186. d
187. c
188. d
189. a
190. a, c
191. a, b
192. b, c, d
193. b
194. d
195. a
196. c
197. b
198. a
199. d

True or false (pp. 189-192)

200. F
201. F
202. T
203. F

204. T
205. F
206. F
207. F
208. T
209. F
210. F
211. T
212. F
213. F
214. T
215. F
216. F
217. T
218. T
219. F
220. F
221. T
222. F
223. F
224. T
225. T
226. T
227. F
228. T
229. T
230. T
231. F
232. T
233. F
234. T

List (p. 192)

235. a. No bone formation and decreased resorption
b. No bone formation and normal resorption
c. No bone formation and increased resorption
d. Decreased bone formation and normal resorption
e. Normal bone formation and increased resorption
f. Increased bone formation and increased resorption
236. a. Water and osmotic diuretics, urea
b. Acid-forming salts; ammonium chloride

c. Inhibition of renal tubular transport; Thiomerin
237. a. Anemia
b. Protein deficiency
c. Age of patient
d. Edema
e. Vitamin C deficiency
f. Anticoagulants
238. a. Foreign body implants
b. Repeated osteotomy
c. Vascular alteration
d. Neurologic alteration
e. Diathermy
f. Administration of growth hormone
239. a. Gross appearance
b. Viscosity
c. Cytology
d. Mucin precipitation
e. Bacteriology
f. Glucose
g. Polarizing microscopy
h. Tetracycline-retention test
240. a. Simple diffusion
b. Facilitated diffusion
c. Exchange diffusion
d. Active transport
e. Pinocytosis
241. a. Adequate intake
b. Vitamin D
c. Chronic bowel disease
d. Celiac disease
e. Parathyroid hormone levels
242. a. Mucosal lining cells of the intestine
b. Kidney
c. Bone tissue level
243. a. Bone tissue level number of osteoclasts
b. Kidney proximal convoluted tubule
c. Bowel wall
d. Breast
244. a. Temperature
b. Blood supply
c. Recurrent trauma
d. Hematoma or seroma
e. Infection

f. Foreign body

245. a. Presence of Bence Jones proteins in urine
  b. Hypercalcemia and uremia
  c. Reversal of albumin-globulin ratio
  d. Anemia and increased sedimentation rate
  e. Abnormal electrophoretic pattern of gamma globulins

246. a. Glycine
  b. Proline
  c. Hydroxyproline
  d. Glutamic acid

247. a. Hydraulic fluid pressure phenomenon secondary to microfractures in the articular cortex
  b. Hypervascularity with proliferation of granulation tissue secondary to stimulation by eroded acetabular cartilage
  c. Subchondral inflammatory pannus similar to b, which is seen in rheumatoid arthritis

248. a. Gamma radiation; photons
  b. Beta radiation; high-speed electrons
  c. Alpha radiation; two protons and two neutrons

249. a. Autoradiography
  b. Radioassay
  c. External scanning
  d. Whole body counting

SECTION 9—PROSTHETICS AND ORTHOTICS
Multiple choice, single answer
(pp. 193-204)

1. a
2. b
3. b
4. c
5. b
6. d
7. c
8. d
9. d

10. c
11. b
12. b
13. c
14. d
15. a
16. a
17. b
18. c
19. a
20. b
21. c
22. a
23. b
24. d
25. d
26. a
27. c
28. d
29. d
30. c
31. d
32. d
33. c
34. a
35. c
36. c
37. a
38. b
39. d
40. d
41. d
42. d
43. a
44. a
45. b
46. b
47. d
48. b
49. a
50. d
51. c
52. d
53. c
54. d
55. d
56. b
57. b
58. b

59. b
60. b

Multiple choice, multiple answers
(pp. 204-211)

61. a, b, c, d
62. b, d
63. c, d
64. a, b, c, d
65. a, b, c, d
66. b
67. a, c
68. d
69. b, c
70. a, b, c, d
71. b, c, d
72. a, b, c, d
73. a, d
74. b, c, d
75. b, c
76. a, d
77. b, d
78. a, b, c, d
79. c, d
80. b, c, d
81. a, b, c
82. a, d
83. b, c
84. c, d
85. c
86. b, c
87. a, c
88. b, d
89. b, d
90. a, b, d
91. b
92. a, b, d
93. a, b, c
94. a, c, d
95. a, b, c

Situation and progressive thought
(pp. 211-217)

96. c, d
97. c
98. c
99. c
100. c

101. d
102. c
103. c
104. e
105. d
106. c
107. c
108. b
109. b
110. a, b, c, d
111. c
112. c
113. c
114. a
115. a

True or false (pp. 217-219)

116. F
117. T
118. F
119. T
120. F
121. F
122. F
123. F
124. T
125. F
126. T
127. T
128. T
129. F
130. F
131. F
132. T
133. F
134. F
135. T
136. F
137. T
138. T
139. T
140. F

List (pp. 219-220)

141. a. Figure-of-eight basic
harness or shoulder saddle
b. Elbow lock control strap
c. Terminal device and elbow
control strap

142. a. Knuckle-bender splint
b. Reverse knuckle-bender splint
c. Cock-up wrist splint
d. Pancake splint
e. Spreading-hand splint

143. a. Myoelectric sensors
b. Skin displacement sensors
c. Strap-controlled position switches

144. a. Reduction of pain and edema
b. Facilitation of healing
c. Confidence and prosthetic adaption gained through early use
d. Minimization of time until use of permanent prosthesis

145. a. Thoracic
b. Lumbar
c. Shoulder sling
d. Shoulder ring
e. Kyphosis
f. Sternal

146. a. Suction socket
b. Suprapatellar cuff suspension
c. Supracondylar fit with medial wedge insert
d. Lacers or corsets
e. Pelvic belt
f. Silesian bandage
g. Suspenders

147. a. Tilting table
b. Saucer type
c. Canadian type

148. a. Klenzak
b. Pearlstein or Pope
c. Caliper
d. Phelps
e. Limited motion

149. a. Lack of motivation or senility
b. Impending gangrene of opposite leg
c. Class IV cardiac condition
d. Severe neurologic disorders or balance disorders
e. Irreparable stump problems
f. Known inadequate life expectancy

150. a. Constant friction, with and without locks
b. Variable friction, with and without locks
c. Hydraulic
d. Polycentric

SECTION 10—SURGICAL PRINCIPLES
Multiple choice, single answer
(pp. 221-224)

1. e
2. e
3. b
4. c
5. c
6. b
7. c
8. d
9. c
10. b
11. c
12. c
13. b
14. d
15. c
16. c
17. e
18. e

Multiple choice, multiple answers
(pp. 224-226)

19. a, b
20. b, c, e
21. a, d
22. e
23. a, b, c, d
24. a, b
25. a, b, e
26. c, e
27. d, e, c
28. b, c

Situation and progressive thought
(pp. 226-227)

29. d
30. a
31. d

32. a, d
33. b, c

True or false (p. 227)

34. T
35. F
36. F
37. T
38. T
39. T
40. F
41. F
42. F
43. T

List (p. 228)

44. a. The free ends are more easily found.
    b. Any branches that are still functioning in the scar will not be damaged or destroyed.
45. a. Mobilization of the nerve ends
    b. Positioning of the extremity to relax the nerve
    c. Transplantation
    d. Bone resection
    e. Bulb suture and nerve stretching, followed by secondary neurorrhaphy
46. a. Inadequate immobilization
    b. Pseudarthrosis or infection
    c. Failure of initial alignment of the foot and ankle
    d. Persistent muscle imbalance
    e. Loss of position at the time of casting
    f. Operation before sufficient bone maturity
47. a. Soft tissue reefing
    b. Arthrodesis
    c. Arthroplasty
    d. Bone block procedures
48. a. Excision of the focus cf infection
    b. Excision of the entire involved bone

c. Arthrodesis
    d. Drainage and curettage of abscesses
    e. Amputation
49. a. Open traumatic wounds
    b. Open fractures
    c. Excessive operating time
    d. Large operating field
    e. Operation in a contaminated area
50. a. Simple excision and closure
    b. Z plasty
    c. Excision and skin grafting
    d. Excision and closure with a pedicle or flap
51. a. In a patient who has been on steroid therapy
    b. When all other methods of shock therapy (blood replacement, plasma expanders, vasopressors, etc.) have failed
52. a. To fill cavities or defects in bone
    b. To affect arthrodesis
    c. To bridge major defects in long bones
    d. To limit joint motion
    e. For use in promoting union in fresh fractures, malunions, nonunions, osteotomies, or congenital pseudarthroses
53. a. Excessive pressure
    b. Excessive time of inflation
    c. Hemorrhagic infiltration of nerves
    d. Disregard of the anatomy above, under, or below the tourniquet

SECTION 11—TRAUMA
Multiple choice, single answer
(pp. 229-240)

1. c
2. a
3. d
4. b
5. d

6. a	54. b
7. c	55. d
8. c	56. b
9. c	57. c
10. b	58. a
11. c	59. b
12. d	60. d
13. d	61. a
14. c	62. d
15. c	63. b
16. d	64. d
17. d	65. c
18. c	66. d
19. a	67. d
20. e	68. e
21. c	69. c
22. c	70. a
23. a	71. b
24. c	72. a
25. e	73. b
26. c	74. a
27. d	75. d
28. d	

Multiple choice, multiple answers
(pp. 240-247)

29. b	76. b, d
30. d	77. b, d
31. d	78. e, a
32. a	79. b, c
33. c	80. a, c
34. d	81. a, c, e
35. c	82. b, e
36. c	83. a, b, c, d
37. e	84. a, d
38. e	85. b, e
39. b	86. a, c
40. a	87. a, c
41. c	88. b, c
42. b	89. a, b, c
43. c	90. a, e
44. c	91. a, e
45. c	92. a, e
46. c	93. b, d
47. d	94. a, b, c, d
48. b	95. b, d
49. d	96. c, e
50. e	97. b, d
51. b	98. a, b, c
52. d	
53. a	

99. a, c
100. a, e
101. a, d
102. b, d
103. c
104. a, b, c, d
105. a, c, d
106. a, b
107. a, d
108. b, c, d
109. b, d
110. a, c, e
111. c, d
112. b, e
113. a, c
114. b
115. a, b, d

Situation and progressive thought
(pp. 247-252)

116. c, d
117. b, e
118. b
119. d
120. b
121. c
122. b
123. a, b, d
124. a
125. d
126. d, e
127. c
128. b, c
129. d
130. e
131. b
132. d
133. a
134. d
135. b, d

True or false (pp. 252-254)

136. F
137. F
138. T
139. F
140. F
141. F
142. T
143. F
144. T
145. F
146. T
147. F
148. T
149. T
150. T
151. F
152. F
153. F
154. F
155. T
156. T
157. T
158. F
159. T
160. T
161. F
162. T
163. T
164. T
165. F

List (pp. 254-255)

166. a. Arthrodesis
    b. Arthrodesis with supra-malleolar osteotomy
    c. Osteotomy at the fracture site
    d. Supramalleolar osteotomy
    e. Correction of a diastasis with or without refracture

167. a. Tear of the quadriceps muscle; young adults and children
    b. Avulsion of the quadriceps tendon; middle-aged to elderly persons
    c. Transverse or comminuted fractures of the patella; adults and adolescents
    d. Patellar dislocations; adolescents and adults
    e. Avulsion of the ligamentum patellae; youths
    f. Avulsion of the tibial tubercle; adolescents

168. a. Fracture of the scaphoid
     b. Fracture of the radial head
     c. Dislocation of the elbow
     d. Fracture of the distal humerus
     e. Fracture of the surgical neck of the humerus
     f. Shoulder dislocation
169. a. Viable femoral head
     b. Free movement of the femoral head
     c. Little or no bone absorption at the neck
     d. Normal radiographic density of both fragments
     e. Strong fibrous union with little displacement of the distal fragment
170. a. Compounding or unwarranted open reduction
     b. Infection
     c. Impaired blood supply to a segmental fracture
     d. Comminution due to severe trauma
     e. Insecure fixation or inadequate immobilization
     f. Distraction by internal fixation devices or interposing tissue
     g. Anticoagulants
171. a. Tear of the acromioclavicular ligaments
     b. Tear of the conoid and trapezoid ligaments
     c. Tear of the clavicular attachment of the deltoid
     d. Posterior splitting of the trapezius
172. a. Decreased amplitude of the heart sounds
     b. Decreased blood pressure
     c. Increased venous pressure
173. a. Arthrodesis of the distal radius, lunate, capitate, navicular, and greater multangular bones

b. Excision of the navicular bone
     c. Bone grafting of the navicular bone
     d. Radial styloidectomy
174. a. Pneumothorax due to laceration of a lung or bronchus
     b. Hemothorax due to lung laceration or rupture of vessels
     c. Hemopericardium
     d. Traumatic asphyxia
     e. Diaphragmatic rupture and hernia
175. a. Pathologic dislocation
     b. Osteomyelitis with or without metastatic infection
     c. Persistent local infection
     d. Pelvic abscess
     e. Degenerative arthritis
176. a. Extreme soft tissue damage about the fracture site
     b. Penetration of the shaft through a small hole in the periosteum
     c. Displacement of the biceps tendon into the fracture site
     d. Interposition of a portion of the deltoid or subscapularis between the fragments
177. a. Mutilating trauma or thermal injuries
     b. Infection
     c. Malignant tumor
     d. Nerve injuries
     e. Peripheral vascular disease
     f. Congenital anomalies or structural deformities
178. a. To eliminate deformity
     b. To allow joint mobility
     c. To provide better coverage of vulnerable structures
     d. To relieve pain
     e. For cosmesis
179. a. When the femoral head has become caught in the pelvis
     b. When fragments of bone are interposed between the

femoral head and the weight-bearing surface of the acetabulum

c. Displacement of one or more fragments despite traction

d. When traction cannot be used because of a femoral shaft fracture

180. a. Kirschner wire transfixation of the joint
b. Wire loop fixation of the joint
c. Resection of the outer one third of the clavicle
d. Bosworth screw fixation
e. Braided wire fixation of the clavicle to the coracoid

181. a. Mauck
b. Augustine
c. Hey-Groves
d. Sage

182. a. Age of the patient
b. Period of immobilization
c. Severity of the injury causing the initial dislocation

183. a. Shortening of the radius with decreased range of motion and deformity
b. Late extensor tendon rupture
c. Sudek's atrophy
d. Decreased range of motion at the distal radioulnar joint with pain
e. Growth disturbance with subsequent deformity (in young persons)

184. a. Allis method
b. Stimson method
c. Bigelow method

185. a. Kocher method
b. Traction leverage
c. Gravity traction
d. Operative

186. a. Traction and external rotation of the arm with the elbow at the patient's side
b. Adduction of the arm

c. Internal rotation of the arm

187. a. Inadequate reduction
b. Incorrect length and positioning of the fixation device
c. Pauwels' type III fracture
d. Comminution of the cortex either inferiorly or posteriorly
e. Long inferior beak attached to the proximal fragment
f. Capsular interposition

188. a. Scar formation with resultant pain
b. Spur formation
c. Neuromas
d. Insufficient stump length
e. Bony overgrowth
f. Phantom limb pain

189. a. Tear of the articular disc
b. Dislocation or subluxation
c. Discrepancy in radial or ulnar length
d. Rupture of the distal radioulnar ligaments
e. Rupture of the ulnar collateral ligament

190. a. If the medical condition of the patient will allow only one operative procedure
b. Neurologic disease of a spastic or athetotic nature
c. Diagnosed malignancy either elsewhere or in the hip
d. A fracture that cannot be securely reduced or nailed
e. A preexisting lesion in the hip, that is, Charcot's joint or aseptic necrosis

191. a. Multiple fractures
b. Subdural hematoma
c. Failure to thrive
d. Soft tissue swelling and/or skin bruising
e. Sudden unexplained death with the type and degree of injury inconsistent with the history